Fungal Biofilms 2020

Fungal Biofilms 2020

Editors

Célia F. Rodrigues
Jesus A. Romo

MDPI • Basel • Beijing • Wuhan • Barcelona • Belgrade • Manchester • Tokyo • Cluj • Tianjin

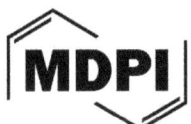

Editors
Célia F. Rodrigues
LEPABE - Dep. Chemical
Engineering
University of Porto
Porto
Portugal

Jesus A. Romo
Department of Molecular
Biology and Microbiology
Tufts University
Boston, MA
United States

Editorial Office
MDPI
St. Alban-Anlage 66
4052 Basel, Switzerland

This is a reprint of articles from the Special Issue published online in the open access journal *Journal of Fungi* (ISSN 2309-608X) (available at: www.mdpi.com/journal/jof/special_issues/biofilms_2020).

For citation purposes, cite each article independently as indicated on the article page online and as indicated below:

LastName, A.A.; LastName, B.B.; LastName, C.C. Article Title. *Journal Name* **Year**, *Volume Number*, Page Range.

ISBN 978-3-0365-5418-1 (Hbk)
ISBN 978-3-0365-5417-4 (PDF)

© 2022 by the authors. Articles in this book are Open Access and distributed under the Creative Commons Attribution (CC BY) license, which allows users to download, copy and build upon published articles, as long as the author and publisher are properly credited, which ensures maximum dissemination and a wider impact of our publications.

The book as a whole is distributed by MDPI under the terms and conditions of the Creative Commons license CC BY-NC-ND.

Contents

About the Editors vii

Célia F. Rodrigues and Jesus A. Romo
Fungal Biofilms 2020
Reprinted from: *J. Fungi* 2021, 7, 603, doi:10.3390/jof7080603 1

Tomasz M. Karpiński, Marcin Ożarowski, Agnieszka Seremak-Mrozikiewicz, Hubert Wolski and Artur Adamczak
Plant Preparations and Compounds with Activities against Biofilms Formed by *Candida* spp.
Reprinted from: *J. Fungi* 2021, 7, 360, doi:10.3390/jof7050360 3

Carmélia Isabel Vitorino Lobo, Ana Carolina Urbano de Araújo Lopes and Marlise Inêz Klein
Compounds with Distinct Targets Present Diverse Antimicrobial and Antibiofilm Efficacy against *Candida albicans* and *Streptococcus mutans*, and Combinations of Compounds Potentiate Their Effect
Reprinted from: *J. Fungi* 2021, 7, 340, doi:10.3390/jof7050340 17

Emilia Gómez-Molero, Iker De-la-Pinta, Jordan Fernández-Pereira, Uwe Groß, Michael Weig and Guillermo Quindós et al.
Candida parapsilosis Colony Morphotype Forecasts Biofilm Formation of Clinical Isolates
Reprinted from: *J. Fungi* 2021, 7, 33, doi:10.3390/jof7010033 33

Angela Maione, Elisabetta de Alteriis, Federica Carraturo, Stefania Galdiero, Annarita Falanga and Marco Guida et al.
The Membranotropic Peptide gH625 to Combat Mixed *Candida albicans*/*Klebsiella pneumoniae* Biofilm: Correlation between In Vitro Anti-Biofilm Activity and In Vivo Antimicrobial Protection
Reprinted from: *J. Fungi* 2021, 7, 26, doi:10.3390/jof7010026 45

Matthew B. Lohse, Craig L. Ennis, Nairi Hartooni, Alexander D. Johnson and Clarissa J. Nobile
A Screen for Small Molecules to Target *Candida albicans* Biofilms
Reprinted from: *J. Fungi* 2020, 7, 9, doi:10.3390/jof7010009 61

Teresa D. Rebaza, Yvette Ludeña, Ilanit Samolski and Gretty K. Villena
Gene Expression Analysis of Non-Clinical Strain of *Aspergillus fumigatus* (LMB-35Aa): Does Biofilm Affect Virulence?
Reprinted from: *J. Fungi* 2020, 6, 376, doi:10.3390/jof6040376 73

Lívia S. Ramos, Laura N. Silva, Marta H. Branquinha and André L. S. Santos
Susceptibility of the *Candida haemulonii* Complex to Echinocandins: Focus on Both Planktonic and Biofilm Life Styles and a Literature Review
Reprinted from: *J. Fungi* 2020, 6, 201, doi:10.3390/jof6040201 87

Renátó Kovács and László Majoros
Fungal Quorum-Sensing Molecules: A Review of Their Antifungal Effect against *Candida* Biofilms
Reprinted from: *J. Fungi* 2020, 6, 99, doi:10.3390/jof6030099 103

Lívia S. Ramos, Thaís P. Mello, Marta H. Branquinha and André L. S. Santos
Biofilm Formed by *Candida haemulonii* Species Complex: Structural Analysis and Extracellular Matrix Composition
Reprinted from: *J. Fungi* **2020**, *6*, 46, doi:10.3390/jof6020046 . . . . **117**

Austin M. Perry, Aaron D. Hernday and Clarissa J. Nobile
Unraveling How *Candida albicans* Forms Sexual Biofilms
Reprinted from: *J. Fungi* **2020**, *6*, 14, doi:10.3390/jof6010014 . . . . **135**

About the Editors

Célia F. Rodrigues

Celia F. Rodrigues (PharmD, PhD) is a *Candida* spp. expert, with extensive know-how in susceptibility assays, biofilm development, antimicrobial drugs, molecular techniques, alternative and novel treatments, and biomaterials. Presently, she is an invited assistant professor at CESPU, where she teaches future pharmacists, and she is a PhD member of TOXRUN (Toxicology Research Unit - CESPU). She has also worked at LEPABE, Faculty of Engineering, the University of Porto on a project related to microorganisms, FISH, and microfluidics, where she maintains a close collaboration. Celia is a reviewer for more than 50 international journals and has co-supervised/mentored MSc, PhD Students, and Post-Doctoral researchers, organized research conferences/seminars, and has been a jury of grants and congress. Finally, Celia has won several grants and awards from portuguese and international entities. (https://www.researchgate.net/profile/Celia Rodrigues2; Ciencia ID: 5F12-D3E1-E028).

Jesus A. Romo

Dr. Jesus Romo is originally from Mexico but moved to Texas at an early age. He received his PhD in Cell and Molecular Biology (Microbiology and Immunology Track) from The University of Texas at San Antonio, where his research focused on developing anti-virulence therapies for the treatment of fungal infections caused by opportunistic pathogenic fungi from the genus Candida. More specifically, he focused on inhibiting biofilm formation and preventing the development of drug resistance. Currently, he is an NIH IRACDA postdoctoral scholar at Tufts University School of Medicine in the department of Molecular Biology and Microbiology studying the role of fungal colonizers of the gastrointestinal tract during infection by the bacterial pathogen *Clostridioides difficile*. Jesus is pursuing a career in academia because of his passion for research and love for teaching and mentoring the next generation of underrepresented scientists.

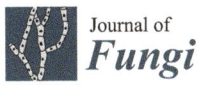

Editorial

Fungal Biofilms 2020

Célia F. Rodrigues [1,*] and Jesus A. Romo [2,*]

1. LEPABE—Laboratory for Process Engineering, Environment, Biotechnology and Energy, Faculty of Engineering, University of Porto, Rua Dr. Roberto Frias, 4200-465 Porto, Portugal
2. Department of Molecular Biology and Microbiology, Tufts University School of Medicine, Boston, MA 02111, USA
* Correspondence: c.fortunae@gmail.com (C.F.R.); jesus.romo@tufts.edu (J.A.R.)

Citation: Rodrigues, C.F.; Romo, J.A. Fungal Biofilms 2020. *J. Fungi* 2021, 7, 603. https://doi.org/10.3390/jof7080603

Received: 22 July 2021
Accepted: 23 July 2021
Published: 26 July 2021

Publisher's Note: MDPI stays neutral with regard to jurisdictional claims in published maps and institutional affiliations.

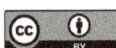

Copyright: © 2021 by the authors. Licensee MDPI, Basel, Switzerland. This article is an open access article distributed under the terms and conditions of the Creative Commons Attribution (CC BY) license (https://creativecommons.org/licenses/by/4.0/).

Fungal infections are an important and increasing global threat, carrying not only high morbidity and mortality rates, but also extraordinary healthcare costs. Without an effective response, it is predicted that 10 million people will die per year because of multidrug-resistant pathogens. A high percentage of the mortalities caused by fungi are known to have a biofilm etiology [1–4]. In fact, biofilms are the predominant mode of fungal growth. They have several ecologic benefits, for example higher nutrient availability, metabolic cooperation, protection from the environmental stresses, and acquisition of new and advantageous features. Besides, single-species and mixed-species biofilms are particularly problematic to eradicate, being, thus, the foundation of chronic infections, particularly if medical devices are existent [5].

A total of ten papers were published in this Special Issue including three reviews and six original articles. These cover a wide range of topics with original research on polymicrobial biofilms of fungi and bacteria, small molecule screening, characterization of the impact of current antifungals on biofilms of non-*albicans* species, characterization of non-*albicans* species biofilm matrix, and biofilms of *Aspergillus fumigatus*. Additionally, review articles cover the antifungal effect of *quorum sensing* molecules on *Candida* biofilms, sexual biofilms of *Candida albicans*, and a compilation of plant derived compounds and their activities against biofilms formed by *Candida* species.

The reports describe original research in the area of antimicrobials and include work involving individual and combinatorial efficacy of compounds with specific activity against fungi, bacteria, or both within polymicrobial biofilms [6], a screen of a small molecule library alone or in combination with current antifungals in search of compounds with anti-biofilm and pre-formed biofilm activities [7], characterization of the effect of echinocandins against planktonic and biofilm lifestyles of clinical isolates from the *Candida haemulonii* complex [8], and the use of a membranotropic peptide to disrupt polymicrobial biofilms of *Candida albicans* and *Klebsiella pneumoniae* [9]. Additional reports phenotypically characterized colonies from *Candida parapsilosis* clinical isolates as a way to predict their biofilm formation capabilities [10], conducted analyses of the biofilm matrix composition from the *Candida haemulonii* species complex [11], and investigated the virulence and biofilm capabilities of an *Aspergillus fumigatus* environmental isolate with interest in the role of this isolate in the textile industry [12].

The reviews in this Special Issue covered recent developments in the area of *Candida albicans* sexual biofilms specifically focusing on how they are formed, their physical characteristics, and their role in *Candida* biology [13], the properties of the quorum sensing molecules farnesol and tyrosol secreted by *Candida* and their effect as anti-biofilm agents [14], and an extensive compilation of plant derived compounds with activities against biofilms of distinct *Candida* species [15]. Overall, this Special Issue is a great resource highlighting novel work on fungal biofilms.

Acknowledgments: C.F.R. would like to acknowledge the UID/EQU/00511/2020 Project—Laboratory of Process Engineering, Environment, Biotechnology and Energy (LEPABE)—financed by national funds through FCT/MCTES (PIDDAC).

Conflicts of Interest: The authors declare no conflict of interest.

References

1. Ivanova, K.; Ramon, E.; Hoyo, J.; Tzanov, T. Innovative Approaches for Controlling Clinically Relevant Biofilms: Current Trends and Future Prospects. *Curr. Top. Med. Chem.* **2017**, *17*, 1889–1914. [CrossRef]
2. Costerton, J.W.; Cheng, K.J.; Geesey, G.G.; Ladd, T.I.; Nickel, J.C.; Dasgupta, M.; Marrie, T.J. Bacterial biofilms in nature and disease. *Annu. Rev. Microbiol.* **1987**, *41*, 435–464. [CrossRef]
3. Costerton, J.W.; Stewart, P.S.; Greenberg, E.P. Bacterial biofilms: A common cause of persistent infections. *Science* **1999**, *284*, 1318–1322. [CrossRef] [PubMed]
4. Hall-Stoodley, L.; Costerton, J.W.; Stoodley, P. Bacterial biofilms: From the natural environment to infectious diseases. *Nat. Rev. Microbiol.* **2004**, *2*, 95–108. [CrossRef] [PubMed]
5. Santos, A.; Galdino, A.C.M.; Mello, T.P.; Ramos, L.S.; Branquinha, M.H.; Bolognese, A.M.; Columbano Neto, J.; Roudbary, M. What are the advantages of living in a community? A microbial biofilm perspective! *Mem. Inst. Oswaldo Cruz* **2018**, *113*, e180212. [CrossRef] [PubMed]
6. Lobo, C.I.V.; Lopes, A.; Klein, M.I. Compounds with Distinct Targets Present Diverse Antimicrobial and Antibiofilm Efficacy against Candida albicans and Streptococcus mutans, and Combinations of Compounds Potentiate Their Effect. *J. Fungi* **2021**, *7*, 340. [CrossRef] [PubMed]
7. Lohse, M.B.; Ennis, C.L.; Hartooni, N.; Johnson, A.D.; Nobile, C.J. A Screen for Small Molecules to Target Candida albicans Biofilms. *J. Fungi* **2020**, *7*, 9. [CrossRef] [PubMed]
8. Ramos, L.S.; Silva, L.N.; Branquinha, M.H.; Santos, A.L.S. Susceptibility of the Candida haemulonii Complex to Echinocandins: Focus on Both Planktonic and Biofilm Life Styles and a Literature Review. *J. Fungi* **2020**, *6*, 201. [CrossRef] [PubMed]
9. Maione, A.; de Alteriis, E.; Carraturo, F.; Galdiero, S.; Falanga, A.; Guida, M.; Di Cosmo, A.; Maselli, V.; Galdiero, E. The Membranotropic Peptide gH625 to Combat Mixed Candida albicans/Klebsiella pneumoniae Biofilm: Correlation between In Vitro Anti-Biofilm Activity and In Vivo Antimicrobial Protection. *J. Fungi* **2021**, *7*, 26. [CrossRef] [PubMed]
10. Gomez-Molero, E.; De-la-Pinta, I.; Fernandez-Pereira, J.; Groß, U.; Weig, M.; Quindos, G.; de Groot, P.W.J.; Bader, O. Candida parapsilosis Colony Morphotype Forecasts Biofilm Formation of Clinical Isolates. *J. Fungi* **2021**, *7*, 33. [CrossRef] [PubMed]
11. Ramos, L.S.; Mello, T.P.; Branquinha, M.H.; Santos, A.L.S. Biofilm Formed by Candida haemulonii Species Complex: Structural Analysis and Extracellular Matrix Composition. *J. Fungi* **2020**, *6*, 46. [CrossRef] [PubMed]
12. Rebaza, T.D.; Ludena, Y.; Samolski, I.; Villena, G.K. Gene Expression Analysis of Non-Clinical Strain of Aspergillus fumigatus (LMB-35Aa): Does Biofilm Affect Virulence? *J. Fungi* **2020**, *6*, 376. [CrossRef] [PubMed]
13. Perry, A.M.; Hernday, A.D.; Nobile, C.J. Unraveling How Candida albicans Forms Sexual Biofilms. *J. Fungi* **2020**, *6*, 14. [CrossRef] [PubMed]
14. Kovacs, R.; Majoros, L. Fungal Quorum-Sensing Molecules: A Review of Their Antifungal Effect against Candida Biofilms. *J. Fungi* **2020**, *6*, 99. [CrossRef]
15. Karpinski, T.M.; Ozarowski, M.; Seremak-Mrozikiewicz, A.; Wolski, H.; Adamczak, A. Plant Preparations and Compounds with Activities against Biofilms Formed by Candida spp. *J. Fungi* **2021**, *7*, 360. [CrossRef] [PubMed]

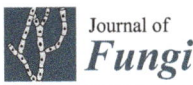

Review

Plant Preparations and Compounds with Activities against Biofilms Formed by *Candida* spp.

Tomasz M. Karpiński [1,*], Marcin Ożarowski [2], Agnieszka Seremak-Mrozikiewicz [3,4,5], Hubert Wolski [3,6] and Artur Adamczak [7]

1. Department of Medical Microbiology, Poznań University of Medical Sciences, Wieniawskiego 3, 61-712 Poznań, Poland
2. Department of Biotechnology, Institute of Natural Fibres and Medicinal Plants, National Research Institute, Wojska Polskiego 71b, 60-630 Poznań, Poland; marcin.ozarowski@iwnirz.pl
3. Division of Perinatology and Women's Diseases, Poznań University of Medical Sciences, Polna 33, 60-535 Poznań, Poland; asm@data.pl (A.S.-M.); hubertwolski@wp.pl (H.W.)
4. Laboratory of Molecular Biology in Division of Perinatology and Women's Diseases, Poznań University of Medical Sciences, Polna 33, 60-535 Poznań, Poland
5. Department of Pharmacology and Phytochemistry, Institute of Natural Fibres and Medicinal Plants, National Research Institute, Kolejowa 2, 62-064 Plewiska, Poland
6. Division of Gynecology and Obstetrics, Podhale Multidisciplinary Hospital, Szpitalna 14, 34-400 Nowy Targ, Poland
7. Department of Botany, Breeding and Agricultural Technology of Medicinal Plants, Institute of Natural Fibres and Medicinal Plants, National Research Institute, Kolejowa 2, 62-064 Plewiska, Poland; artur.adamczak@iwnirz.pl
* Correspondence: tkarpin@ump.edu.pl; Tel.: +48-61-854-61-38

Citation: Karpiński, T.M.; Ożarowski, M.; Seremak-Mrozikiewicz, A.; Wolski, H.; Adamczak, A. Plant Preparations and Compounds with Activities against Biofilms Formed by *Candida* spp. *J. Fungi* **2021**, *7*, 360. https://doi.org/10.3390/jof7050360

Academic Editors: Célia F. Rodrigues and Jesus A. Romo

Received: 20 March 2021
Accepted: 1 May 2021
Published: 5 May 2021

Publisher's Note: MDPI stays neutral with regard to jurisdictional claims in published maps and institutional affiliations.

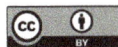

Copyright: © 2021 by the authors. Licensee MDPI, Basel, Switzerland. This article is an open access article distributed under the terms and conditions of the Creative Commons Attribution (CC BY) license (https://creativecommons.org/licenses/by/4.0/).

Abstract: Fungi from the genus *Candida* are very important human and animal pathogens. Many strains can produce biofilms, which inhibit the activity of antifungal drugs and increase the tolerance or resistance to them as well. Clinically, this process leads to persistent infections and increased mortality. Today, many *Candida* species are resistant to drugs, including *C. auris*, which is a multiresistant pathogen. Natural compounds may potentially be used to combat multiresistant and biofilm-forming strains. The aim of this review was to present plant-derived preparations and compounds that inhibit *Candida* biofilm formation by at least 50%. A total of 29 essential oils and 16 plant extracts demonstrate activity against *Candida* biofilms, with the following families predominating: Lamiaceae, Myrtaceae, Asteraceae, Fabaceae, and Apiacae. *Lavandula dentata* (0.045–0.07 mg/L), *Satureja macrosiphon* (0.06–8 mg/L), and *Ziziphora tenuior* (2.5 mg/L) have the best antifungal activity. High efficacy has also been observed with *Artemisia judaica*, *Lawsonia inermis*, and *Thymus vulgaris*. Moreover, 69 plant compounds demonstrate activity against *Candida* biofilms. Activity in concentrations below 16 mg/L was observed with phenolic compounds (thymol, pterostilbene, and eugenol), sesquiterpene derivatives (warburganal, polygodial, and ivalin), chalconoid (lichochalcone A), steroidal saponin (dioscin), flavonoid (baicalein), alkaloids (waltheriones), macrocyclic bisbibenzyl (riccardin D), and cannabinoid (cannabidiol). The above compounds act on biofilm formation and/or mature biofilms. In summary, plant preparations and compounds exhibit anti-biofilm activity against *Candida*. Given this, they may be a promising alternative to antifungal drugs.

Keywords: *Candida*; biofilm; treatment; antifungals; natural compounds; essential oil; extract; minimal inhibitory concentration (MIC)

1. Introduction

The genus *Candida* contains about 150 species; however, most are environmental organisms. The most medically important is *Candida albicans*, which accounts for about 80% of infections. *C. albicans* causes more than 400,000 cases of bloodstream life-threatening infections annually, with a mortality rate of about 42% [1]. *Candida* non-*albicans* species that are mainly responsible for infections are *C. glabrata*, *C. parapsilosis*, *C. tropicalis*, *C. krusei*, and *C. dubliniensis* [2]. Less frequently identified are *C. guilliermondii*, *C. lusitaniae*, *C. rugosa*, *C. orthopsilosis*, *C. metapsilosis*, *C. famata*, *C. inconspicua*, and *C. kefyr* [3].

C. albicans is a member of the commensal microflora. It colonizes the oral mucosal surface of 30–50% of healthy people. The rate of carriage increases with age and in persons with dental prostheses up to 60% [4–6]. Opportunistic infection caused by *Candida* species is termed candidiasis. At least one episode of vulvovaginal candidiasis (or thrush) concerns 50 to 75% of women of childbearing age [7]. Candidiasis can also affect the oral cavity, penis, skin, nails, cornea, and other parts of the body. In immunocompromised persons, untreated candidiasis poses the risk of systemic infection and fungemia [5,8]. *Candida* can be an important etiological factor in the infection of chronic wounds that are difficult to treat; this is mainly related to the production of biofilm [9].

Treatment of candidiasis depends on the infection site and the patient's condition. According to guidelines, vulvovaginal candidiasis should be treated with oral or topical fluconazole; however, regarding *C. glabrata* infection, topical boric acid, nystatin, or flucytosine is suggested. In oropharyngeal candidiasis, the treatment options include clotrimazole, miconazole, or nystatin, and in severe disease, fluconazole or voriconazole. In candidemia and invasive candidiasis, the drugs of choice are echinocandins (caspofungin, micafungin, anidulafungin), fluconazole, or voriconazole; in resistant strains, amphoteticin B is used. In selected cases of candidemia caused by *C. krusei*, voriconazole is recommended [10–12]. More details can be found in the Guidelines of the Infectious Diseases Society of America [12] and the European Society of Clinical Microbiology and Infectious Diseases [11]. Increasingly, *Candida* species are becoming resistant to drugs. Marak and Dhanashree [13] tested the resistance of 90 *Candida* strains isolated from different clinical samples, such as pus, urine, blood, and body fluid. Their study revealed that about 41% of *C. albicans* strains are resistant to fluconazole and voriconazole. Simultaneously, about 41% of *C. tropicalis* strains are resistant to voriconazole and about 36% of strains to fluconazole. In strains of *C. krusei*, about 23% are resistant to fluconazole and about 18% to voriconazole. Rudramurthy et al. [14] studied resistance in *C. auris*, which is considered a multiresistant pathogen. Among 74 strains obtained from patients with candidemia, over 90% of strains were resistant to fluconazole and about 73% to voriconazole. Virulence factors of *Candida* species include the secretion of hydrolases, the transition of yeast to hyphae, phenotypic switching, and biofilm formation [15,16]. All microorganisms in biofilm form are more resistant to antimicrobial and host factors, which leads to difficulties in eradication [17]. It has also been shown that resistance to drugs increases significantly in the case of *Candida* biofilm occurrence. Biofilm prevents the spread of antifungals; moreover, fluconazole is bound by the biofilm matrix [18]. The formation of a *Candida* biofilm during infection increases mortality, length of hospital stay, and cost of antifungal therapy [19].

Due to the above, new antifungal drugs are sought that could effectively combat not only planktonic fungi but also fungal biofilms. The natural compounds offer promise, with many acting on *Candida* species or biofilms in vitro [20].

The aim of this review was to present plant-derived natural compounds that have an effect against biofilms formed by *Candida* species.

2. Materials and Methods

In this review, publications available in PubMed and Scopus databases and through the Google search engine were taken into account. The following keywords and their combinations were used: "antifungal," "Candida," "anti-biofilm," "biofilm," "plant," "compound," "extract," and "essential oil." The principal inclusion criterion was the inhibition of biofilm formation by at least 50%. We focused on biofilm inhibition assays, in which the time of culture allowed for *Candida* biofilm maturation was at least 24 hours. Articles from the year 2000 to the present were taken into account. All articles published in predatory journals were rejected.

3. Results and Discussion

3.1. Plant Preparations That Display Activity against Candida Biofilms

The present review includes 60 articles in which *Candida* biofilm formation was inhibited by at least 50%. It has been shown that preparations from 34 plants demonstrate activity against *Candida* biofilms. Among them were 29 essential oils and 16 extracts. The plants from the following families dominated: Lamiaceae (6 species in 5 genera), Myrtaceae (5 species in 4 genera), Asteraceae (4 species in 4 genera), Fabaceae (4 species in 3 genera), and Apiacae (4 species in 2 genera).

Plants from the Lamiaceae family had the best antifungal activity, including *Lavandula dentata* (0.045–0.07 mg/L) [21], *Satureja macrosiphon* (0.06–8 mg/L) [22], and *Ziziphora tenuior* (2.5 mg/L) [23]. *Artemisia judaica* (2.5 mg/L) from the Asteraceae family [24], *Lawsonia inermis* (2.5–12.5 mg/L) from the Lythraceae family [25], and *Thymus vulgaris* (12.5 mg/L) from the Lamiaceae family [26] likewise exhibited good antifungal activity (Table 1). All preparations were essential oils, with the exception of *Lawsonia inermis*, which was an extract. Most of the plant preparations presented in Table 1 acted on biofilm formation and/or mature biofilms.

Table 1. Antifungal (MICs) and anti-biofilm (inhibition >50%) activity of plant preparations (essential oils or extracts).

Name of Plant (Family)	Main Compounds Presented in the Reference (EO: Essential Oil)	Targeted Species of *Candida*	MICs (mg/L; mL/L)	Inhibition of Biofilm Formation by at Least 50% (mg/L; mL/L)	Inhibited Stage of Biofilm; Method of Biofilm Detection	Ref.
Acorus calamus var. *angustatus* Besser = *A. tatarinowii* Schott (Acoraceae)	EO: asaraldehyde, 1-(2,4,5-trimethoxyphenyl)-1,2-propanediol, α-asarone, β-asarone, γ-asarone, acotatarone C	*C. albicans*	51.2	50–200	Mature biofilm; crystal violet and fluorescence microscopy	[27]
Allium sativum L. (Amaryllidaceae)	Extract: allicin	*C. albicans*	400	60	Biofilm formation; XTT	[28]
Aloysia gratissima (Aff & Hook).Tr (Verbenaceae)	EO: E-pinocamphone (16.07%), β-pinene (12.01%), guaiol (8.53%), E-pinocarveol acetate (8.19%)	*C. albicans*	15	500	Biofilm formation; crystal violet	[29]
Artemisia judaica L. (Asteraceae)	EO: piperitone (30.4%), camphor (16.1%), ethyl cinnamate (11.0%), chrysanthenone (6.7%)	*C. albicans*	1.25	2.5	Mature biofilm; XTT	[24]
		C. guillermondii	1.25	2.5		
		C. krusei	1.25	2.5		
		C. parapsilosis	1.25	2.5		
		C. tropicalis	1.25	2.5		
Buchenavia tomentosa Eichler (Combretaceae)	Extract: gallic acid, kaempferol, epicatechin, ellagic acid, vitexin, and corilagin	*C. albicans*	625	312.5	Biofilm formation and mature biofilm; culture	[30]
Chamaecostus cuspidatus (Nees & Mart.) C.Specht & D.W.Stev. (Costaceae)	Extract: dioscin, aferoside A, aferoside C	*C. albicans*	250	15.62	Biofilm formation and mature biofilm; MTT	[31]
Cinnamomum verum J. Presl (Lauraceae)	EO: eugenol (77.22%), benzyl benzoate (4.53%), trans-caryophyllene (3.39%), acetyl eugenol (2.75%), linalool 2.11%	*C. albicans*	1000	150	Biofilm adhesion; XTT	[32]
		C. dubliniensis	1000	200		
		C. tropicalis	1000	350		
Citrus limon (L.) Osbeck (Rutaceae)	EO: limonene (53.4%), neral (11%), geraniol (9%), trans-limonene oxide (7%), nerol (6%)	*C. albicans*	500	2000	Biofilm formation and mature biofilm; XTT	[33]
		C. glabrata	250	1000		
		C. krusei	500	125		
		C. orthopsilosis	500	1000		
		C. parapsilosis	500	2000		
		C. tropicalis	250	2000		
Copaifera paupera (Herzog) Dwyer (Fabaceae)	Extract: galloylquinic acids, quercetrin, afzelin	*C. glabrata*	5.89	46.87	Biofilm formation and mature biofilm; XTT	[34]
Copaifera reticulata Ducke (Fabaceae)	Extract: galloylquinic acids, quercetrin, afzelin	*C. glabrata*	5.89	46.87	Biofilm formation and mature biofilm; XTT	[34]
Coriandrum sativum L. (Apiaceae)	EO: 1-decanol (33.91%), E-2-decen-1-ol (23.59%), 2-dodecen-1-ol (13.06%), E-2-tetradecen-1-ol (5.46%)	*C. albicans*	7	250	Biofilm formation; crystal violet	[29]
	EO: decanal (19.09%), trans-2-decenal (17.54%), 2-decen-1-ol (12.33%), cyclodecane (12.15%)	*C. albicans*	15.6	62.5–125	Biofilm adhesion; crystal violet	[35]
		C. dubliniensis	31.2	62.5–125		
		C. rugosa	15.6	62.5		
		C. tropicalis	31.2	31.25–250		

Table 1. Cont.

Name of Plant (Family)	Main Compounds Presented in the Reference (EO: Essential Oil)	Targeted Species of Candida	MICs (mg/L; mL/L)	Inhibition of Biofilm Formation by at Least 50% (mg/L; mL/L)	Inhibited Stage of Biofilm; Method of Biofilm Detection	Ref.
Croton eluteria (L.) W.Wright (Euphorbiaceae)	EO: α-pinene (29.37%), β-pinene (19.35%), camphene (10.31%), 1,8-cineole (9.68%)	C. albicans	4000	5–500	Biofilm formation; confocal laser microscopy	[36]
Cupressus sempervirens L. (Cupressaceae)	EO: sabinene (20.3%), citral (20%), terpinene-4-ol (15.4%), α-pinene (8%)	C. albicans	250	1000	Biofilm formation and mature biofilm; XTT	[33]
		C. glabrata	31.25	250		
		C. krusei	62.5	62.5		
		C. orthopsilosis	31.25	125		
		C. parapsilosis	62.5	500		
		C. tropicalis	250	500		
Cymbopogon citratus (DC.) Stapf (Poaceae)	EO: no composition	C. albicans	180–360	22.5–180	Biofilm formation; XTT	[37]
Cymbopogon martini (Roxb.) W.Watson (Poaceae)	EO: no composition	C. albicans	16,800	800	Biofilm formation; XTT	[38]
Cymbopogon nardus (L.) Rendle (Poaceae)	EO: citronellal (27.87%), geraniol (22.77%), geranial (14.54%), citronellol (11.85%), neral (11.21%)	C. albicans	1000	2500–5000	Biofilm adhesion; XTT	[39]
		C. krusei	250–500	2500		
		C. parapsilosis	500–1000	5000–10,000		
Cyperus articulatus L. (Cyperaceae)	EO: α-pinene (5.72%), mustakone (5.66%), α-bulnesene (5.02%), α-copaene (4.97%)	C. albicans	125	250	Biofilm formation; crystal violet	[29]
Eucalyptus sp. (Myrtaceae)	EO: no composition	C. albicans	8	8	Mature biofilm; luminescence	[40]
Eucalyptus globulus Labill. (Myrtaceae)	EO: 1,8-cineole (75.8%), p-cymene (7.5%), α-pinene (7.4%), limonene (6.4%)	C. albicans	219	11,250–22,500	Mature biofilm; atomic force microscopy	[41]
		C. glabrata	219	11,250–22,500		
		C. tropicalis	885	11,250–22,500		
	EO: no composition	C. albicans	8400	500	Biofilm formation; XTT	[38]
Eugenia brasiliensis Lam. (Myrtaceae)	Extract: no composition	C. albicans	15.62–31.25	156	Mature biofilm; scanning electron microscopy	[42]
Eugenia leitonii Legrand nom. inval. (Myrtaceae)	Extract: no composition	C. albicans	15.62–250	156	Mature biofilm; scanning electron microscopy	[42]
Helichrysum italicum (Roth) G.Don (Asteraceae)	EO: α-pinene (27.64%), γ-elemene (23.84%), β-caryophyllene (13.05%), α-longipinene (11.25%)	C. albicans	6000	10–500	Biofilm formation; confocal laser microscopy	[36]
Laserpitium latifolium L. (Apiaceae)	Extract: laserpitine	C. albicans	1250	6300	Mature biofilm; luminescence	[43]
		C. krusei	1250	6300		
Laserpitium ochridanum Micevski (Apiaceae)	Extract: isomontanolide, montanolide, tarolide	C. albicans	5000	10,000	Mature biofilm; luminescence	[43]
		C. krusei	5000	10,000		
Laserpitium zernyi Hayek = L. siler subsp. zernyi (Hayek) Tutin (Apiaceae)	Extract: isomontanolide, montanolide, tarolide	C. albicans	7500	15,000	Mature biofilm; luminescence	[43]
		C. krusei	7500	37,500		
Lavandula dentata L. (Lamiaceae)	EO: eucalyptol (42.66%), β-pinene (8.59%), trans-α-bisabolene (6.34%), pinocarveol (6.3%)	C. albicans	0.15–0.18	0.045–0.07	Mature biofilm; XTT	[21]
Lawsonia inermis L. (Lythraceae)	Extract: no composition	C. albicans	10	2.5–12.5	Mature biofilm; MTT	[25]
Lippia sidoides Cham. (Verbenaceae)	EO: thymol (65.76%), p-cymene (17.28%), α-caryophyllene (10.46%), cyclohexanone (6.5%)	C. albicans	250	500	Biofilm formation; crystal violet	[29]
Litsea cubeba (Lour.) Pers. (Lauraceae)	EO: limonene (37%), neral (31.4%), citral (12%), linalool (4%)	C. albicans	500	2000	Biofilm formation and mature biofilm; XTT	[33]
		C. glabrata	250	2000		
		C. krusei	62.5	250		
		C. orthopsilosis	250	2000		
		C. parapsilosis	500	1000		
		C. tropicalis	1000	2000		
Mentha × piperita L. (Lamiaceae)	EO: menthol (32.93%), menthone (24.41%), 1,8-cineole (7.89%)	C. albicans	1–10	10	Biofilm formation; MTT	[44]
	EO: no composition	C. albicans	11,600	800	Biofilm formation; XTT	[38]
Mikania glomerata Spreng (Asteraceae)	EO: germacrene D (38.29%), α-caryophyllene (9.49%), bicyclogermacrene (7.98%), caryophyllene oxide (4.28%)	C. albicans	250	500	Biofilm formation; crystal violet	[29]

Table 1. Cont.

Name of Plant (Family)	Main Compounds Presented in the Reference (EO: Essential Oil)	Targeted Species of Candida	MICs (mg/L; mL/L)	Inhibition of Biofilm Formation by at Least 50% (mg/L; mL/L)	Inhibited Stage of Biofilm; Method of Biofilm Detection	Ref.
Myrtus communis L. (Myrtaceae)	EO: α-pinene (39.8%), 1,8-cineole (24.8%), limonene (10.7%), linalool (6.4%)	*C. albicans*	1250–10,000	None or 1250	No data; no data	[45]
		C. parapsilosis	1250 to >16,000	1250		
		C. tropicalis	1250–16,000	1250		
Ononis spinosa L. (Fabaceae)	Extract: kaempferol-O-dihexoside, kaempferol-O-hexoside-pentoside, kaempferol-O-hexoside, quercetin-O-hexoside-pentoside, acetylquercetin-O-hexoside	*C. albicans*	620	10,000	Mature biofilm; luminescence	[46]
		C. krusei	620	5000		
		C. tropicalis	310	10,000		
Pelargonium graveolens L'Hér. (Geraniaceae)	EO: geraniol (42.3%), linalool (20.1%), citronellol (11.1%), menthone (8.0%)	*C. albicans*	125	4000–8000	Mature biofilm; XTT	[47]
Piper claussenianum (Miq.) C. DC. (Piperaceae)	EO: nerolidols	*C. albicans*	4100–9600	2400–12,600	Mature biofilm; MTT	[48]
Portulaca oleracea L. (Portulacaceae)	Extract: no composition	*C. albicans*	10	12.5	Mature biofilm; MTT	[25]
Punica granatum L. (Lythraceae)	Extract: ellagic acid	*C. albicans*	1000	100–750	Biofilm formation and mature biofilm; crystal violet	[49]
Santolina impressa Hoffmanns. & Link (Asteraceae)	EO: β-pinene (22.5%), 1,8-cineole (10.0%), limonene (9.1%), camphor (8.1%), β-phellandrene (8.0%)	*C. albicans*	540	70–1050	Biofilm formation; XTT	[50]
Satureja hortensis L. (Lamiaceae)	EO: thymol (45.9%), gamma-terpinen (16.71%), carvacrol (12.81%), p-cymene (9.61%)	*C. albicans*	200–400	400–4800	Biofilm adhesion, formation, and mature biofilm; MTT	[51]
Satureja macrosiphon (Coss.) = *Micromeria macrosiphon* Coss. (Lamiaceae)	EO: linalool (28.46%), borneol (16.22%), terpinene-4-ol (14.58%), *cis*-sabinene hydrate (12.96%)	*C. albicans*	0.06–4	0.06–8	Biofilm formation; XTT	[22]
		C. dubliniensis	0.25–4	2–8		
Syzygium aromaticum (L.) Merr. & L.M.Perry = *Eugenia caryophyllus* (Spreng.) Bullock & S.G.Harrison (Myrtaceae)	EO: no composition	*C. albicans*	100–200	50	Biofilm formation; XTT	[37]
	EO: no composition	*C. albicans*	48,000	3300	Biofilm formation; XTT	[38]
Thymus vulgaris L. (Lamiaceae)	EO: thymol (54.73%), carvacrol (12.42%), terpineol (4.00%), nerol acetate (2.86%), fenchol (0.5%)	*C. albicans*	1.56–25	12.5	Biofilm formation; absorbance, crystal violet, and scanning electron microscopy	[26]
		C. tropicalis	25–50	12.5		
Warburgia ugandensis Sprague (Canellaceae)	Extract: ugandenial A, warburganal, polygodial, alpha-linolenic acid ALA	*C. albicans*	Lack of data	1000	Biofilm formation and mature biofilm; XTT and confocal laser microscopy	[52]
		C. glabrata	Lack of data	1000		
Ziziphora tenuior L. (Lamiaceae)	EO: pulegone (46.8%), p-menth-3-en-8-ol (12.5%), isomenthone (6.6%), 8-hydroxymenthone (6.2%), isomenthol (4.7%)	*C. albicans*	1.25	2.5	Mature biofilm; XTT	[23]
Zuccagnia punctata L. (Fabaceae)	Extract: no composition	*C. albicans*	400	100	Biofilm formation and mature biofilm; XTT and crystal violet	[53]

Legend: MIC—minimal inhibitory concentration; XTT—reduction assay of 2,3-bis(2-methoxy-4-nitro-5-sulfophenyl)-5-[carbonyl(phenylamino)]-2H-tetrazolium hydroxide; MTT—reduction assay of 3-(4,5-dimethylthiazol-2-yl)-2,5-diphenyltetrazolium bromide [54,55].

Antibiofilm activity may vary between plants in the same family. For example, in the Lamiaceae family, essential oil from *Lavandula dentata* acted against *C. albicans* biofilm at concentrations of 0.045–0.07 μL/mL [21], while essential oil from *Satureja hortensis* acted against the same biofilm at concentrations of 400–4800 mg/L [51]. There may also be large differences within the same species, due to various reasons. This may be influenced by, for example, different research methodologies, the use of different strains of fungi, and different chemical compositions depending on the plant variety, country, and season of harvest. A notable example of such a difference is observed with *Mentha* × *piperita*. In studies by Benzaid et al. [44], essential oil of *M. piperita* acted against *Candida* biofilm at a concentration of 10 μL/mL. However, the work of Agarwal et al. [38] showed that the same essential oil was active at 800 μL/mL.

Changes in the content of active substances were described by Gonçalves et al. [56]. They showed that in essential oil from *Mentha cervina* collected in August, the amount of isomenthone was 8.7% and pulegone was 75.1%. However, in essential oil collected in February, the ratio of the two compounds reversed and amounted to 77.0% for isomenthone and 12.9% for pulegone. The method of obtaining the compounds likewise had an influence on their content in the final essential oil. In a study by Ćavar et al. [57], the composition of essential oils of *Calamintha glandulosa* differed depending on the extraction method. The level of menthone was 3.3% using aqueous reflux extraction, 4.7% using hydrodistillation, and 8.3% using steam distillation, while the concentration of shisofuran was only 0.1% using hydrodistillation and steam distillation, while aqueous reflux yielded 9.7%.

3.2. Plant Compounds That Display Activity against Candida Biofilm

It has been shown that 69 compounds obtained from plants demonstrate activity against *Candida* biofilms (Table 2). Among these, the most common are monoterpenes (20), followed by sesquiterpene lactones (7) and sesquiterpenes (6). Another big group is also phenolic compounds, including phenols (6), phenolic acids (5), phenolic aldehydes (2), polyphenols (2), and phenolic alcohol (1).

In terms of activity, large differences were found, depending on the authors cited. Eugenol and thymol serve as good examples. Both compounds exhibited excellent activity in some studies (from 12.5 mg/L for eugenol [58] and 1.56 mg/L for thymol [26]), and in other studies, the activity was very poor (up to 80,000 for both [59]). These differences may be related, for example, to a different purity of the compound, a different fungal suspension density, or even to the use of other *Candida* strains with different sensitivities to chemical substances. A number of other factors, such as the type of culture medium, pH of the medium, incubation time, and temperature may likewise influence the antimicrobial activity [20].

According to the European Committee on Antimicrobial Susceptibility Testing (EUCAST), the antifungal clinical breakpoints are between 0.001 mg/L and 16 mg/L [60]. Using EUCAST guidelines in this review, the most active compounds that inhibit (>50%) *Candida* biofilm formation are lichochalcone A (from 0.2 mg/L) [61], thymol (from 3.12 mg/L) [26], dioscin (from 3.9 mg/L) [31], baicalein (from 4 mg/L) [62], warburganal (4.5 mg/L) [52], pterostilbene, waltheriones and riccardin D (both from 8 mg/L) [63–65], polygodial (10.8 mg/L) [52], cannabidiol and eugenol (both from 12.5 mg/L) [58,66], and ivalin (15.4 mg/L) [67]. It is interesting that monoterpenes, which represent the highest percentage of substances listed in Table 2, are not the most active compounds. The two larger groups with the best activity are phenolic compounds (thymol, pterostilbene, and eugenol), and sesquiterpene derivatives (warburganal, polygodial, and ivalin). Single compounds with the highest observed activity belong to chalconoids (lichochalcone A), steroidal saponins (dioscin), flavonoids (baicalein), alkaloids (waltheriones), macrocyclic bisbibenzyls (riccardin D), and cannabinoids (cannabidiol). Most of the compounds presented in Table 2 acted on biofilm formation and/or mature biofilm.

Table 2. Antifungal and antibiofilm activity of plant compounds.

Active Compound	Example of Plant Origin	Targeted Fungus	MICs (mg/L, mL/L)	Inhibition of Biofilm Formation by at Least 50% (mg/L, mL/L)	Inhibited Stage of Biofilm; Method of Biofilm Detection	Ref.
Antidesmone (alkaloid)	*Waltheria indica*, *W. brachypetala*	C. albicans	32	16	Mature biofilm; XTT	[63]
		C. glabrata	>32	16		
		C. krusei	16	16		
		C. parapsilosis	4	16		
		C. tropicalis	>32	16		
Anisaldehyde (phenolic aldehyde)	*Pimpinella anisum*, *Foeniculum vulgare*	C. albicans	500	500	Mature biofilm; XTT, crystal violet, and inverted light microscopy	[68]
Anisic acid (phenolic acid)	*Pimpinella anisum*	C. albicans	4000	4000	Mature biofilm; XTT, crystal violet, and inverted light microscopy	[68]
Anisyl alcohol (phenolic alcohol)	*Pimpinella anisum*	C. albicans	31	500	Mature biofilm; XTT, crystal violet, and inverted light microscopy	[68]
Baicalein (flavonoid)	*Scutellaria baicalensis*, *S. lateriflora*	C. albicans	No data	4–32	Biofilm formation; XTT	[62]

Table 2. Cont.

Active Compound	Example of Plant Origin	Targeted Fungus	MICs (mg/L, mL/L)	Inhibition of Biofilm Formation by at Least 50% (mg/L, mL/L)	Inhibited Stage of Biofilm; Method of Biofilm Detection	Ref.
Camphene (monoterpene)	Croton eluteria, Cinnamomum verum	C. albicans	No data	500	Biofilm formation; confocal laser microscopy	[36]
		C. albicans	1000	2000	Mature biofilm; XTT, crystal violet, and inverted light microscopy	[69]
Camphor (bicyclic monoterpene)	Cinnamomum camphora, Artemisia annua	C. albicans	125–250	Not or 62.5–250	Biofilm formation; crystal violet and absorbance	[70]
		C. glabrata	175	Not		
		C. krusei	350	Not		
		C. parapsilosis	125	Not		
		C. tropicalis	175	175		
Cannabidiol (cannabinoid)	Cannabis sativa	C. albicans	No data	12.5–100	Biofilm formation; confocal microscopy	[66]
Carvacrol (phenol)	Thymus serpyllum, Carum carvi, Origanum vulgare	C. albicans	250	500	Mature biofilm; XTT, crystal violet, and inverted light microscopy	[69]
			100–20,000	300–1250	Mature biofilm; XTT	[71]
			1000	750–1500	Biofilm formation; MTT	[72]
		C. glabrata	100–20,000	300–1250	Mature biofilm; XTT	[71]
		C. parapsilosis	100–20,000	300–1250		
Carvene/Limonene (monoterpene)	Citrus × aurantium, Citrus limon	C. albicans	1000	4000	Mature biofilm; XTT, crystal violet, and inverted light microscopy	[69]
Carvone/Carvol (monoterpene)	Carum carvi, Mentha spicata	C. albicans	>4000	250	Mature biofilm; XTT, crystal violet, and inverted light microscopy	[69]
β-Caryophyllene (sesquiterpene)	Helichrysum italicum, Caryophyllusaromaticus	C. albicans	No data	100–500	Biofilm formation; confocal microscopy	[36]
1,4-Cineole (monoterpene)	Rosmarinus officinalis, Thymus vulgaris	C. albicans	>4000	4000	Mature biofilm; XTT, crystal violet, and inverted light microscopy	[69]
1,8-Cineole/Eucalyptol (monoterpene)	Eucalyptus globulus, Salvia officinalis, Pinus sylvestris	C. albicans	4000	4000	Mature biofilm; XTT, crystal violet, and inverted light microscopy	[69]
			8	4	Mature biofilm; luminescence	[40]
			3000–23,000	Not or 3000–23,000	Biofilm formation; crystal violet and absorbance	[70]
		C. glabrata	2000	Not		
		C. krusei	4000	2000–4000		
		C. parapsilosis	2000	1000–2000		
		C. tropicalis	4000	2000–4000		
Cinnamaldehyde (aldehyde)	Cinnamomum sp., Apium graveolens	C. albicans	62	125	Mature biofilm; XTT, crystal violet, and inverted light microscopy	[68]
			50–400	25–200	Mature biofilm; XTT	[58]
Cinnamic acid (phenolic acid)	Cinnamomum sp.	C. albicans	2000	4000	Mature biofilm; XTT, crystal violet, and inverted light microscopy	[68]
Citral (monoterpene)	Melissa officinalis, Backhousia citriodora	C. albicans	500	1000	Mature biofilm; XTT, crystal violet, and inverted light microscopy	[69]
Citronellal (monoterpene)	Cymbopogon citratus, Melissa officinalis	C. albicans	500	1000	Mature biofilm; XTT, crystal violet, and inverted light microscopy	[69]
β-Citronellol (monoterpene)	Melissa officinalis, Pelargonium roseum	C. albicans	500	1000	Mature biofilm; XTT, crystal violet, and inverted light microscopy	[69]
Cuminaldehyde (monoterpene)	Carum carvi, Cinnamomum verum	C. albicans	1000 to >4000	6000–7000	Biofilm formation; MTT	[72]
p-Cymene (monoterpene)	Thymus vulgaris, Eucalyptus sp.	C. albicans	2000	4000	Mature biofilm; XTT, crystal violet, and inverted light microscopy	[69]
8-Deoxoantidesmone (alkaloid)	Waltheria indica	C. albicans	16	32	Mature biofilm; XTT	[63]
		C. glabrata	>32	32		
		C. krusei	32	32		
		C. parapsilosis	32	32		
		C. tropicalis	>32	32		
2′,4′-Dihydroxy-3′-methoxychalcone (chalcone)	Zuccagnia punctata, Oxytropis falcata	C. albicans	100	25	Biofilm formation and mature biofilm; XTT and crystal violet	[53]
Dioscin (steroidal saponin)	Dioscorea sp., Chamaecostus	C. albicans	3.9–15.62	3.9–31.25	Biofilm formation and mature biofilm; MTT	[31]
Ellagic acid (polyphenol)	Punica granatum L.	C. albicans	75–100	25–40	Biofilm formation and mature biofilm; crystal violet	[49]
Emodin (anthraquinone)	Rheum palmatum, Frangula alnus	C. albicans	12.5–50	Not or 100–400	Biofilm adhesion; MTT	[73]

Table 2. Cont.

Active Compound	Example of Plant Origin	Targeted Fungus	MICs (mg/L, mL/L)	Inhibition of Biofilm Formation by at Least 50% (mg/L, mL/L)	Inhibited Stage of Biofilm; Method of Biofilm Detection	Ref.
4α,5α-Epoxy-10α,14H-1-epi-inuviscolide (sesquiterpene lactone)	Carpesium macrocephalum	C. albicans	>128	38	Biofilm formation and mature biofilm; XTT	[67]
Eugenol (phenol)	Syzygium aromaticum, Cinnamomum sp.	C. albicans	50–400	12.5–200	Mature biofilm; XTT	[58]
			250	500	Mature biofilm; XTT, crystal violet, and inverted light microscopy	[69]
			500	500	Mature biofilm; XTT, crystal violet, and inverted light microscopy	[68]
			1200	10,000–80,000	Mature biofilm; XTT	[59]
Farnesol (sesquiterpene)	Tilia sp., Cymbopogon sp.	C. albicans	1000	500	Mature biofilm; XTT, crystal violet, and inverted light microscopy	[68]
			1000	500	Mature biofilm; XTT, crystal violet, and inverted light microscopy	[69]
Gallic acid (phenolic acid)	Polygonum sp., Buchenavia tomentosa	C. albicans	5000	2500	Biofilm formation and mature biofilm; culture	[30]
Geraniol (monoterpene)	Pelargonium graveolens, Rosa sp.	C. albicans	1000	1000	Mature biofilm; XTT, crystal violet, and inverted light microscopy	[69]
		C. albicans	100–20,000	300–1250	Mature biofilm; XTT	[71]
		C. albicans	No data	1000–8000	Mature biofilm; XTT	[47]
		C. glabrata	100–20,000	300–1250	Mature biofilm; XTT	[71]
		C. parapsilosis	100–20,000	300–1250		
Guaiacol (phenol)	Guaiacum officinale, Apium graveolens	C. albicans	500	1000	Mature biofilm; XTT, crystal violet, and inverted light microscopy	[68]
Hydroxychavicol (phenol)	Piper betle	C. albicans	125–500	125–1000	Biofilm formation and mature biofilm; XTT	[74]
β-Ionone (carotenoid)	Lawsonia inermis, Camellia sinensis	C. albicans	250	250	Mature biofilm; XTT, crystal violet, and inverted light microscopy	[69]
Isomontanolide (sesquiterpenic lactone)	Laserpitium ochridanum, L. zernyi	C. albicans	50	250	Mature biofilm; luminescence	[43]
		C. krusei	200	250		
Isopulegol (monoterpene)	Mentha rotundifolia, Melissa officinalis	C. albicans	>4000	250	Mature biofilm; XTT, crystal violet, and inverted light microscopy	[69]
Ivalin (sesquiterpene lactone)	Geigeria aspera, Carpesium macrocephalum	C. albicans	>128	15.4	Biofilm formation and mature biofilm; XTT	[67]
Laserpitine (sesquiterpene lactone)	Laserpitium latifolium, Laserpitiumhalleri	C. albicans	200	400	Mature biofilm; luminescence	[43]
		C. krusei	200	400		
Lichochalcone A (chalconoid)	Glycyrrhiza sp.	C. albicans	6.25–12.5	0.2–20	Biofilm formation; crystal violet	[61]
Linalool (monoterpene)	Lavandula officinalis, Pelargonium graveolens	C. albicans	No data	100–500	Biofilm formation; confocal laser microscopy	[36]
			2000	1000	Mature biofilm; XTT, crystal violet, and inverted light microscopy	[69]
			No data	1000–8000	Mature biofilm; XTT	[47]
α-Longipinene (sesquiterpene)	Croton eluteria, Helichrysum italicum	C. albicans	No data	100–500	Biofilm formation; confocal laser microscopy	[36]
Menthol (monoterpene)	Mentha spp.	C. albicans	>4000	2000	Mature biofilm; XTT, crystal violet, and inverted light microscopy	[69]
			2500	10,000–80,000	Mature biofilm; XTT	[59]
Montanolide (sesquiterpene lactone)	Laserpitium ochridanum, L. zernyi	C. albicans	200	400	Mature biofilm; luminescence	[43]
		C. krusei	200	400		
Morin (flavonoid)	Prunus dulcis, Morus alba	C. albicans	150	37.5–600	Biofilm formation; crystal violet	[75]
Myrcene (monoterpene)	Humulus lupulus, Cannabis sativa	C. albicans	1000	2000	Mature biofilm; XTT, crystal violet, and inverted light microscopy	[69]
Nerol (monoterpene)	Citrus × aurantium, Humulus lupulus	C. albicans	2000	500	Mature biofilm; XTT, crystal violet, and inverted light microscopy	[69]
Nerolidols (sesquiterpene)	Citrus × aurantium, Piper claussenianum	C. albicans	18,600–62,500	2500–10,000	Mature biofilm; MTT	[48]
α-Pinene (monoterpene)	Pinus sylvestris, Picea abies	C. albicans	3125	3125	Biofilm formation; XTT	[76]
β-Pinene (monoterpene)	Pinus sylvestris, Picea abies	C. albicans	2000	4000	Mature biofilm; XTT, crystal violet, and inverted light microscopy	[69]
			187	187	Biofilm formation; XTT	[76]
Polygodial (sesquiterpene)	Warburgia ugandensis, Polygonum hydropiper	C. albicans	4.1	10.8	Biofilm formation and mature biofilm; XTT and confocal laser microscopy	[52]
		C. glabrata	94.1	50.6–61.9		

Table 2. Cont.

Active Compound	Example of Plant Origin	Targeted Fungus	MICs (mg/L, mL/L)	Inhibition of Biofilm Formation by at Least 50% (mg/L, mL/L)	Inhibited Stage of Biofilm; Method of Biofilm Detection	Ref.
Pterostilbene (polyphenol)	Pterocarpus marsupium, Pterocarpus santalinus, Vitis vinifera	C. albicans	No data	8–32	Biofilm formation and mature biofilm; XTT	[65]
Riccardin D (macrocyclic bisbibenzyl)	Dumortiera hirsuta	C. albicans	16	8–64	Mature biofilm; XTT	[64]
Salicylaldehyde (phenolic aldehyde)	Filipendula ulmaria, Fagopyrum esculentum	C. albicans	31	125	Mature biofilm; XTT, crystal violet, and inverted light microscopy	[68]
Salicylic acid (phenolic acid)	Salix sp., Filipendula ulmaria	C. albicans	4000	2000	Mature biofilm; XTT, crystal violet, and inverted light microscopy	[68]
Scopoletin (cumarin)	Mitracarpus frigidus, Scopolia carniola	C. tropicalis	50	50	Biofilm adhesion, formation, and mature biofilm; absorbance and digital scanning	[77]
6-Shogaol (phenylalkane)	Zingiber officinale	C. auris	32–64	16–64	Mature biofilm; crystal violet	[78]
Tarolide (sesquiterpene lactone)	Laserpitium ochridanum, L. zernyi	C. albicans	400	1000	Mature biofilm; luminescence	[43]
		C. krusei	400	1000		
Telekin (sesquiterpene lactone)	Carpesium macrocephalum, Telekia speciose	C. albicans	>128	36	Biofilm formation and mature biofilm; XTT	[67]
Terpinolene (terpene)	Cannabis sativa, Citrus limon	C. albicans	2000	4000	Mature biofilm; XTT, crystal violet, and inverted light microscopy	[69]
5,7,3′,4′-Tetramethoxyflavone (flavonoid)	Psiadia punctulate, Kaempferia parviflora	C. albicans	100	40	Biofilm formation; crystal violet	[79]
α-Thujone (monoterpene)	Artemisia absinthium, Tanacetum vulgare	C. albicans	>4000	500	Mature biofilm; XTT, crystal violet, and inverted light microscopy	[69]
Thymol (phenol)	Thymus vulgaris, Trachyspermum copticum	C. albicans	250	250	Mature biofilm; XTT, crystal violet, and inverted light microscopy	[69]
			1.56–50	3.12	Biofilm formation; absorbance, crystal violet, and scanning electron microscopy	[26]
			32–128	128	Biofilm adhesion and mature biofilm; XTT	[80]
			100–20,000	300–1250	Mature biofilm; XTT	[71]
			125	125–250	Biofilm formation and mature biofilm; XTT	[81]
			1200	5000–80,000	Mature biofilm; XTT	[59]
		C. tropicalis	1.56–50	12.5	Biofilm formation; absorbance, crystal violet, and scanning electron microscopy	[26]
		C. glabrata	100–20,000	300–1250	Mature biofilm; XTT	[71]
		C. parapsilosis	100–20,000	300–1250		
Tn-AFP1 (protein)	Trapa natans	C. tropicalis	32	16	Mature biofilm; XTT	[82]
5,6,8-Trihydroxy-7,4′ dimethoxy flavone (flavonoid)	Thymus membranaceus subsp. membranaceus, Dodonaea viscosa var. angustifolia	C. albicans	390	390	Biofilm formation and mature biofilm; MTT	[83]
5(R)-Vanessine (alkaloid)	Waltheria indica	C. albicans	32	16	Mature biofilm; XTT	[63]
		C. glabrata	>32	16		
		C. krusei	32	16		
		C. parapsilosis	>32	16		
		C. tropicalis	>32	16		
Vanillic acid (phenolic acid)	Angelica sinensis, Solanum tuberosum	C. albicans	>4000	4000	Mature biofilm; XTT, crystal violet, and inverted light microscopy	[68]
Vanillin (phenol)	Vanilla planifolia	C. albicans	1000	500	Mature biofilm; XTT, crystal violet, and inverted light microscopy	[68]
Waltheriones (alkaloid)	Waltheria indica, W. viscosissima	C. albicans	4–32	8–32	Mature biofilm; XTT	[63]
		C. glabrata	32 or >32	8–32		
		C. krusei	16–32 or >32	8–32		
		C. parapsilosis	2–32 or >32	8–32		
		C. tropicalis	32 or >32	8–32		
Warburganal (sesquiterpene)	Warburgia sp.	C. albicans	4	4.5	Biofilm formation and mature biofilm; XTT and confocal laser microscopy	[52]
		C. glabrata	72–72.6	49.1–55.9		

Legend: MIC—minimal inhibitory concentration; XTT—reduction assay of 2,3-bis(2-methoxy-4-nitro-5-sulfophenyl)-5-[carbonyl(phenylamino)]-2H-tetrazolium hydroxide; MTT—reduction assay of 3-(4,5-dimethylthiazol-2-yl)-2,5-diphenyltetrazolium bromide [54,55].

4. Conclusions

Plant preparations (essential oils and extracts) and pure compounds exhibit anti-biofilm activity against *Candida* species. Some of them are characterized by high activity in concentrations below 16 mg/L. Given this activity at relatively low concentrations, some may prove to be promising alternatives to antifungal drugs, especially in the cases of resistant or multiresistant strains of *Candida*. Moreover, the simple chemical structures involved and relative ease of extraction from natural sources warrant further research into the development of new, promising, and much-needed plant-based antifungals.

Author Contributions: Conceptualization, T.M.K. and M.O.; methodology, T.M.K.; analysis of results, T.M.K. and M.O.; writing—original draft preparation, T.M.K., M.O., A.S.-M., H.W., and A.A.; writing—review and editing, T.M.K. and M.O.; supervision, T.M.K.; funding acquisition, T.M.K. and H.W. All authors have read and agreed to the published version of the manuscript.

Funding: This research received no external funding.

Institutional Review Board Statement: Not applicable.

Informed Consent Statement: Not applicable.

Acknowledgments: We are very grateful to Mark Stasiewicz for English language corrections.

Conflicts of Interest: The authors declare no conflict of interest.

References

1. Brown, G.D.; Denning, D.W.; Gow, N.A.R.; Levitz, S.M.; Netea, M.G.; White, T.C. Hidden Killers: Human Fungal Infections. *Sci. Transl. Med.* **2012**, *4*, 165rv13. [CrossRef]
2. Ciurea, C.N.; Kosovski, I.-B.; Mare, A.D.; Toma, F.; Pintea-Simon, I.A.; Man, A. *Candida* and Candidiasis-Opportunism Versus Pathogenicity: A Review of the Virulence Traits. *Microorganisms* **2020**, *8*, 857. [CrossRef] [PubMed]
3. Moran, G.; Coleman, D.; Sullivan, D. An Introduction to the Medically Important Candida Species. In *Candida and Candidiasis*, 2nd ed.; Wiley: Hoboken, NJ, USA, 2012; pp. 11–25.
4. Buranarom, N.; Komin, O.; Matangkasombut, O. Hyposalivation, Oral Health, and *Candida* Colonization in Independent Dentate Elders. *PLoS ONE* **2020**, *15*, e0242832. [CrossRef] [PubMed]
5. Arya, N.R.; Naureen, R.B. Candidiasis. In *StatPearls*; StatPearls Publishing: Treasure Island, FL, USA, 2021.
6. Millet, N.; Solis, N.V.; Swidergall, M. Mucosal IgA Prevents Commensal *Candida Albicans* Dysbiosis in the Oral Cavity. *Front. Immunol.* **2020**, *11*, 555363. [CrossRef] [PubMed]
7. Sobel, J.D. Vulvovaginal Candidosis. *Lancet* **2007**, *369*, 1961–1971. [CrossRef]
8. Vila, T.; Sultan, A.S.; Montelongo-Jauregui, D.; Jabra-Rizk, M.A. Oral Candidiasis: A Disease of Opportunity. *J. Fungi* **2020**, *6*, 15. [CrossRef] [PubMed]
9. Karpiński, T.; Sopata, M.; Mańkowski, B. The Antimicrobial Effectiveness of Antiseptics as a Challenge in Hard to Heal Wounds. *Leczenie Ran* **2020**, *17*, 88–94. [CrossRef]
10. Bhattacharya, S.; Sae-Tia, S.; Fries, B.C. Candidiasis and Mechanisms of Antifungal Resistance. *Antibiotics* **2020**, *9*, 312. [CrossRef]
11. Cornely, O.A.; Bassetti, M.; Calandra, T.; Garbino, J.; Kullberg, B.J.; Lortholary, O.; Meersseman, W.; Akova, M.; Arendrup, M.C.; Arikan-Akdagli, S.; et al. ESCMID* Guideline for the Diagnosis and Management of *Candida* Diseases 2012: Non-Neutropenic Adult Patients. *Clin. Microbiol. Infect.* **2012**, *18* (Suppl. 7), 19–37. [CrossRef]
12. Pappas, P.G.; Kauffman, C.A.; Andes, D.R.; Clancy, C.J.; Marr, K.A.; Ostrosky-Zeichner, L.; Reboli, A.C.; Schuster, M.G.; Vazquez, J.A.; Walsh, T.J.; et al. Clinical Practice Guideline for the Management of Candidiasis: 2016 Update by the Infectious Diseases Society of America. *Clin. Infect. Dis.* **2016**, *62*, e1–e50. [CrossRef]
13. Marak, M.B.; Dhanashree, B. Antifungal Susceptibility and Biofilm Production of *Candida* Spp. Isolated from Clinical Samples. *Int. J. Microbiol.* **2018**, *2018*, 7495218. [CrossRef] [PubMed]
14. Rudramurthy, S.M.; Chakrabarti, A.; Paul, R.A.; Sood, P.; Kaur, H.; Capoor, M.R.; Kindo, A.J.; Marak, R.S.K.; Arora, A.; Sardana, R.; et al. *Candida auris* Candidaemia in Indian ICUs: Analysis of Risk Factors. *J. Antimicrob. Chemother.* **2017**, *72*, 1794–1801. [CrossRef] [PubMed]
15. Mayer, F.L.; Wilson, D.; Hube, B. *Candida Albicans* Pathogenicity Mechanisms. *Virulence* **2013**, *4*, 119–128. [CrossRef] [PubMed]
16. Łaska, G.; Sienkiewicz, A. Antifungal Activity of the Rhizome Extracts of *Pulsatilla Vulgaris* against *Candida Glabrata*. *Eur. J. Biol. Res.* **2019**, *9*, 93–103.
17. Gebreyohannes, G.; Nyerere, A.; Bii, C.; Sbhatu, D.B. Challenges of Intervention, Treatment, and Antibiotic Resistance of Biofilm-Forming Microorganisms. *Heliyon* **2019**, *5*, e02192. [CrossRef]
18. Pereira, R.; Dos Santos Fontenelle, R.O.; de Brito, E.H.S.; de Morais, S.M. Biofilm of *Candida Albicans*: Formation, Regulation and Resistance. *J. Appl. Microbiol.* **2020**. [CrossRef] [PubMed]

19. Tumbarello, M.; Fiori, B.; Trecarichi, E.M.; Posteraro, P.; Losito, A.R.; De Luca, A.; Sanguinetti, M.; Fadda, G.; Cauda, R.; Posteraro, B. Risk Factors and Outcomes of Candidemia Caused by Biofilm-Forming Isolates in a Tertiary Care Hospital. *PLoS ONE* **2012**, *7*, e33705. [CrossRef]
20. Karpiński, T.M. Essential Oils of Lamiaceae Family Plants as Antifungals. *Biomolecules* **2020**, *10*, 103. [CrossRef]
21. Müller-Sepúlveda, A.; Chevecich, C.C.; Jara, J.A.; Belmar, C.; Sandoval, P.; Meyer, R.S.; Quijada, R.; Moura, S.; López-Muñoz, R.; Díaz-Dosque, M.; et al. Chemical Characterization of *Lavandula Dentata* Essential Oil Cultivated in Chile and Its Antibiofilm Effect against *Candida Albicans*. *Planta Med.* **2020**, *86*, 1225–1234. [CrossRef]
22. Motamedi, M.; Saharkhiz, M.J.; Pakshir, K.; Amini Akbarabadi, S.; Alikhani Khordshami, M.; Asadian, F.; Zareshahrabadi, Z.; Zomorodian, K. Chemical Compositions and Antifungal Activities of *Satureja Macrosiphon* against *Candida* and *Aspergillus* Species. *Curr. Med. Mycol.* **2019**, *5*, 20–25. [CrossRef]
23. Abu-Darwish, M.S.; Cabral, C.; Gonçalves, M.J.; Cavaleiro, C.; Cruz, M.T.; Paoli, M.; Tomi, F.; Efferth, T.; Salgueiro, L. *Ziziphora Tenuior*, L. Essential Oil from Dana Biosphere Reserve (Southern Jordan); Chemical Characterization and Assessment of Biological Activities. *J. Ethnopharmacol.* **2016**, *194*, 963–970. [CrossRef] [PubMed]
24. Abu-Darwish, M.S.; Cabral, C.; Gonçalves, M.J.; Cavaleiro, C.; Cruz, M.T.; Zulfiqar, M.; Khan, I.A.; Efferth, T.; Salgueiro, L. Chemical Composition and Biological Activities of *Artemisia Judaica* Essential Oil from Southern Desert of Jordan. *J. Ethnopharmacol.* **2016**, *191*, 161–168. [CrossRef]
25. Soliman, S.S.M.; Semreen, M.H.; El-Keblawy, A.A.; Abdullah, A.; Uppuluri, P.; Ibrahim, A.S. Assessment of Herbal Drugs for Promising Anti-*Candida* Activity. *BMC Complement. Altern. Med.* **2017**, *17*, 257. [CrossRef]
26. Jafri, H.; Ahmad, I. *Thymus Vulgaris* Essential Oil and Thymol Inhibit Biofilms and Interact Synergistically with Antifungal Drugs against Drug Resistant Strains of *Candida Albicans* and *Candida Tropicalis*. *J. Mycol. Med.* **2020**, *30*, 100911. [CrossRef] [PubMed]
27. Wang, Z.-J.; Zhu, Y.-Y.; Yi, X.; Zhou, Z.-S.; He, Y.-J.; Zhou, Y.; Qi, Z.-H.; Jin, D.-N.; Zhao, L.-X.; Luo, X.-D. Bioguided Isolation, Identification and Activity Evaluation of Antifungal Compounds from *Acorus Tatarinowii* Schott. *J. Ethnopharmacol.* **2020**, *261*, 113119. [CrossRef]
28. Said, M.M.; Watson, C.; Grando, D. Garlic Alters the Expression of Putative Virulence Factor Genes SIR2 and ECE1 in Vulvovaginal C. Albicans Isolates. *Sci. Rep.* **2020**, *10*, 3615. [CrossRef]
29. Bersan, S.M.F.; Galvão, L.C.C.; Goes, V.F.F.; Sartoratto, A.; Figueira, G.M.; Rehder, V.L.G.; Alencar, S.M.; Duarte, R.M.T.; Rosalen, P.L.; Duarte, M.C.T. Action of Essential Oils from Brazilian Native and Exotic Medicinal Species on Oral Biofilms. *BMC Complement. Altern. Med.* **2014**, *14*, 451. [CrossRef]
30. Teodoro, G.R.; Gontijo, A.V.L.; Salvador, M.J.; Tanaka, M.H.; Brighenti, F.L.; Delbem, A.C.B.; Delbem, Á.C.B.; Koga-Ito, C.Y. Effects of Acetone Fraction From *Buchenavia Tomentosa* Aqueous Extract and Gallic Acid on *Candida Albicans* Biofilms and Virulence Factors. *Front. Microbiol.* **2018**, *9*, 647. [CrossRef] [PubMed]
31. Barros Cota, B.; Batista Carneiro de Oliveira, D.; Carla Borges, T.; Cristina Catto, A.; Valverde Serafim, C.; Rogelis Aquiles Rodrigues, A.; Kohlhoff, M.; Leomar Zani, C.; Assunção Andrade, A. Antifungal Activity of Extracts and Purified Saponins from the Rhizomes of *Chamaecostus Cuspidatus* against *Candida* and *Trichophyton* Species. *J. Appl. Microbiol.* **2021**, *130*, 61–75. [CrossRef] [PubMed]
32. Wijesinghe, G.K.; Maia, F.C.; de Oliveira, T.R.; de Feiria, S.N.B.; Joia, F.; Barbosa, J.P.; Boni, G.C.; de Cássia Orlandi Sardi, J.; Rosalen, P.L.; Höfling, J.F. Effect of *Cinnamomum Verum* Leaf Essential Oil on Virulence Factors of *Candida* Species and Determination of the In-Vivo Toxicity with Galleria Mellonella Model. *Mem. Inst. Oswaldo. Cruz.* **2020**, *115*, e200349. [CrossRef]
33. Pedroso, R.D.S.; Balbino, B.L.; Andrade, G.; Dias, M.C.P.S.; Alvarenga, T.A.; Pedroso, R.C.N.; Pimenta, L.P.; Lucarini, R.; Pauletti, P.M.; Januário, A.H.; et al. In Vitro and In Vivo Anti-*Candida* Spp. Activity of Plant-Derived Products. *Plants* **2019**, *8*, 494. [CrossRef]
34. Andrade, G.; Orlando, H.C.S.; Scorzoni, L.; Pedroso, R.S.; Abrão, F.; Carvalho, M.T.M.; Veneziani, R.C.S.; Ambrósio, S.R.; Bastos, J.K.; Mendes-Giannini, M.J.S.; et al. Brazilian *Copaifera* Species: Antifungal Activity against Clinically Relevant *Candida* Species, Cellular Target, and In Vivo Toxicity. *J. Fungi* **2020**, *6*, 153. [CrossRef]
35. de Almeida Freires, I.; Murata, R.M.; Furletti, V.F.; Sartoratto, A.; de Alencar, S.M.; Figueira, G.M.; de Oliveira Rodrigues, J.A.; Duarte, M.C.T.; Rosalen, P.L. *Coriandrum Sativum* L. (Coriander) Essential Oil: Antifungal Activity and Mode of Action on *Candida* spp., and Molecular Targets Affected in Human Whole-Genome Expression. *PLoS ONE* **2014**, *9*, e99086. [CrossRef]
36. Manoharan, R.K.; Lee, J.-H.; Kim, Y.-G.; Kim, S.-I.; Lee, J. Inhibitory Effects of the Essential Oils α-Longipinene and Linalool on Biofilm Formation and Hyphal Growth of *Candida Albicans*. *Biofouling* **2017**, *33*, 143–155. [CrossRef] [PubMed]
37. Khan, M.S.A.; Ahmad, I. Biofilm Inhibition by *Cymbopogon Citratus* and *Syzygium Aromaticum* Essential Oils in the Strains of *Candida Albicans*. *J. Ethnopharmacol.* **2012**, *140*, 416–423. [CrossRef] [PubMed]
38. Agarwal, V.; Lal, P.; Pruthi, V. Prevention of *Candida Albicans* Biofilm by Plant Oils. *Mycopathologia* **2008**, *165*, 13–19. [CrossRef] [PubMed]
39. De Toledo, L.G.; Ramos, M.A.D.S.; Spósito, L.; Castilho, E.M.; Pavan, F.R.; Lopes, É.D.O.; Zocolo, G.J.; Silva, F.A.N.; Soares, T.H.; Dos Santos, A.G.; et al. Essential Oil of *Cymbopogon Nardus* (L.) Rendle: A Strategy to Combat Fungal Infections Caused by *Candida* Species. *Int. J. Mol. Sci.* **2016**, *17*, 1252. [CrossRef]
40. Hendry, E.R.; Worthington, T.; Conway, B.R.; Lambert, P.A. Antimicrobial Efficacy of *Eucalyptus* Oil and 1,8-Cineole Alone and in Combination with Chlorhexidine Digluconate against Microorganisms Grown in Planktonic and Biofilm Cultures. *J. Antimicrob. Chemother.* **2009**, *64*, 1219–1225. [CrossRef]

41. Quatrin, P.M.; Verdi, C.M.; de Souza, M.E.; de Godoi, S.N.; Klein, B.; Gundel, A.; Wagner, R.; de Almeida Vaucher, R.; Ourique, A.F.; Santos, R.C.V. Antimicrobial and Antibiofilm Activities of Nanoemulsions Containing *Eucalyptus Globulus* Oil against *Pseudomonas Aeruginosa* and *Candida* spp. *Microb. Pathog.* **2017**, *112*, 230–242. [CrossRef] [PubMed]
42. Sardi, J.d.C.O.; Freires, I.A.; Lazarini, J.G.; Infante, J.; de Alencar, S.M.; Rosalen, P.L. Unexplored Endemic Fruit Species from Brazil: Antibiofilm Properties, Insights into Mode of Action, and Systemic Toxicity of Four *Eugenia* spp. *Microb. Pathog.* **2017**, *105*, 280–287. [CrossRef]
43. Popović, V.; Stojković, D.; Nikolić, M.; Heyerick, A.; Petrović, S.; Soković, M.; Niketić, M. Extracts of Three *Laserpitium* L. Species and Their Principal Components Laserpitine and Sesquiterpene Lactones Inhibit Microbial Growth and Biofilm Formation by Oral *Candida* Isolates. *Food. Funct.* **2015**, *6*, 1205–1211. [CrossRef]
44. Benzaid, C.; Belmadani, A.; Djeribi, R.; Rouabhia, M. The Effects of *Mentha* × *Piperita* Essential Oil on *C. Albicans* Growth, Transition, Biofilm Formation, and the Expression of Secreted Aspartyl Proteinases Genes. *Antibiotics* **2019**, *8*, 10. [CrossRef] [PubMed]
45. Cannas, S.; Molicotti, P.; Usai, D.; Maxia, A.; Zanetti, S. Antifungal, Anti-Biofilm and Adhesion Activity of the Essential Oil of *Myrtus Communis* L. against *Candida* Species. *Nat. Prod. Res.* **2014**, *28*, 2173–2177. [CrossRef]
46. Stojković, D.; Dias, M.I.; Drakulić, D.; Barros, L.; Stevanović, M.; C F R Ferreira, I.; D Soković, M. Methanolic Extract of the Herb *Ononis Spinosa* L. Is an Antifungal Agent with No Cytotoxicity to Primary Human Cells. *Pharmaceuticals* **2020**, *13*, 78. [CrossRef] [PubMed]
47. Souza, C.M.C.; Pereira Junior, S.A.; Moraes, T.d.S.; Damasceno, J.L.; Amorim Mendes, S.; Dias, H.J.; Stefani, R.; Tavares, D.C.; Martins, C.H.G.; Crotti, A.E.M.; et al. Antifungal Activity of Plant-Derived Essential Oils on *Candida Tropicalis* Planktonic and Biofilms Cells. *Med. Mycol.* **2016**, *54*, 515–523. [CrossRef] [PubMed]
48. Curvelo, J.A.R.; Marques, A.M.; Barreto, A.L.S.; Romanos, M.T.V.; Portela, M.B.; Kaplan, M.A.C.; Soares, R.M.A. A Novel Nerolidol-Rich Essential Oil from *Piper Claussenianum* Modulates *Candida Albicans* Biofilm. *J. Med. Microbiol.* **2014**, *63*, 697–702. [CrossRef] [PubMed]
49. Bakkiyaraj, D.; Nandhini, J.R.; Malathy, B.; Pandian, S.K. The Anti-Biofilm Potential of Pomegranate (*Punica Granatum* L.) Extract against Human Bacterial and Fungal Pathogens. *Biofouling* **2013**, *29*, 929–937. [CrossRef] [PubMed]
50. Alves-Silva, J.M.; Zuzarte, M.; Gonçalves, M.J.; Cruz, M.T.; Cavaleiro, C.; Salgueiro, L. Unveiling the Bioactive Potential of the Essential Oil of a Portuguese Endemism, *Santolina Impressa*. *J. Ethnopharmacol.* **2019**, *244*, 112120. [CrossRef]
51. Sharifzadeh, A.; Khosravi, A.R.; Ahmadian, S. Chemical Composition and Antifungal Activity of *Satureja Hortensis* L. Essentiall Oil against Planktonic and Biofilm Growth of *Candida Albicans* Isolates from Buccal Lesions of HIV(+) Individuals. *Microb. Pathog.* **2016**, *96*, 1–9. [CrossRef]
52. Kipanga, P.N.; Liu, M.; Panda, S.K.; Mai, A.H.; Veryser, C.; Van Puyvelde, L.; De Borggraeve, W.M.; Van Dijck, P.; Matasyoh, J.; Luyten, W. Biofilm Inhibiting Properties of Compounds from the Leaves of *Warburgia Ugandensis* Sprague Subsp. *Ugandensis* against *Candida* and Staphylococcal Biofilms. *J. Ethnopharmacol.* **2020**, *248*, 112352. [CrossRef] [PubMed]
53. Gabriela, N.; Rosa, A.M.; Catiana, Z.I.; Soledad, C.; Mabel, O.R.; Esteban, S.J.; Veronica, B.; Daniel, W.; Ines, I.M. The Effect of *Zuccagnia Punctata*, an Argentine Medicinal Plant, on Virulence Factors from *Candida* Species. *Nat. Prod. Commun.* **2014**, *9*, 933–936. [CrossRef]
54. Karpiński, T.M. Efficacy of Octenidine against *Pseudomonas Aeruginosa* Strains. *Eur. J. Biol. Res.* **2019**, *9*, 135–140.
55. Loures, F.V.; Levitz, S.M. XTT Assay of Antifungal Activity. *Bio. Protoc.* **2015**, *5*, e1543. [CrossRef] [PubMed]
56. Gonçalves, M.J.; Vicente, A.M.; Cavaleiro, C.; Salgueiro, L. Composition and Antifungal Activity of the Essential Oil of *Mentha Cervina* from Portugal. *Nat. Prod. Res.* **2007**, *21*, 867–871. [CrossRef]
57. Ćavar, S.; Vidic, D.; Maksimović, M. Volatile Constituents, Phenolic Compounds, and Antioxidant Activity of *Calamintha Glandulosa* (Req.) Bentham. *J. Sci. Food Agric.* **2013**, *93*, 1758–1764. [CrossRef]
58. Khan, M.S.A.; Ahmad, I. Antibiofilm Activity of Certain Phytocompounds and Their Synergy with Fluconazole against *Candida Albicans* Biofilms. *J. Antimicrob. Chemother.* **2012**, *67*, 618–621. [CrossRef]
59. Pemmaraju, S.C.; Pruthi, P.A.; Prasad, R.; Pruthi, V. *Candida Albicans* Biofilm Inhibition by Synergistic Action of Terpenes and Fluconazole. *Indian J. Exp. Biol.* **2013**, *51*, 1032–1037.
60. EUCAST: Breakpoints for Antifungals. Available online: https://eucast.org/astoffungi/clinicalbreakpointsforantifungals/ (accessed on 19 March 2021).
61. Messier, C.; Grenier, D. Effect of Licorice Compounds Licochalcone A, Glabridin and Glycyrrhizic Acid on Growth and Virulence Properties of *Candida Albicans*. *Mycoses* **2011**, *54*, e801–e806. [CrossRef] [PubMed]
62. Cao, Y.; Dai, B.; Wang, Y.; Huang, S.; Xu, Y.; Cao, Y.; Gao, P.; Zhu, Z.; Jiang, Y. In Vitro Activity of Baicalein against *Candida Albicans* Biofilms. *Int. J. Antimicrob. Agents* **2008**, *32*, 73–77. [CrossRef] [PubMed]
63. Cretton, S.; Dorsaz, S.; Azzollini, A.; Favre-Godal, Q.; Marcourt, L.; Ebrahimi, S.N.; Voinesco, F.; Michellod, E.; Sanglard, D.; Gindro, K.; et al. Antifungal Quinoline Alkaloids from *Waltheria Indica*. *J. Nat. Prod.* **2016**, *79*, 300–307. [CrossRef]
64. Cheng, A.; Sun, L.; Wu, X.; Lou, H. The Inhibitory Effect of a Macrocyclic Bisbibenzyl Riccardin D on the Biofilms of *Candida Albicans*. *Biol. Pharm. Bull.* **2009**, *32*, 1417–1421. [CrossRef] [PubMed]
65. Hu, D.-D.; Zhang, R.-L.; Zou, Y.; Zhong, H.; Zhang, E.-S.; Luo, X.; Wang, Y.; Jiang, Y.-Y. The Structure-Activity Relationship of Pterostilbene Against *Candida Albicans* Biofilms. *Molecules* **2017**, *22*, 360. [CrossRef]

66. Feldman, M.; Sionov, R.V.; Mechoulam, R.; Steinberg, D. Anti-Biofilm Activity of Cannabidiol against *Candida Albicans*. *Microorganisms* **2021**, *9*, 441. [CrossRef] [PubMed]
67. Xie, C.; Sun, L.; Meng, L.; Wang, M.; Xu, J.; Bartlam, M.; Guo, Y. Sesquiterpenes from *Carpesium Macrocephalum* Inhibit *Candida Albicans* Biofilm Formation and Dimorphism. *Bioorg. Med. Chem. Lett.* **2015**, *25*, 5409–5411. [CrossRef] [PubMed]
68. Raut, J.S.; Shinde, R.B.; Chauhan, N.M.; Karuppayil, S.M. Phenylpropanoids of Plant Origin as Inhibitors of Biofilm Formation by *Candida Albicans*. *J. Microbiol. Biotechnol.* **2014**, *24*, 1216–1225. [CrossRef] [PubMed]
69. Raut, J.S.; Shinde, R.B.; Chauhan, N.M.; Karuppayil, S.M. Terpenoids of Plant Origin Inhibit Morphogenesis, Adhesion, and Biofilm Formation by *Candida Albicans*. *Biofouling* **2013**, *29*, 87–96. [CrossRef] [PubMed]
70. Ivanov, M.; Kannan, A.; Stojković, D.S.; Glamočlija, J.; Calhelha, R.C.; Ferreira, I.C.F.R.; Sanglard, D.; Soković, M. Camphor and Eucalyptol-Anticandidal Spectrum, Antivirulence Effect, Efflux Pumps Interference and Cytotoxicity. *Int. J. Mol. Sci.* **2021**, *22*, 483. [CrossRef] [PubMed]
71. Dalleau, S.; Cateau, E.; Bergès, T.; Berjeaud, J.-M.; Imbert, C. In Vitro Activity of Terpenes against *Candida* Biofilms. *Int. J. Antimicrob. Agents* **2008**, *31*, 572–576. [CrossRef] [PubMed]
72. Touil, H.F.Z.; Boucherit, K.; Boucherit-Otmani, Z.; Khoder, G.; Madkour, M.; Soliman, S.S.M. Optimum Inhibition of Amphotericin-B-Resistant *Candida Albicans* Strain in Single- and Mixed-Species Biofilms by *Candida* and Non-*Candida* Terpenoids. *Biomolecules* **2020**, *10*, 342. [CrossRef]
73. Janeczko, M.; Masłyk, M.; Kubiński, K.; Golczyk, H. Emodin, a Natural Inhibitor of Protein Kinase CK2, Suppresses Growth, Hyphal Development, and Biofilm Formation of *Candida Albicans*. *Yeast* **2017**, *34*, 253–265. [CrossRef] [PubMed]
74. Ali, I.; Khan, F.G.; Suri, K.A.; Gupta, B.D.; Satti, N.K.; Dutt, P.; Afrin, F.; Qazi, G.N.; Khan, I.A. In Vitro Antifungal Activity of Hydroxychavicol Isolated from *Piper Betle* L. *Ann. Clin. Microbiol. Antimicrob.* **2010**, *9*, 7. [CrossRef] [PubMed]
75. Abirami, G.; Alexpandi, R.; Durgadevi, R.; Kannappan, A.; Veera Ravi, A. Inhibitory Effect of Morin Against *Candida Albicans* Pathogenicity and Virulence Factor Production: An in Vitro and in Vivo Approaches. *Front. Microbiol.* **2020**, *11*, 561298. [CrossRef] [PubMed]
76. Rivas da Silva, A.C.; Lopes, P.M.; Barros de Azevedo, M.M.; Costa, D.C.M.; Alviano, C.S.; Alviano, D.S. Biological Activities of α-Pinene and β-Pinene Enantiomers. *Molecules* **2012**, *17*, 6305–6316. [CrossRef] [PubMed]
77. Lemos, A.S.O.; Florêncio, J.R.; Pinto, N.C.C.; Campos, L.M.; Silva, T.P.; Grazul, R.M.; Pinto, P.F.; Tavares, G.D.; Scio, E.; Apolônio, A.C.M.; et al. Antifungal Activity of the Natural Coumarin Scopoletin Against Planktonic Cells and Biofilms From a Multidrug-Resistant *Candida Tropicalis* Strain. *Front. Microbiol.* **2020**, *11*, 1525. [CrossRef]
78. Kim, H.-R.; Eom, Y.-B. Antifungal and Anti-Biofilm Effects of 6-Shogaol against *Candida Auris*. *J. Appl. Microbiol.* **2020**. [CrossRef] [PubMed]
79. Dal Piaz, F.; Bader, A.; Malafronte, N.; D'Ambola, M.; Petrone, A.M.; Porta, A.; Ben Hadda, T.; De Tommasi, N.; Bisio, A.; Severino, L. Phytochemistry of Compounds Isolated from the Leaf-Surface Extract of *Psiadia Punctulata* (DC.) Vatke Growing in Saudi Arabia. *Phytochemistry* **2018**, *155*, 191–202. [CrossRef] [PubMed]
80. Shu, C.; Sun, L.; Zhang, W. Thymol Has Antifungal Activity against *Candida Albicans* during Infection and Maintains the Innate Immune Response Required for Function of the P38 MAPK Signaling Pathway in *Caenorhabditis Elegans*. *Immunol. Res.* **2016**, *64*, 1013–1024. [CrossRef] [PubMed]
81. Braga, P.C.; Culici, M.; Alfieri, M.; Dal Sasso, M. Thymol Inhibits *Candida Albicans* Biofilm Formation and Mature Biofilm. *Int. J. Antimicrob. Agents* **2008**, *31*, 472–477. [CrossRef]
82. Mandal, S.M.; Migliolo, L.; Franco, O.L.; Ghosh, A.K. Identification of an Antifungal Peptide from *Trapa Natans* Fruits with Inhibitory Effects on *Candida Tropicalis* Biofilm Formation. *Peptides* **2011**, *32*, 1741–1747. [CrossRef] [PubMed]
83. Patel, M.; Srivastava, V.; Ahmad, A. Dodonaea Viscosa Var Angustifolia Derived 5,6,8-Trihydroxy-7,4' Dimethoxy Flavone Inhibits Ergosterol Synthesis and the Production of Hyphae and Biofilm in *Candida Albicans*. *J. Ethnopharmacol.* **2020**, *259*, 112965. [CrossRef]

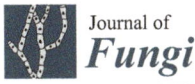

Article

Compounds with Distinct Targets Present Diverse Antimicrobial and Antibiofilm Efficacy against *Candida albicans* and *Streptococcus mutans*, and Combinations of Compounds Potentiate Their Effect

Carmélia Isabel Vitorino Lobo, Ana Carolina Urbano de Araújo Lopes and Marlise Inêz Klein *

Department of Dental Materials and Prosthodontics, School of Dentistry, São Paulo State University (Unesp), Araraquara. Rua Humaitá, 1680, Araraquara, São Paulo 14801-903, Brazil; carmelialobo@gmail.com (C.I.V.L.); carolina.urbano@unesp.br (A.C.U.d.A.L.)
* Correspondence: marlise.klein@unesp.br; Tel.: +55-16-3301-6410

Abstract: *Candida albicans* and *Streptococcus mutans* interact synergistically in biofilms associated with a severe form of dental caries. Their synergism is driven by dietary sucrose. Thus, it is necessary to devise strategies to hinder the development of those biofilms and prevent cavities. Six compounds [tt-farnesol (sesquiterpene alcohol that decreases the bacterium acidogenicity and aciduricity and a quorum sensing fungal molecule), myricetin (flavonoid that interferes with *S. mutans* exopolysaccharides production), two 2'-hydroxychalcones and 4'-hydroxychalcone (intermediate metabolites for flavonoids), compound 1771 (inhibitor of lipoteichoic synthase in Gram-positive bacteria)] with targets in both fungus and bacterium and their products were investigated for their antimicrobial and antibiofilm activities against single-species cultures. The compounds and concentrations effective on single-species biofilms were tested alone and combined with or without fluoride to control initial and pre-formed dual-species biofilms. All the selected treatments eliminated both species on initial biofilms. In contrast, some combinations eliminated the bacterium and others the fungus in pre-formed biofilms. The combinations 4'-hydroxychalcone+tt-farnesol+myricetin, 4'-hydroxychalcone+tt-farnesol+fluoride, and all compounds together with fluoride were effective against both species in pre-formed biofilms. Therefore, combinations of compounds with distinct targets can prevent *C. albicans* and *S. mutans* dual-species biofilm build-up in vitro.

Keywords: biofilm; *Candida albicans*; *Streptococcus mutans*; extracellular matrix; antimicrobial agents; antibiofilm agents

Citation: Lobo, C.I.V.; Lopes, A.C.U.d.A.; Klein, M.I. Compounds with Distinct Targets Present Diverse Antimicrobial and Antibiofilm Efficacy against *Candida albicans* and *Streptococcus mutans*, and Combinations of Compounds Potentiate Their Effect. *J. Fungi* **2021**, *7*, 340. https://doi.org/10.3390/jof7050340

Academic Editors: Célia F. Rodrigues and Jesus A. Romo

Received: 31 March 2021
Accepted: 25 April 2021
Published: 28 April 2021

Publisher's Note: MDPI stays neutral with regard to jurisdictional claims in published maps and institutional affiliations.

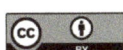

Copyright: © 2021 by the authors. Licensee MDPI, Basel, Switzerland. This article is an open access article distributed under the terms and conditions of the Creative Commons Attribution (CC BY) license (https://creativecommons.org/licenses/by/4.0/).

1. Introduction

Several human diseases are caused by dysbiotic biofilms, including tooth decay, periodontal diseases, and oral candidiasis [1]. *Candida albicans* is an opportunistic species that, when associated with *Streptococcus mutans*, contributes to forming a complex and organized biofilm that is more tolerant to environmental stresses, including antimicrobial [2]. The interaction between these two species is synergistic in the presence of dietary sucrose and leads to severe dental caries lesions [3]. Therefore, it is necessary to devise strategies to hinder the development of those biofilms.

Within the complex oral microbiota, *S. mutans* is a producer of the extracellular matrix and modulates cariogenic biofilm formation when sucrose from the host's diet is available [4]. This bacterium is acidogenic and aciduric but not the most numerous species in the mouth, and there are other acidogenic and aciduric microorganisms [5,6]. However, its exoenzymes glucosyltransferases (Gtfs) and fructosyltransferase (Ftf) use sucrose as a substrate for the synthesis of exopolysaccharides (α-glucans and fructans), important components of biofilm construction [4]. Gtfs also adsorb on the surface of other oral microorganisms, converting them into glucan producers [4]. *C. albicans* is one of the microorganisms to which Gtfs binds and form high amounts of exopolysaccharides [7]. This fungus is also acidogenic and aciduric [8], and oral biofilms could serve as reservoirs for it.

The extracellular matrix of *C. albicans* biofilms contains extracellular DNA, β-glucans, mannans, proteins, and lipids [9–12]. This matrix has been associated with resistance against antifungals [13,14]. Moreover, the biogenesis of this matrix is coordinated extracellularly, reflecting cooperative actions in the biofilm community [14]. Therefore, the production of exopolysaccharides synthesized on surfaces in situ allows adhesion and microbial accumulation [4] and contributes to the construction of the 3D matrix that surrounds and supports cells, forming an environment with acidic niches and limited diffusion [6,15]. Thus, strategies that control the matrix formation could prevent pathogenic biofilms development [13] and perhaps control the amount of *C. albicans* in oral biofilms that could flourish when conditions are favorable.

The therapeutic modalities for controlling dental biofilm formation are still limited. Chlorhexidine is a broad-spectrum antimicrobial agent that suppresses microorganisms levels in saliva but is not effective against mature biofilms, and its daily and continuous use is not recommended [16]. Fluoride is the mainstay of caries prevention, but its protection against the disease is incomplete [17]. Therefore, an attractive and superior strategy would be to use or include bioactive agents targeting virulence factors and the mechanisms for biofilm development.

Several studies have prioritized finding new antibiofilm agents, including natural substances [18–20]. Among the promising agents, *tt*-farnesol (a membrane-targeting sesquiterpenoid) and myricetin (a flavonoid) hinder the development of cariogenic biofilm formed by *S. mutans*. Myricetin inhibits the *gtfs* gene expression and Gtfs activity, thereby hindering the exopolysaccharides synthesis in situ [18,19]. *tt*-farnesol targets the cellular membrane, affecting the tolerance of *S. mutans* to acid stress. Both agents have a moderate biocidal effect [18,19], and their combination with fluoride results in fewer and less severe carious lesions [19]. In addition, *tt*-farnesol is a derivative of the sterol biosynthesis pathway in eukaryotic cells and a *quorum-sensing* molecule of *C. albicans* [21], which keeps the fungus in yeast form. However, it appears not to affect *S. mutans* in concentrations produced when both microorganisms are co-cultivated in biofilms, possible due to the thickness and amount of biomass of these biofilms [2,3]. Additionally, at concentrations above the threshold (i.e., the physiological concentration of the species), *tt*-farnesol can induce apoptosis in planktonic cultures of *C. albicans* cells [22]. Therefore, the antibiofilm effect of *tt*-farnesol and myricetin against *C. albicans* and *S. mutans* biofilms still needs to be investigated [23].

Hydroxychalcones are precursor metabolic intermediates for flavonoids and isoflavonoids. These agents inhibit the streptococcal Gtfs activity [24], impair *S. mutans* survival in planktonic culture [25]; thus, possibly impairing the structure of biofilms. In addition, flavonoids interfere with *C. albicans* cell wall formation, cause disruption of the plasma membrane and mitochondrial dysfunction, affect cell division, protein synthesis, and the efflux-mediated pumping system [26]. Also, synthetic hydroxychalcones were shown to have anti-*Candida* activity [25,27]. Nevertheless, the efficacy of hydroxychalcones on dual-species *S. mutans* and *C. albicans* biofilms is unexplored.

Also, the interference in the metabolism of lipoteichoic acids (LTA) would affect the development of biofilms by Gram-positive bacteria. The compound 1771 targets LtaS, an LTA synthase enzyme in *S. aureus* [28] and *Enterococcus faecium* [29]. This compound also hinders *S. mutans* biofilm formation [30]. However, the effect of compound 1771 on *C. albicans* is unknown.

Thus, considering the virulence and difficulty of controlling mature biofilms, this study evaluated the antimicrobial and antibiofilm activities of six compounds (*tt*-farnesol, myricetin, two 2'-hydroxychalcones, 4'-hydroxychalcone, and compound 1771) against *C. albicans* and *S. mutans* single- and dual-species settings.

2. Materials and Methods

2.1. Experimental Design

Antimicrobial activity was evaluated using planktonic cultures of *C. albicans* and *S. mutans* in microdilution assay to determine the minimum inhibitory concentration (MIC) and minimum fungicidal and bactericidal concentrations (MFC and MBC). Next, single-species biofilms were used to investigate the antibiofilm activities of compounds during initial biofilm formation (24 h) and against pre-formed biofilms (48 h). Finally, promising compounds (and their corresponding concentrations) on both species were combined to analyze the antibiofilm activity on dual-species biofilms formed by *C. albicans* and *S. mutans* on initial biofilm formation (24 h) and pre-formed biofilms (48 h). At that time, fluoride was also added, and groups with and without fluoride were evaluated. All tests were performed using a 96-polystyrene microplate to determine viable microbial population (colony forming units or CFU). At least three independent experiments were performed in triplicate for the antimicrobial and antibiofilm tests ($n = 9$). The data were statistically analyzed according to the factorial design of this study, considering each microplate well as a statistical block. The hypothesis was that elimination or reduction of at least 50% of microbial cells (of both species) from biofilm using the proposed agents and their combinations substantially affect the development of dual-species biofilms.

2.2. Test Agents

An in vitro study with *C. albicans* and *S. mutans* was conducted to investigate the antimicrobial and antibiofilm activity of six compounds: *tt*-farnesol or (E,E)-3,7,11-Trimethyl-2,6,10-dodecatrien-1-ol, trans,trans-3,7,11-Trimethyl-2,6,10-dodecatrien-1-ol (Sigma-Aldrich Co., St Louis, MO, USA; Cat.#46193; 96% purity), myricetin or 3,5,7-trihydroxy-2-(3,4,5-trihydroxyphenyl)-4H-chromen-4-one (AK Scientific, Inc., Union City, CA, USA; Cat.#J10595; 95% purity), three hydroxychalcones [2'-hydroxichalcone or 1-(2-hydroxyphenyl)-3-phenylprop-2-en-1-one (Angene, Hong Kong, China; Cat.#AGN-PC-015IM; 95% purity), 2'-hydroxichalcone or (2E)-1-(2-hydroxyphenyl)-3-phenylprop-2-en-1-one (AK Scientific, Inc.; Cat.#R815; 98% purity), 4'-hydroxichalcone or (2E)-1-(4-hydroxyphenyl)-3-phenylprop-2-en-1-one (AK Scientific, Inc.; Cat.#C135; 98% purity)], and compound 1771 [(5-phenyl-1,3,4-oxadiazol-2-yl)carbamoyl]methyl 2-{naphtho[2,1-b]furan-1-yl}acetate)] (UkrOrgSynthesis Ltd., Kiev, Ukraine; Cat.#PB25353228; purity not available). The compounds were diluted with 84.15% ethanol (EtOH; Sigma-Aldrich; Cat.#E7023) and 15% dimethyl sulfoxide (DMSO; Sigma-Aldrich; Cat.#D8418) to have stock solutions at 15 mg/mL, except for compound 1771 that was used at 2 mg/mL. The concentration for compound 1771 was lower than the other agents because of solubility issues. Also, sodium fluoride was prepared at 5000 ppm (Sigma-Aldrich; Cat.# 71519). These stock solutions were diluted to distinct concentrations for assays. For antimicrobial assays, the agents with stock concentration at 15 mg/mL were tested using concentrations of 1250, 1000, 500, 250, 125, 62.5, 31.25, 15.625 µg/mL. For compound 1771 (stock concentration at 2 mg/mL), the concentrations used were 250, 125, 62.5, 31.25, 15.625, 7.813, 3.906, 1.953, 0.977, 0.488, 0.244 µg/mL.

2.3. Microbial Strain and Growth Conditions

C. albicans SC5314 and *S. mutans* UA159 (serotype c; ATCC 700610) strains preserved in a freezer $-80\ °C$ were thaw, platted on a blood agar plate (5% sheep's blood; Laborclin, Pinhais, PR, Brazil), and incubated (48 h, 37 °C, 5% CO_2; Steri-Cult™ Thermo Scientific, Waltham, MA, USA). Next, five colonies of each microorganism were inoculated into a liquid culture medium (2.5% tryptone with 1.5% yeast extract or TY, pH 7.0; Becton, Dickinson and Company (BD), Sparks, MD, USA) containing 1% of glucose (w/v) (TY+1% glucose) and incubated (16 h, 37 °C, 5% CO_2). After that, the starter cultures were diluted 1:20 in the same culture medium and grown until mid-log growth phase: *S. mutans* $OD_{562\ nm}$ 0.500 (± 0.100) and *C. albicans* OD_{562nm} 0.482 (± 0.058) (ELISA plate reader, Biochrom Ez, Cambourne, UK). These cultures were diluted in TY+1% glucose for each microorganism inoculum with 2×10^6 colony-forming units per milliliter (CFU/mL) for antimicrobial evaluation. However, the mid-log growth phase cultures were diluted in TY+1% sucrose (w/v) to yield 2×10^6 CFU/mL for single-species antibiofilm assays.

2.4. Antimicrobial Activity

The antimicrobial activity was evaluated by determining the minimum inhibitory concentration (MIC) and minimum fungicidal and bactericidal concentration (MFC and MBC, respectively) using broth microdilution following the Clinical and Laboratory Standards Institute [31–33], with some modifications [34]. The compounds were evaluated according their stock concentration ranging from 0 to 1250 µg/mL (when stock concentration 15 mg/mL) and 0 to 250 µg/mL (for compound 1771 with stock concentration at 2 mg/mL). Of note, 0 µg/mL was the vehicle-control. For most of the newest compounds, MIC has been described with some caveats, as when the visual inspection and the optical density are compromised by precipitation, for example [35]. Here, most agents complexed when in contact with the culture medium, making visual inspection subjective and interfering with optical density readings, and most of them did not present a clear dose-dependent effect. Therefore, the abbreviation IC_{50} was defined as the inhibitory concentration of the agent that inhibited the growth of the microorganism by 50% [34], considering microbial growth as the CFU/mL counts. Thus, MIC abbreviation was not employed to state the outcomes.

All selected compounds [*tt*-farnesol, myricetin, 2′-hydroxychalcone (AGN), 2′-hydroxychalcone (R815), 4′-hydroxychalcones (C135), and compound 1771 (1771)] were tested against *S. mutans* planktonic culture. However, only the effective compounds against the bacterium (*tt*-farnesol, myricetin, C135, and compound 1771) were used for *C. albicans* because when both species are together, they form robust biofilms mediated primarily by the exopolysaccharides produced by the bacterium in a rich-sucrose environment [3].

The inoculum culture (100 µL of bacterium or fungus) was transferred to 96-well plates containing TY+1% glucose and distinct concentrations of agents were arranged from the highest to the lowest for a final volume of 200 µL (yielding 1×10^6 CFU/mL for each species). As controls for each experiment, wells containing only culture medium, only inoculum (growth control without treatment), and inoculum plus vehicle (final concentration of 7% EtOH and 1.25% DMSO) were added to rule out any effect of the vehicle on microbial cells. The assembled plates were incubated (24 h, 37 °C, 5% CO_2), followed visual inspection (turbidity: microbial growth, clear: no growth), and $OD_{562\,nm}$ readings (ELISA plate reader). Next, the plates were incubated to homogenize the cultures (5 min, 75 rpm, 37 °C) (Quimis, São Paulo, Brazil). After that, an aliquot from each well was removed for serial dilution in saline solution (0.89% NaCl; Synth, Diadema, SP, Brazil), plating (undiluted and 10^{-1} to 10^{-5}), and incubation (48 h, 37 °C, 5% CO_2) to determine CFU/mL quantification and inhibitory concentration (IC_{50}). The MBC and MFC were measured by CFU/mL count and defined as the lowest compound concentration that inhibited microbial growth (or absence of colony growth on agar). However, for some compounds that may target the extracellular matrix production in biofilms, the concentrations that inhibited at least 50% of microbial growth (i.e., 50% of CFU/mL reduction vs. vehicle) were considered promising antimicrobial activity [34,35].

2.5. Antibiofilm Activity

This analysis was conducted after determining antimicrobial activity and was performed using single- and dual-species settings and different exposure to compounds: activity against initial biofilm formation (24 h) and pre-formed biofilms (48 h). For initial biofilm formation, the agents were introduced at the time 0 h, and biofilms were evaluated at 24 h of development. For pre-formed biofilms, biofilms were grown for 24 h and then treated, being evaluated at 48 h of growth. Thus, it was evaluated the inhibition of biofilm formation for biofilms at 24 h and the eradication of biofilm growth for 48 h-old biofilms. The measurement was considered effective when the CFU/mL count was reduced by 50% (vs. vehicle) for 24 and 48 h-old biofilms [34,36].

The strains were grown and prepared using the methodology described above. However, the culture medium and inoculum of the experiments were prepared using TY+1% sucrose. The selected compounds and their concentrations were based on antimicrobial data: C135 (from 1250 to 62.5 µg/mL), myricetin (from 1250 to 125 µg/mL), tt-farnesol (from 1250 to 31.25 µg/mL), and compound 1771 (from 250 to 1.953 µg/mL). Previous studies evaluated the antibiofilm activity of myricetin, compound 1771, and tt-farnesol for *S. mutans* [18,19,30], but here distinct concentrations were tested. Tests with compound 1771 for *C. albicans* and C135 for both species will be presented for the first time.

Initially, single-species biofilm to prevent initial biofilm formation (24 h) were analyzed. On a 96-well plate, 100 µL of final inoculum with 2×10^6 CFU/mL (for both species) were added to each well, containing test concentrations and culture medium (TY+1% sucrose), totalizing 200 µL (1×10^6 CFU/mL). Controls of experiments were also added (wells containing only culture medium, wells containing only the inoculum of the experiment, and wells containing the inoculum plus vehicle or 0 µg/mL). The plate was incubated (24 h, 37 °C, 5% CO_2). After incubation, visual inspection was performed, followed by orbital incubation (5 min, 75 rpm, 37 °C). The remaining biofilms on the wells were rinsed three times with 200 µL of 0.89% NaCl solution to remove any loose material. Next, these biofilms were scraped with pipet tips five times (5X) with 200 µL of 0.89% NaCl, totalizing 1 mL of biofilm suspension (from each well). This biofilm suspension was placed in a microtube, subjected to serial dilutions (10^{-1} to 10^{-5}), which were plated, as were the undiluted suspensions. The plates were incubated (48 h, 37 °C, 5% CO_2), and the CFU/mL was calculated. Next, the microbial growth inhibition of each concentration was compared to vehicle control.

Subsequently, prevention of build-up pre-formed biofilm (48 h) was evaluated [36]. Here, 96-well plates were assembled using 100 µL final inoculum of *C. albicans* or *S. mutans* (2×10^6 CFU/mL) and 100 µL of TY+1% sucrose (to reach 1×10^6 CFU/mL). The microplate was incubated (24 h, 37 °C, 5% CO_2) without any treatment or vehicle control. After incubation and biofilm formation, visual inspection was performed, followed by culture medium removal and washing of remaining biofilms (three times with 200 µL 0.89% NaCl solution). Next, fresh culture medium TY+1% sucrose and test concentrations of agents or the vehicle were added. The microplate was incubated again (24 h, 37 °C, 5% CO_2). After incubation (when biofilms were 48 h-old), the same processing protocol applied for 24 h-old biofilms was conducted until obtaining 1 mL of biofilm suspension. The biofilm suspensions were sonicated (30 s at 7 w, Sonicator QSonica, Q125, Newtown, CT, USA), subjected to serial dilutions (10^{-1} to 10^{-5}), and plated. The undiluted suspensions were also plated. The CFU/mL counts were evaluated and compared to vehicle control.

Finally, the antibiofilm activity for dual-species biofilms of *C. albicans* and *S. mutans* was also performed at 24 and 48 h. These analyzes were performed with the same methodology used for single-species biofilms (24 and 48 h). However, the inoculum of the dual-species culture was prepared with 2×10^6 CFU/mL of *S. mutans* and 2×10^4 CFU/mL of *C. albicans* [3] to reach 1×10^6 CFU/mL of *S. mutans* and 1×10^4 CFU/mL of *C. albicans* after adding culture medium or treatments.

The concentrations of agents with better results against each species in the single-species biofilm setting were selected: 125 µg/mL (C135 and tt-farnesol), 500 µg/mL (myricetin), and 3.906 µg/mL (1771). Then, compounds with selected concentrations were combined with each other and with or without sodium fluoride (250 ppm) or F totalizing 16 groups. The elected combinations included groups without fluoride (C135, C135+tt-farnesol, C135+1771, C135+myricetin, C135+tt-farnesol+1771, C135+tt-farnesol+myricetin, C135+myricetin+1771, C135+tt-farnesol+1771+myricetin, 1771+myricetin, tt-farnesol+1771+myricetin) and groups with fluoride (250 ppm) (C135+fluoride, C135+tt-farnesol+fluoride, C135+1771+fluoride, C135+myricetin+fluoride, C135+tt-farnesol+1771+myricetin+fluoride). The concentration of fluoride was selected based on the commercially available fluoride-based mouth rinse [19,37].

2.6. Statistical Analyses

The statistical analyses for CFU/mL values were performed using descriptive and inferential statistics. Normality was evaluated with the Shapiro-Wilk test employing a significance level of 5%. The data were non-parametric; thus, the data were evaluated with Kruskal–Wallis test, followed by Dunn's post-test, considering $\alpha = 0.05$ (Prism 9 software, GraphPad Software, Inc. 2021). The microbial growth inhibition of each agent and concentration was compared to vehicle control. In addition, the CFU/mL data were transformed to $\log_{10}$ or log to verify the log reduction.

3. Results
3.1. Antimicrobial Activity
3.1.1. S. mutans

Three compounds (AGN, C135, R815) complexed with the culture medium, making the visual inspection analysis inaccurate; turbidity was also present for myricetin (but in minor proportion than for the three aforementioned compounds), and compound 1771 (at concentrations equal of more than 31.25 µg/mL). The observation of culture medium turbidity occurred immediately after adding the compound into the culture media, without microbial inoculation and incubation (controls per each concentration tested). The compound that did not complex with culture medium was tt-farnesol, and the absence of visual growth was observed at 31.25 µg/mL, which was also its IC_{50}.

Regarding MBC, as per CLSI definition, the absence of colony growth on an agar plate was found for tt-farnesol and compound 1771, as 62.5 µg/mL and 250 µg/mL, respectively. Thus, a potential antimicrobial activity was achieved for the compounds when the compound at a specific concentration yielded a 50% reduction of CFU/mL counts compared to the vehicle control (IC_{50}), as follows.

For C135, the lowest concentration that yielded 50% reduction was 62.5 µg/mL, but the same reduction was observed for 125, 250, and 500 µg/mL (Figure 1). Thus, the antibacterial activity of C135 was not dose-dependent.

There was an absence of expressive effect on growth inhibition for all concentrations of AGN and R815 (vs. vehicle). However, some concentrations of R815 showed statistical differences and some inhibition of growth at 500 and 250 µg/mL (2 and 1 log reduction, respectively), 125 and 62.5 µg/mL (0.5 log reduction). These reductions were not dose-dependent and are not within the cutoff established for an effective compound (Figure 1). Thus, AGN and R815 were not used in the downstream assays.

Three concentrations of myricetin presented statistical differences compared to the vehicle (250, 500, and 1000 µg/mL) but were not dose-dependent. However, a better effect was obtained for 500 µg/mL, which was considered the IC_{50}.

For compound 1771, the IC_{50} was 7.813 µg/mL; higher concentrations also demonstrated significative statistical differences (at least 4 log reduction vs. vehicle) and, as mentioned above, 250 µg/mL rendered absence of CFU/mL quantification on agar (MBC).

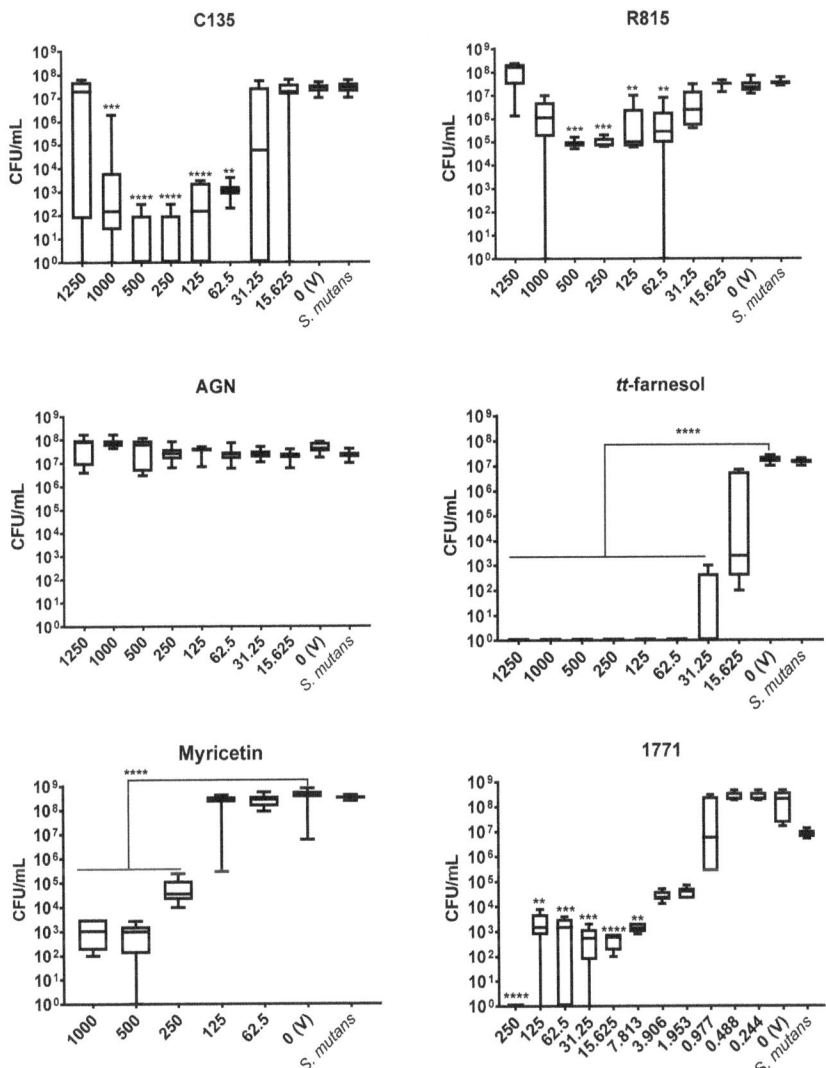

Figure 1. Antimicrobial activity of *S. mutans* using six compounds: C135, R815, AGN, *tt*-farnesol, myricetin and 1771. Data represents median and interquartile ranges ($n = 9$). Statistical differences are represented with ** ($p < 0.05$), *** ($p < 0.001$), and **** ($p < 0.0001$) (Kruskal Wallis, followed by Dunn's test). The tabulated results are in Table S1.

3.1.2. *C. albicans*

The antimicrobial activity of *C. albicans* was analyzed using four agents (C135, *tt*-farnesol, myricetin, and compound 1771) that were selected based on the effective antimicrobial activity founded for *S. mutans*. Among them, only *tt*-farnesol did not complex with the culture medium; the absence of visual growth was observed at 125 µg/mL, which was also its IC_{50}.

C135 and *tt*-farnesol presented a dose-dependent effect on viable fungal growth. C135 was the most effective in inhibiting fungal viability (Figure 2). All its concentrations above 31.25 µg/mL hindered colony growth on agar plates; thus, its IC_{50} and MFC were determined as 62.5 µg/mL (absence of colony growth on agar plates). The MFC for *tt*-farnesol was 1000 µg/mL (Figure 2). Both myricetin and compound 1771 did not demonstrate significant antimicrobial activities as per the cutoff of 50% colony growth reduction (IC$_{50}$), although statistical differences were observed, as depicted in Figure 2.

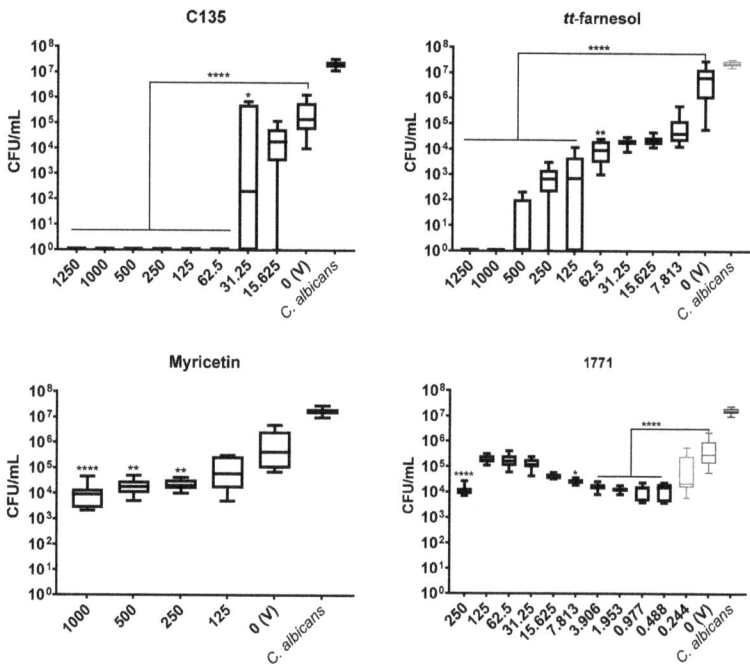

Figure 2. Antimicrobial activity of *C. albicans* with compounds: C135, *tt*-farnesol, myricetin and 1771. Data represents median and interquartile ranges ($n = 9$). Statistical differences are represented with * (C135 $p = 0.048$; 1771 $p = 0.013$), ** ($p < 0.05$) and **** ($p < 0.0001$) (Kruskal Wallis, followed by Dunn's test). The tabulated results are in Table S2.

3.2. Antibiofilm Activity

3.2.1. Single-Species *S. mutans* Biofilm

On 24 h biofilm (initial biofilm formation), all concentrations of tested compounds (C135, myricetin, *tt*-farnesol, and compound 1771) demonstrated antibiofilm activity, specially myricetin and *tt*-farnesol concentrations that eliminated bacterial growth (Figure 3). C135 eliminated the bacterium at 62.5, 125, and 250 µg/mL, but not at higher concentrations. Also, all concentrations of compound 1771 reduced about 5 logs of bacterium growth (vs. vehicle).

However, on *S. mutans* pre-formed biofilms (48 h) a greater inhibitory effect was achieved with *tt*-farnesol; where concentrations of 62.5 µg/mL and higher eliminated the bacterium. For C135 the best concentration was 125 µg/mL with 5 logs reduction (vs. vehicle). In contrast, a lower inhibitory activity was observed for myricetin and compound 1771 (although they presented statistical differences, the reduction was about 1 log vs. vehicle) (Figure 3).

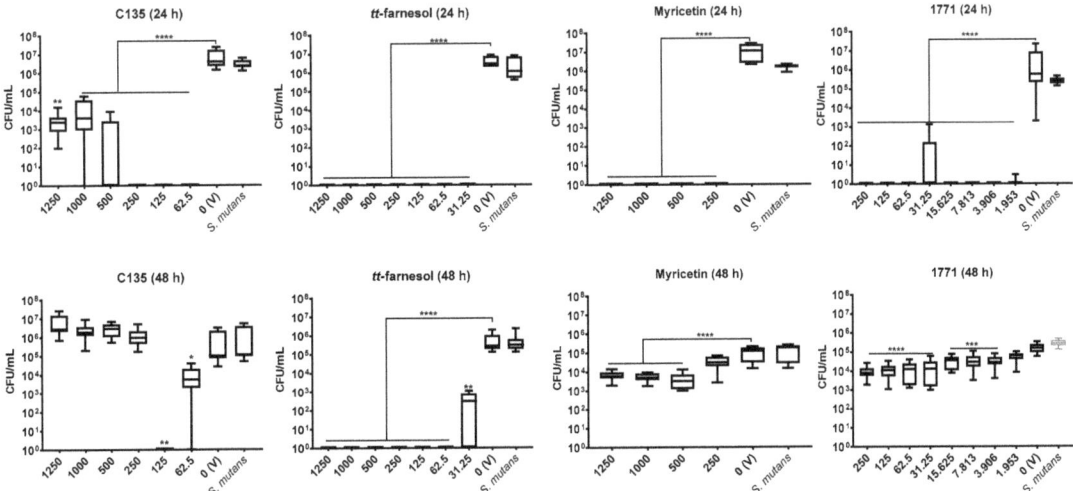

Figure 3. Antibiofilm activity of *S. mutans* with compounds: C135, *tt*-farnesol, myricetin, and 1771. On the first line are presented data of 24 h biofilm (initial biofilm formation); and right below are the data of pre-formed biofilms (48 h). The data represents median and interquartile ranges ($n = 9$). Statistical differences are represented with * ($p = 0.026$), ** ($p < 0.05$), *** ($p < 0.001$), and **** ($p < 0.0001$) (Kruskal Wallis, followed by Dunn's test). The tabulated results are in Table S3.

3.2.2. Single-Species *C. albicans* Biofilm

The best antibiofilm activity for *C. albicans* 24 h biofilm was observed for C135 and *tt*-farnesol; both eliminated the fungus, except at 31.25 µg/mL of *tt*-farnesol that reduced 4 logs (vs. vehicle). Compound 1771 reduced 3 logs from 3.906 µg/mL to higher concentrations. However, the lowest antibiofilm effect was observed for myricetin with about 1 log reduction (vs. vehicle) in all tested concentrations, although statistical differences were observed (Figure 4).

The antibiofilm activity against *C. albicans* pre-formed biofilm (48 h) was achieved effectively only by C135. C135 eliminated the fungus at 125, 500, and 1250 µg/mL; it also decreases CFU/mL counts by 4 logs (62.5 µg/mL) and 5 logs (250 and 1000 µg/mL) (vs. vehicle). A weak activity was observed using *tt*-farnesol, where concentrations above 125 µg/mL presented about 2 log reduction (vs. vehicle). However, no effect was observed using myricetin and compound 1771 (except 1771 at 250 µg/mL with 2 logs reduction vs. vehicle) (Figure 4).

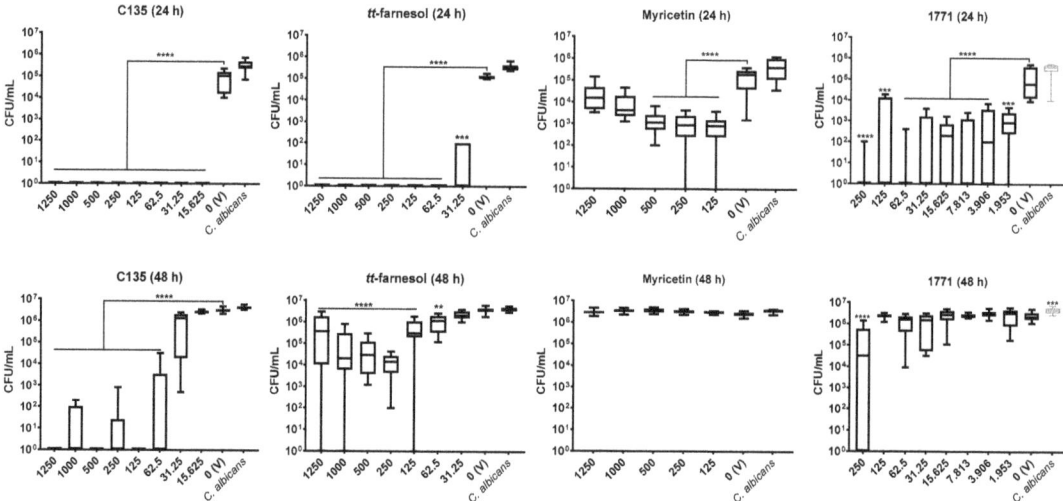

Figure 4. Antibiofilm activity of *C. albicans* with compounds: C135, *tt*-farnesol, myricetin, and 1771. On the first line are presented data of 24 h biofilm (initial biofilm formation); and right below are the data of pre-formed biofilms (48 h). The data represents median and interquartile ranges (n = 9). Statistical differences are represented with ** (p = 0.002), *** ($p \leq 0.0003$), and **** ($p \leq 0.0001$) (Kruskal Wallis, followed by Dunn's test). The tabulated results are in Table S4.

3.2.3. Dual-Species *C. albicans* and *S. mutans* Biofilms.

Based on the previously presented data, compounds and their most effective concentrations were selected for combinations of compounds tested on dual-species *C. albicans* and *S. mutans* biofilms (see data summarized in Table 1). The selected concentrations were: 125 µg/mL for C135 and *tt*-farnesol, 500 µg/mL for myricetin, and 3.906 µg/mL for compound 1771. In addition, C135 was used alone or combined with the other agents with and without sodium fluoride because it was the most effective agent against the fungus growth.

Table 1. Summary of antimicrobial and antibiofilm activity on single-species cultures for selection of compounds concentrations (µg/mL) to test against dual-species biofilms.

Compound	Antimicrobial Activity				Antibiofilm Activity (Single-Species)			
	S. mutans		*C. albicans*		*S. mutans*		*C. albicans*	
	IC_{50}	MBC	IC_{50}	MFC	24 h	48 h	24 h	48 h
C135	62.5	-	62.5	62.5	62.5	125	15.625	125
tt-farnesol	31.25	62.5	125	1000	31.25	62.5	62.5	125 *
Myricetin	500	-	-	-	250	500 *	500 *	-
1771	7.813	250	-	-	3.906	3.906 *	3.906 *	250 *

* represent selected concentrations that did not reduce 50% of CFU/mL but had a significative statistical reduction vs. vehicle between all tested concentrations. IC_{50}: the inhibitory concentration of the agent that inhibited the growth of the microorganism by 50%, considering microbial growth as the CFU/mL counts. MBC: minimum bactericidal concentration. MFC: minimum fungicidal concentration. 24 h: 24 h-old biofilms. 48 h: 48 h-old biofilms.

For 24 h-old biofilms (initial biofilm formation), all 16 formulations were effective, impeding the growth of both species (bacterium and fungus) (Figure 5). However, the microbial growth inhibition of pre-formed (48 h-old biofilms) was different between treatments and species (Figure 5). Among the 16 formulations tested, three inhibited the growth of both species completely: C135+*tt*-farnesol+myricetin, C135+*tt*-farnesol+fluoride, and C135+*tt*-farnesol+1771+myricetin+fluoride (all compounds combined with fluoride).

Furthermore, considering the total inhibition of bacterial growth in the dual-species setting, four formulations were effective (C135+*tt*-farnesol+1771+myricetin, C135+fluoride, C135+1771+fluoride, and C135+myricetin+fluoride). Considering the total inhibition of fungal growth in the dual-species setting, four treatments were effective (C135, C135+*tt*-farnesol, C135+1771, and C135+myricetin). Also, some formulations reduced at least 50% CFU/mL (vs. vehicle) of *S. mutans* (C135+*tt*-farnesol, C135+*tt*-farnesol+1771), or *C. albicans* (C135+*tt*-farnesol+1771+myricetin and C135+myricetin+fluoride).

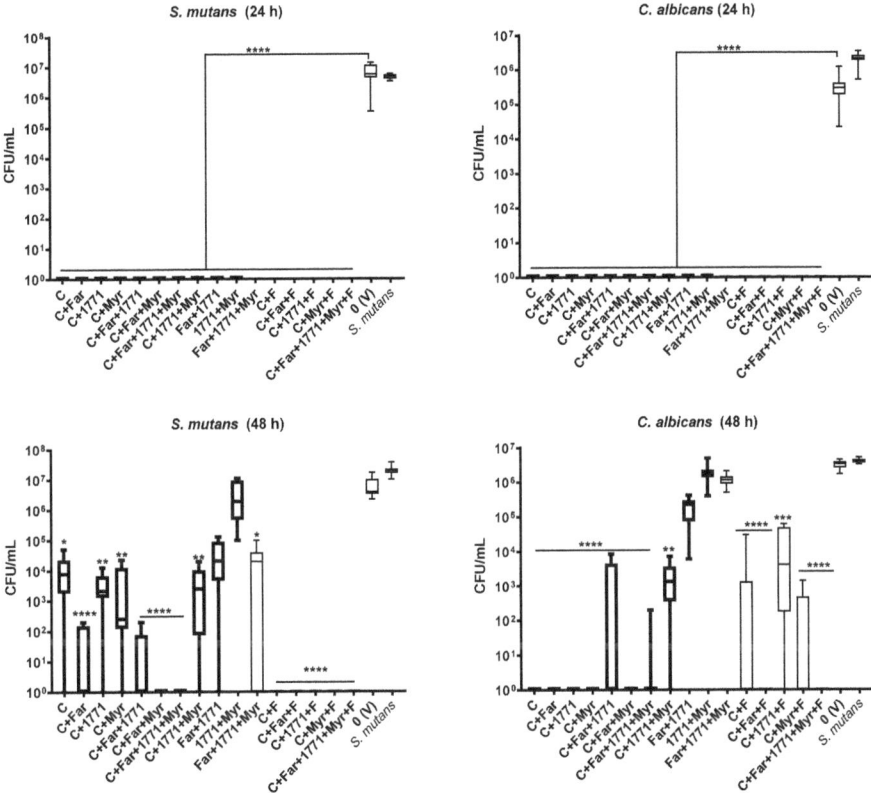

Figure 5. Antibiofilm activity of dual-species *S. mutans* and *C. albicans* biofilms with combined compounds (with and without sodium fluoride): C135 (C), *tt*-farnesol (Far), myricetin (Myr), 1771, and sodium fluoride (F). The top graphs presented data of 24 h biofilm (initial biofilm formation). The bottom graphs depict data of pre-formed biofilms (48 h). The data represents median and interquartile ranges ($n = 9$). Statistical differences are represented with * ($p = 0.04$), ** ($p \leq 0.002$), *** ($p = 0.0007$), and **** ($p \leq 0.0001$) (Kruskal Wallis, followed by Dunn's test). The tabulated results are in Table S5.

4. Discussion

Several strategies can be used to control biofilms to prevent oral diseases. The classical strategies for oral biofilm control include brushing/flossing (mechanical removal of biofilms) and restricting dietary sugar intake (mainly frequency) to prevent biofilm build-up. Both diet restriction and brushing/flossing require behavioral compliance, which can be challenging. In addition, fluoride is used to avoid teeth demineralization and promote remineralization as part of oral hygiene products (toothpaste and mouthwashes) and/or supplied in tap drinking water. However, they may not be appropriate to all individuals, such as those without adequate dexterity (e.g., young children, elderly, people with disabilities, people in ICUs), which may require supervision for brushing/flossing and aids to weaken the overall biofilm structure to facilitate its mechanical removal, or even substances to enhance biofilm control.

Single targets for biofilm prevention and antimicrobial control can be difficult and limit the treatment options. Thus, combining agents with distinct targets can be an effective approach to access different sites in biofilms, which present complex biological traits and protected niches [1,19]. Therefore, this study evaluated the antimicrobial and antibiofilm activities of six compounds [tt-farnesol, myricetin, two 2′-hydroxychalcones (AGN and R815), 4′-hydroxychalcone (C135), and compound 1771] with different targets against C. albicans and S. mutans single- and dual-species settings.

Of note, an antimicrobial substance/molecule may not be an antibiofilm agent, and a compound with antibiofilm activity may not be an antimicrobial per se (e.g., molecules that affect extracellular enzymes responsible for the extracellular matrix construction). This scenario is depicted by the findings in both antimicrobial and antibiofilm assays performed as some agents were effective against the microorganisms in planktonic cultures and were not in the biofilms' settings. Also, the effect of compounds was mostly non-dose-dependent for both C. albicans and S. mutans.

The antimicrobial outcome for S. mutans showed the lowest IC_{50} value for compound 1771 (7.813 µg/mL), followed by tt-farnesol (31.25 µg/mL), C135 (62.5 µg/mL), while the highest value was observed for myricetin (500 µg/mL). However, IC_{50} values for C. albicans were C135 (62.5 µg/mL) and tt-farnesol (125 µg/mL). Furthermore, tt-farnesol eliminated CFU/mL count of both species reaching a MBC (62.5 µg/mL) and a MFC (1000 µg/mL). The compound 1771 presented MBC (250 µg/mL) and C135 reached MFC (62.5 µg/mL). The findings for C135 for both species and 1771 for C. albicans are presented for the first time here. Thus, C135 presented a promising antimicrobial effect for both species, and compound 1771 did not inhibit C. albicans growth.

A previous study with S. mutans using different concentrations of compound 1771 did not eliminate the bacterium [30], but the total elimination of CFU/mL count was observed here using the greatest concentration. In the same study [30], the antimicrobial activity of myricetin for S. mutans was at a lower concentration than the one found here. The antimicrobial effect of tt-farnesol on both species corroborates previous findings [18,22]. Among the three chalcones tested, the antimicrobial activity was better for C135, a 4′-hydroxychalcone. The other two 2′-hydroxychalcones (AGN and R815) did not present antimicrobial effect for S. mutans. These results can be explained by the differences between the chemical structure of the selected hydroxychalcones, suggesting that the presence of hydroxyl groups on the ring of the 4′-hydroxychalcone scaffold is crucial for the growth inhibition [24,38,39].

The presence of an extracellular matrix is essential for the existence of biofilm and the complete expression of virulence by microbial pathogens and pathobionts, hindering the action of antimicrobial agents and preventing their access to microbial cells [40]. Sucrose can modulate microbial synergism and ecology of the oral microbiota because its hexoses (glucose and fructose) are used for exopolysaccharides and organic acid production that influences the structure and composition of dental biofilms [1,6]. Cariogenic biofilms promote interactions and mechanisms that control dysbiosis [1,6] as observed on dual-species biofilms of S. mutans and C. albicans in vitro [2,3]. Therefore, it is important to understand the mechanisms of possible antibiofilm compounds.

Myricetin and some hydroxychalcones inhibit S. mutans F-ATPase activity (acid tolerance mechanism) [19], glycolysis (organic acid production or acidogenicity) [19], and synthesis of extracellular matrix glucans (by interfering with gtfs gene expression and Gtfs activity) [19,24]. The deficit in glucan production can compromise the integrity and 3D structure biofilms [4], facilitating their disruption. These findings can explain the antibiofilm effect of myricetin on S. mutans initial biofilms (24 h) and the greatest potential of C135 (4′-hydroxychalcone) on initial (24 h) and mature S. mutans biofilm (48 h). The weaker inhibition of myricetin on pre-formed biofilms (48 h—biofilm eradication) can be promoted by the presence of pre-formed microcolonies and their 3D extracellular matrix.

tt-farnesol eliminated the bacterium in 24- and 48 h-old single-species biofilms (at 62.5 µg/mL and higher concentrations). The antimicrobial and antibiofilm effect of this compound can be related to the targets on *S. mutans* cytoplasmatic membrane, altering its proton permeability, decreasing its tolerance to acid stress [18]. Compound 1771 also had a promising antibiofilm effect for the bacterium, especially on initial biofilm (24 h-old single-species biofilms). This compound inhibits the LTA synthesis [28], interfering with the cell wall composition, making the cytoplasmatic membrane an easy target for environmental stresses. Also, LTA from the cell wall are released in the matrix and interact with exopolysaccharides during the development and maturation of biofilms [41]; hence, interfering with LTA metabolism can impair cell wall and extracellular matrix composition. Thus, *tt*-farnesol and compound 1771 hindered *S. mutans* biofilms by promoting antimicrobial and antibiofilm activities.

Hydroxychalcones inhibit the cell wall formation of *C. albicans* cells [42,43], while *tt*-farnesol keeps the fungus in its yeast form [21]. However, it is unknown whether myricetin inhibits *C. albicans* biofilm formation or its extracellular matrix development or whether compound 1771 could target this fungus or its metabolism. The effect on the extracellular matrix components and construction could make the fungal cells more susceptible to antimicrobial agents. Here, single-species *C. albicans* biofilms were not greatly affected by myricetin. However, the 4′-hydroxychalcone C135 presented a promising effect in the initial (24 h) and mature (48 h) fungal biofilms. Also, *tt*-farnesol and 1771 were effective on initial fungal biofilm, but only *tt*-farnesol eliminated the fungus (at 62.5 µg/mL and higher concentrations). In addition, *tt*-farnesol had a weak effect, while 1771 had practically no effect on fungal growth on pre-formed biofilms. Thus, eradication of *C. albicans* biofilm (48 h) was achieved only with C135.

Previous studies with *C. albicans* biofilms demonstrate that chalcones inhibited enzymes involved in resistance pathways [42]. Thus, the effect of C135 on *C. albicans* biofilms can be related to targets on resistance pathways; nevertheless, this hypothesis must be better explained. In addition, as observed on the data above from antimicrobial activity of *tt*-farnesol, this compound can inhibit fungal growth, induce apoptosis in *C. albicans* cells, and inhibit the fungal hyphae [21,22]. As described for initial biofilms (24 h), the treatment was applied at 0 h, so it may be that the effect of *tt*-farnesol (preventing filamentous morphology) supports the inhibition of fungal growth in 24 h while hampered its effect on pre-formed biofilm (48 h). Therefore, combine compounds could improve the effect in mature biofilms. This hypothesis is confirmed by the potentiated effect on *C. albicans* cells in dual-species biofilm (48 h) when C135 and *tt*-farnesol were combined, suggesting inhibition of the resistance mechanisms when both compounds are present.

Altogether, the data from antimicrobial and single-species biofilms assays enabled the selection of specific concentrations of the four compounds (C135, myricetin, *tt*-farnesol, and compound 1771) that were combined, with or without sodium fluoride, to assess the antibiofilm activity of formulations against dual-species *S. mutans* and *C. albicans* biofilm. All formulations without fluoride [(C135, C135+*tt*-farnesol, C135+1771, C135+myricetin, C135+*tt*-farnesol+1771, C135+*tt*-farnesol+myricetin, C135+*tt*-farnesol+1771+myricetin, C135+1771+myricetin, *tt*-farnesol+1771, 1771+myricetin, *tt*-farnesol+1771+myricetin)] and with fluoride [(C135+fluoride, C135+*tt*-farnesol+fluoride, C135+1771+fluoride, C135+J10595+fluoride, C135+*tt*-farnesol+1771+myricetin+fluoride completely inhibited the initial biofilm formation (24 h). These findings showed that there might be a potential synergism between the compounds and a greater effect when they are combined and applied since the beginning of biofilm formation and during the 24 h of dual-species biofilm development. Part of the effect can be because of the antimicrobial effect per se, as microbial cells were exposed to formulations in their free form before adhesion to the surface. Also, the effect on extracellular matrix formation can not be ruled out.

In contrast, dual-species biofilm eradication (48 h) in which both species did not grow occurred for three formulations: C135+*tt*-farnesol+myricetin, C135+*tt*-farnesol+fluoride, and C135+*tt*-farnesol+1771+myricetin+fluoride. Four formulations only eradicated the bacterial growth (C135+*tt*-farnesol+1771+myricetin, C135+fluoride, C135+1771+fluoride, and C135+myricetin+fluoride), while other four formulations eradicated fungal growth (C135, C135+*tt*-farnesol, C135+1771, and C135+myricetin). Of note, the formulations with fluoride exhibited a greater antibiofilm activity (mainly for the bacterium), reinforcing the importance of its inclusion in strategies to prevent and control cariogenic biofilms [18]; fewer and less severe carious lesions were observed using combined treatments and fluoride on a rodent model of dental caries [19]. Fluoride can interfere with microbial metabolism, especially on glycolytic enzymes and proton gradient dissipation on the cell cytoplasmatic membrane (when the extracellular pH is higher than the intracellular pH) [44]. This effect can hamper cell growth. Nevertheless, C135 alone or combined with other agents (even those without pronounced effect on singles-species 48 h-old biofilms) prevented fungal and bacterial growth in dual-species biofilms, making it a promising agent.

The present findings provided insights about: (i) compounds as inhibitors of biofilm formation of single-species biofilm (24 h); (ii) compounds that can eradicate pre-formed biofilm (48 h); and (iii) formulations with combined compounds for biofilm inhibition (24 h) and eradication (48 h) of both species in dual-species biofilms. C135 is a novel compound with possible distinct targets alone or in combination with other agents. The formulations that combined agents with distinct targets prevented *C. albicans* and *S. mutans* dual-species biofilm build-up in vitro. The formulation C135+*tt*-farnesol with or without fluoride may represent a potential alternative approach that deserves further investigation, including cytotoxicity to host [30,45]. Therefore, the outcomes of this study could be applied to future studies using the compound alone or combined as an adjuvant strategy to control oral biofilms using shorter exposure times, as mouthwashes.

Supplementary Materials: The following are available online at https://www.mdpi.com/article/10.3390/jof7050340/s1. Table S1: Antimicrobial activity of *S. mutans* using six compounds: C135, R815, AGN, *tt*-farnesol, myricetin, and 1771. Data shown in Figure 1 as CFU/mL. Table S2: Antimicrobial activity of *C. albicans* with compounds: C135, *tt*-farnesol, myricetin, and 1771. Data shown in Figure 2 as CFU/mL. Table S3: Antibiofilm activity of *S. mutans* with compounds: C135, *tt*-farnesol, myricetin, and 1771 of 24 h biofilm (initial biofilm formation) and pre-formed biofilms (48 h). Data shown in Figure 3 as CFU/mL. Table S4: Antibiofilm activity of *C. albicans* with compounds: C135, *tt*-farnesol, myricetin, and 1771 of 24 h biofilm (initial biofilm formation) and pre-formed biofilms (48 h). Data shown in Figure 4 as CFU/mL. Table S5. Antibiofilm activity of dual-species *S. mutans* and *C. albicans* biofilms with combined compounds (with and without sodium fluoride): C135 (C), *tt*-farnesol (Far), myricetin (Myr), 1771, and sodium fluoride (F). Data shown in Figure 5 as CFU/mL.

Author Contributions: Conceived and designed the experiments: C.I.V.L. and M.I.K. Carried out the experiments: C.I.V.L. Analyzed the data C.I.V.L. and M.I.K. Reagents/materials/analysis tools: M.I.K. Wrote the paper: C.I.V.L., A.C.U.d.A.L., and M.I.K. All authors have read and agreed to the published version of the manuscript.

Funding: This research was supported by a research grant from the National Council for Scientific and Technological Development (CNPq #409668/2018-4 to M.I.K.) and scholarships (the Coordination of Superior Level Staff Improvement—CAPES #001 and CNPq #141316/2020-9 to C.I.V.L.; and CAPES #001 and the São Paulo Research Foundation—FAPESP #2020/02946-2 to A.C.U.A.L.). The funding body had no role in the design of the study or collection, analysis, and interpretation of data and in writing the manuscript.

Institutional Review Board Statement: Not applicable.

Informed Consent Statement: Not applicable.

Data Availability Statement: The data presented in this study are available as supplementary material. Additional data are available on request from the corresponding author.

Acknowledgments: The authors are thankful to CNPq, CAPES, and FAPESP for grant and scholarships funding. The present research will be part of the Ph.D. thesis by C.I.V.L.

Conflicts of Interest: The authors declare that the research was conducted in the absence of any commercial or financial relationships that could be construed as a potential conflict of interest.

References

1. Lamont, R.J.; Koo, H.; Hajishengallis, G. The oral microbiota: Dynamic communities and host interactions. *Nat. Rev. Microbiol.* **2018**, *16*, 745–759. [CrossRef]
2. Lobo, C.I.V.; Rinaldi, T.B.; Christiano, C.M.S.; Leite, L.S.; Barbugli, P.A.; Klein, M.I. Dual-species biofilms of *Streptococcus mutans* and *Candida albicans* exhibit more biomass and are mutually beneficial compared with single-species biofilms. *J. Oral Microbiol.* **2019**, *11*, 1581520. [CrossRef]
3. Falsetta, M.L.; Klein, M.I.; Colonne, P.M.; Scott-Anne, K.; Gregoire, S.; Pai, C.H.; Gonzalez-Begne, M.; Watson, G.; Krysan, D.J.; Bowen, W.H.; et al. Symbiotic relationship between *Streptococcus mutans* and *Candida albicans* synergizes virulence of plaque biofilms in vivo. *Infect. Immun.* **2014**, *82*, 1968–1981. [CrossRef] [PubMed]
4. Bowen, W.H.; Koo, H. Biology of *Streptococcus mutans* Derived Glucosyltransferases: Role in Extracellular Matrix formation of Cariogenic Biofilms. *Caries Res.* **2011**, *45*, 69–86. [CrossRef]
5. Takahashi, N.; Nyvad, B. The role of bacteria in the caries process: Ecological perspectives. *J. Dent. Res.* **2011**, *90*, 294–303. [CrossRef]
6. Bowen, W.H.; Burne, R.A.; Wu, H.; Koo, H. Oral Biofilms: Pathogens, Matrix, and Polymicrobial Interactions in Microenvironments. *Trends Microbiol.* **2018**, *26*, 229–242. [CrossRef] [PubMed]
7. Gregoire, S.; Xiao, J.; Silva, B.B.; Gonzalez, I.; Agidi, P.S.; Klein, M.I.; Ambatipudi, K.S.; Rosalen, P.L.; Bauserman, R.; Waugh, R.E.; et al. Role of glucosyltransferase B in the interactions of *Candida albicans* with *Streptococcus mutans* and experimental pellicle formed on hydroxyapatite surface. *Appl. Environ. Microbiol.* **2011**, *77*, 6357–6367. [CrossRef] [PubMed]
8. Klinke, T.; Kneist, S.; De Soet, J.; Kuhlisch, E.; Mauersberger, S.; Förster, A.; Klimm, W. Acid production by oral strains of *Candida albicans* and lactobacilli. *Caries Res.* **2009**, *43*, 83–91. [CrossRef]
9. Al-Fattani, M.A.; Douglas, L.J. Biofilm matrix of *Candida albicans* and *Candida tropicalis*: Chemical composition and role in drug resistance. *J. Med. Microbiol.* **2006**, *55*, 999–1008. [CrossRef]
10. Lal, P.; Sharma, D.; Pruthi, P.; Pruthi, V. Exopolysaccharide analysis of biofilm-forming *Candida albicans*. *J. Appl. Microbiol.* **2010**, *109*, 128–136. [CrossRef]
11. Nett, J.E.; Sanchez, H.; Cain, M.T.; Andes, D.R. Genetic basis of Candida biofilm resistance due to drug-sequestering matrix glucan. *J. Infect. Dis.* **2010**, *202*, 171–175. [CrossRef]
12. Zarnowski, R.; Westler, W.M.; Lacmbouh, G.A.; Marita, J.M.; Bothe, J.R.; Bernhardt, J.; Sahraoui, A.L.-H.; Fontaine, J.; Sanchez, H.; Hatfield, R.D.; et al. Novel entries in a fungal biofilm matrix encyclopedia. *mBio* **2014**, *5*, e01333-14. [CrossRef]
13. Taff, H.T.; Nett, J.E.; Zarnowski, R.; Ross, K.M.; Sanchez, H.; Cain, M.T.; Hamaker, J.; Mitchell, A.P.; Andes, D.R. A Candida Biofilm-Induced Pathway for Matrix Glucan Delivery: Implications for Drug Resistance. *PLoS Pathog.* **2012**, *8*, e1002848. [CrossRef]
14. Mitchell, K.F.; Zarnowski, R.; Sanchez, H.; Edward, J.A.; Reinicke, E.L.; Nett, J.E.; Mitchell, A.P.; Andes, D.R. Community participation in biofilm matrix assembly and function. *Proc. Natl. Acad. Sci. USA* **2015**, *112*, 4092–4097. [CrossRef] [PubMed]
15. Melvaer, K.L.; Helgeland, K.; Rolla, G. Some physical and chemical properties of 'soluble' and 'insoluble' polysaccharides produced by strains of *Streptococcus mutans* and *sanguis*. *Caries Res.* **1972**, *6*, 79. [PubMed]
16. Brookes, Z.L.S.; Bescos, R.; Belfield, L.A.; Ali, K.; Roberts, A. Current uses of chlorhexidine for management of oral disease: A narrative review. *J. Dent.* **2020**, *103*, 103497. [CrossRef]
17. Ten Cate, J.M. Novel anticaries and remineralizing agents: Prospects for the future. *J. Dent. Res.* **2012**, *91*, 813–815. [CrossRef] [PubMed]
18. Koo, H.; Schobel, B.; Scott-Anne, K.; Watson, G.; Bowen, W.H.; Cury, J.A.; Rosalen, P.L.; Park, Y.K. Apigenin and tt-farnesol with fluoride effects on *S. mutans* biofilms and dental caries. *J. Dent. Res.* **2005**, *84*, 1016–1020. [CrossRef]
19. Falsetta, M.L.; Klein, M.I.; Lemos, J.A.; Silva, B.B.; Agidi, S.; Scott-Anne, K.K.; Koo, H. Novel antibiofilm chemotherapy targets exopolysaccharide synthesis and stress tolerance in *Streptococcus mutans* to modulate virulence expression in vivo. *Antimicrob. Agents Chemother.* **2012**, *56*, 6201–6211. [CrossRef]
20. Bersan, S.M.F.; Galvão, L.C.C.; Goes, V.F.F.; Sartoratto, A.; Figueira, G.M.; Rehder, V.L.G.; Alencar, S.M.; Duarte, R.M.T.; Rosalen, P.L.; Duarte, M.C.T. Action of essential oils from Brazilian native and exotic medicinal species on oral biofilms. *BMC Complement. Altern. Med.* **2014**, *14*, 451. [CrossRef]
21. Hall, R.A.; Turner, K.J.; Chaloupka, J.; Cottier, F.; De Sordi, L.; Sanglard, D.; Levin, L.R.; Buck, J.; Mühlschlegel, F.A. The quorum-sensing molecules farnesol/homoserine lactone and dodecanol operate via distinct modes of action in *Candida albicans*. *Eukaryot. Cell* **2011**, *10*, 1034–1042. [CrossRef]
22. Zhu, J.; Krom, B.P.; Sanglard, D.; Intapa, C.; Dawson, C.C.; Peters, B.M.; Shirtliff, M.E.; Jabra-Rizk, M.A. Farnesol-Induced Apoptosis in *Candida albicans* Is Mediated by Cdr1-p Extrusion and Depletion of Intracellular Glutathione. *PLoS ONE* **2011**, *6*, e28830. [CrossRef]
23. Rocha, G.R.; Florez Salamanca, E.J.; de Barros, A.L.; Lobo, C.I.V.; Klein, M.I. Effect of tt-farnesol and myricetin on in vitro biofilm formed by *Streptococcus mutans* and *Candida albicans*. *BMC Complement. Altern. Med.* **2018**, *18*, 61. [CrossRef]
24. Nijampatnam, B.; Casals, L.; Zheng, R.; Wu Hui Velu, S.E. Hydroxychalcone inhibitors of *Streptococcus mutans* glucosyl transferases and biofilms as potential anticaries agents. *Bioorg. Med. Chem. Lett.* **2016**, *26*, 3508–3513. [CrossRef] [PubMed]
25. Sato, M.; Tsuchiya, H.; Akagiri, M.; Takagi, N.; Iinuma, M. Growth inhibition of oral bacteria related to denture stomatitis by anti-candidal chalcones. *Aust. Dent. J.* **1997**, *42*, 343–346. [CrossRef] [PubMed]

26. Aboody, M.S.A.; Mickymaray, S. Anti-Fungal Efficacy and Mechanisms of Flavonoids. *Antibiotics* **2020**, *9*, 45. [CrossRef] [PubMed]
27. Tsuchiya, H.; Sato, M.; Akagiri, M.; Takagi, N.; Tanaka, T.; Iinuma, M. Anti-Candida activity of synthetic hydroxychalcones. *Die Pharm.* **1994**, *49*, 756–758.
28. Richter, S.G.; Elli, D.; Kim, H.K.; Hendrickx, A.P.A.; Sorg, J.A.; Schneewind, O.; Missiakas, D. Small molecule inhibitor of lipoteichoic acid synthesis is an antibiotic for Gram-positive bacteria. *Proc. Natl. Acad. Sci. USA* **2013**, *110*, 3531–3536. [CrossRef] [PubMed]
29. Paganelli, F.L.; Van De Kamer, T.; Brouwer, E.C.; Leavis, H.L.; Woodford, N.; Bonten, M.J.; Willems, R.J.; Hendrickx, A.P. Lipoteichoic acid synthesis inhibition in combination with antibiotics abrogates growth of multidrug-resistant *Enterococcus faecium*. *Int. J. Antimicrob. Agents* **2017**, *49*, 355–363. [CrossRef] [PubMed]
30. Castillo Pedraza, M.C.; Fratucelli, E.D.O.; Ribeiro, S.M.; Florez Salamanca, E.J.; Colin, J.S.; Klein, M.I. Modulation of lipoteichoic acids and exopolysaccharides prevents *Streptococcus mutans* biofilm accumulation. *Molecules* **2020**, *25*, 2232. [CrossRef]
31. Clinical and Laboratory Standards Institute. CLSI Document M100-S25. In *Performance Standards for Antimicrobial Susceptibility Testing*; Clinical and Laboratory Standards Institute: Wayne, PA, USA, 2015.
32. Clinical and Laboratory Standards Institute. CLSI Document M27: Reference Method for Broth Dilution Antifungal Susceptibility Testing of Yeasts. In *Performance Standards for Antimicrobial Susceptibility Testing*, 4th ed.; Clinical and Laboratory Standards Institute: Wayne, PA, USA, 2017.
33. Clinical and Laboratory Standards Institute. CLSI Document M23: Development of In Vitro Susceptibility Testing Criteria and Quality Control Parameters. In *Performance Standards for Antimicrobial Susceptibility Testing*, 5th ed.; Clinical and Laboratory Standards Institute: Wayne, PA, USA, 2018.
34. Van Dijck, P.; Sjollema, J.; Cammue, B.P.A.; Lagrou, K.; Berman, J.; D'Enfert, C.; Andes, D.R.; Arendrup, M.C.; Brakhage, A.A.; Calderone, R.; et al. Methodologies for in vitro and in vivo evaluation of efficacy of antifungal and antibiofilm agents and surface coatings against fungal biofilms. *Microb. Cell* **2018**, *5*, 300–326. [CrossRef] [PubMed]
35. Eloff, J.N. Avoiding pitfalls in determining antimicrobial activity of plant extracts and publishing the results. *BMC Complement. Altern. Med.* **2019**, *19*, 106. [CrossRef]
36. Saputo, S.; Faustoferri, R.C.; Quivey, R.G., Jr. A drug repositioning approach reveals that *Streptococcus mutans* is susceptible to a diverse range of established antimicrobials and nonantibiotics. *Antimicrob. Agents Chemother.* **2017**, *62*, e01674-17. [CrossRef] [PubMed]
37. Zero, D.T. Dentifrices, mouthwashes, and remineralization/caries arrestment strategies. *BMC Oral Health* **2006**, *6* (Suppl. S1), S9. [CrossRef]
38. Heim, K.E.; Tagliaferro, A.R.; Bobilya, D.J. Flavonoid antioxidants: Chemistry, metabolism and structure-activity relationships. *J. Nutr. Biochem.* **2002**, *13*, 572–584. [CrossRef]
39. Cushnie, T.P.; Lamb, A.J. Antimicrobial activity of flavonoids. *Int. J. Antimicrob. Agents* **2005**, *26*, 343–356. [CrossRef]
40. Flemming, H.C.; Wingender, J. The biofilm matrix. *Nat. Rev. Microbiol.* **2010**, *8*, 623–633. [CrossRef]
41. Castillo Pedraza, M.C.; Rosalen, P.L.; de Castilho, A.R.F.; Freires, I.D.A.; Leite, L.D.S.; Leite, L.D.S.; Faustoferri, R.C.; Quivey, R.G., Jr.; Klein, M.I. Inactivation of *Streptococcus mutans* genes *lytST* and *dltAD* impairs its pathogenicity in vivo. *J. Oral Microbiol.* **2019**, *11*, 1607505. [CrossRef]
42. Batovska, D.; Parushev, S.; Slavova, A.; Bankova, V.; Tsvetkova, I.; Ninova, M.; Najdenski, H. Study on the substituents' effects of a series of synthetic chalcones against the yeast *Candida albicans*. *Eur. J. Med. Chem.* **2007**, *42*, 87–92. [CrossRef] [PubMed]
43. Santana, D.P.; Ribeiro, T.F.; Ribeiro, E.L.; de Aquino, G.L.B.; Faleiro Naves, P.L. Ação de chalconas contra a formação de biofilme de *Candida albicans*. *J. Basic Appl. Pharm. Sci.* **2015**, *36*, 83–90.
44. Marquis, R.E.; Clock, S.A.; Mota-Meira, M. Fluoride and organic weak acids as modulators of microbial physiology. *FEMS Microbiol. Rev.* **2003**, *26*, 493–510. [CrossRef] [PubMed]
45. Seleem, D.; Benso, B.; Noguti, J.; Pardi, V.; Murata, R.M. In Vitro and In Vivo Antifungal Activity of Lichochalcone-A against *Candida albicans* Biofilms. *PLoS ONE* **2016**, *11*, e0157188. [CrossRef] [PubMed]

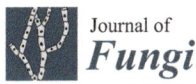

Article

Candida parapsilosis Colony Morphotype Forecasts Biofilm Formation of Clinical Isolates

Emilia Gómez-Molero [1,2], Iker De-la-Pinta [3], Jordan Fernández-Pereira [2], Uwe Groß [1], Michael Weig [1], Guillermo Quindós [3], Piet W. J. de Groot [2,*] and Oliver Bader [1,*]

1. Institute for Medical Microbiology, University Medical Center Göttingen, Kreuzbergring 57, 37075 Göttingen, Germany; emiliagomez803@hotmail.com (E.G.-M.); ugross@gwdg.de (U.G.); mweig@gwdg.de (M.W.)
2. Regional Center for Biomedical Research, Castilla-La Mancha Science & Technology Park, University of Castilla–La Mancha, 02008 Albacete, Spain; Jordan.Fernandez@alu.uclm.es
3. Department of Immunology, Microbiology and Parasitology, School of Medicine and Nursing, Universidad del País Vasco (UPV/EHU), 48940 Bilbao, Spain; iker.delapinta@ehu.eus (I.D.-l.-P.); guillermo.quindos@ehu.eus (G.Q.)
* Correspondence: piet.degroot@uclm.es (P.W.J.d.G.); obader@gwdg.de (O.B.)

Abstract: *Candida parapsilosis* is a frequent cause of fungal bloodstream infections, especially in critically ill neonates or immunocompromised patients. Due to the formation of biofilms, the use of indwelling catheters and other medical devices increases the risk of infection and complicates treatment, as cells embedded in biofilms display reduced drug susceptibility. Therefore, biofilm formation may be a significant clinical parameter, guiding downstream therapeutic choices. Here, we phenotypically characterized 120 selected isolates out of a prospective collection of 215 clinical *C. parapsilosis* isolates, determining biofilm formation, major emerging colony morphotype, and antifungal drug susceptibility of the isolates and their biofilms. In our isolate set, increased biofilm formation capacity was independent of body site of isolation and not predictable using standard or modified European Committee on Antimicrobial Susceptibility Testing (EUCAST) drug susceptibility testing protocols. In contrast, biofilm formation was strongly correlated with the appearance of non-smooth colony morphotypes and invasiveness into agar plates. Our data suggest that the observation of non-smooth colony morphotypes in cultures of *C. parapsilosis* may help as an indicator to consider the initiation of anti-biofilm-active therapy, such as the switch from azole- to echinocandin- or polyene-based strategies, especially in case of infections by potent biofilm-forming strains.

Keywords: *Candida parapsilosis*; biofilm; colony morphology; drug susceptibility

Citation: Gómez-Molero, E.; De-la-Pinta, I.; Fernández-Pereira, J.; Groß, U.; Weig, M.; Quindós, G.; de Groot, P.W.J.; Bader, O. *Candida parapsilosis* Colony Morphotype Forecasts Biofilm Formation of Clinical Isolates. *J. Fungi* **2021**, *7*, 33. https://doi.org/10.3390/jof7010033

Received: 8 December 2020
Accepted: 5 January 2021
Published: 7 January 2021

Publisher's Note: MDPI stays neutral with regard to jurisdictional claims in published maps and institutional affiliations.

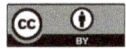

Copyright: © 2021 by the authors. Licensee MDPI, Basel, Switzerland. This article is an open access article distributed under the terms and conditions of the Creative Commons Attribution (CC BY) license (https://creativecommons.org/licenses/by/4.0/).

1. Introduction

Candida parapsilosis was first described as a non-pathogenic yeast with no clinical relevance [1]. However, increased use of medical devices, parenteral nutrition, and nosocomial infections [2] has made *C. parapsilosis* one of the most critical fungal species causing bloodstream infections (BSI) [3], which are of particular relevance in critically ill neonates [4–6] and immunocompromised patients [5,7].

The high infection rate with *C. parapsilosis* among neonates is likely due to the frequent requirement of parenteral nutrition [8] and the concomitant ability of *C. parapsilosis* to utilize fats and fatty acids as major energy sources [9]. In addition, the immature or compromised immune system may favor infections with this species [10].

Another risk factor for acquiring *C. parapsilosis* infections is the use of indwelling catheters and other medical devices onto which *C. parapsilosis* may form biofilms in conjunction with other *Candida* species or bacteria [4]. Primarily, this is attributed to its capacity to attach to the different materials of which medical devices are made [5,11,12]. This feature is highly variable among individual clinical isolates [13]. In *C. parapsilosis*, the formation of biofilms is associated with the ability to form pseudohyphae [14–16] as well as the concomitant change in expression levels of cell wall-localized adhesins such as Als1-7 [17–19] or Rbt1 [20]. Importantly, susceptibility to commonly used azole-based antifungal agents in fungal biofilms on medical devices may be strongly reduced [21,22].

Similar to *C. albicans* (reviewed in [23]), *C. parapsilosis* can have different colony morphotypes on diagnostic agar plates (Figure 1). While mixed-morphology culture plates can be the result of infection with multiple strains [24] in diagnostic procedures, also, the morphologic switching of some strains is a well-described phenomenon [25]. In addition to their role in biofilm formation, pseudohyphae formation and adhesin expression are also key to the visual appearance of fungal colonies on solid agars [26–28], which in turn may well be correlated to the capacity to form biofilms in the host, the incorporation of cell wall proteins (CWP), and, consequently, virulence [15].

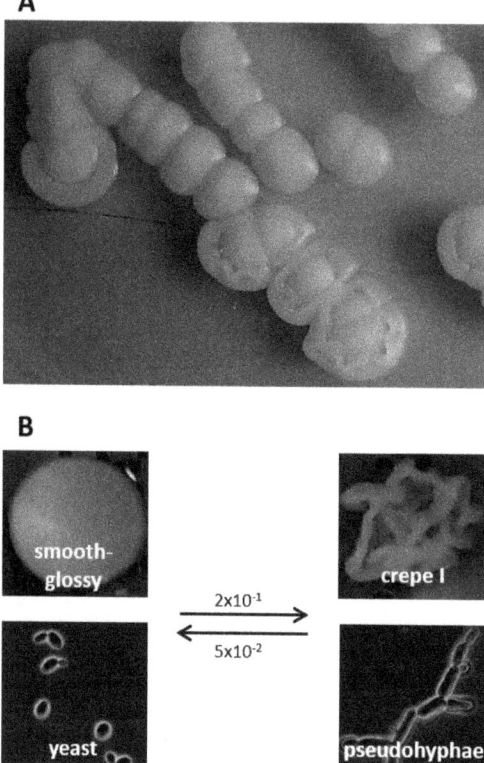

Figure 1. Colony morphotypes formed by *C. parapsilosis*. (**A**) Mixed morphotypes observed on a routine diagnostic plate. (**B**) Cells with distinct morphological colony phenotypes can be subcultured, but some strains (here strain PEU582: smooth-glossy vs. crepe, see below) sometimes undergo switching with strain-dependent frequencies. Smooth colonies are composed mainly of yeast-form cells, whereas non-smooth colonies are composed of pseudohyphal cells or mixtures of both morphologies.

Here, we phenotypically characterized a large collection of clinical *C. parapsilosis* isolates, including the description of novel intermediate morphotypes. We determined if early colony morphology was a potential predictor of biofilm production and pseudohyphal growth and as such might reveal the need to direct the antifungal therapy against biofilms containing *C. parapsilosis*.

2. Materials and Methods

2.1. Clinical Routine Diagnostic and Strain Maintenance

C. parapsilosis clinical isolates were routinely identified using MALDI-TOF (MALDI Biotyper, Bruker Daltonics, Bremen, Germany) according to the protocol described [29]. Mixed cultures were differentiated on YEPD agar (1% yeast extract, 2% peptone, 2% glucose, 2% agar) supplemented with 5 mg/mL phloxine B. On this medium, most tested colonies developed a final morphotype within 48 h of incubation at 30 °C (Figure 1, Supplementary Figures S1 and S2). Cells from colonies with stable morphotypes were transferred onto Sabouraud dextrose agar (SDA, Oxoid, Munich, Germany), regrown, and stored at −70 °C in cryovials (Mast Diagnostica, Reinfeld, Germany) for further analyses.

2.2. Biofilm Quantitation

Biofilm quantification assays on polystyrol were performed as described previously [11,30,31], with adaptations to suit *C. parapsilosis*. Briefly, isolates were grown on phloxine B-containing YEPD agar plates. Inoculum was prepared from single colonies grown to stationary phase in YEPD broth at 30 °C overnight at 220 rpm. A cell suspension adjusted to a cell density of McFarland = 2 was prepared using sterile saline, and 100 µL YEPD medium plus 50 µL aliquots of the cell suspensions were mixed in 96-well polystyrol microtiter plates (Greiner Bio-one) and incubated for 24 h at 37 °C. After removal of the medium by aspiration, the attached biofilms were washed once with 200 µL of distilled water. Cells were stained for 30 min in 100 µL of 0.1% aqueous crystal violet (CV). Excess CV was removed, and the biofilm was washed once with 200 µL of distilled water. To release CV from the cells, 200 µL of 1% SDS in 50% ethanol was added, and the cellular material was resuspended by pipetting. CV absorbance was quantified at 490 nm using a microtiter plate reader (MRX TC Revelation). Data shown are the average of three independent biological experiments, each including four technical repeats, using reference strain CDC317 as inter-experiment quality control.

2.3. Antifungal Drug Susceptibility Testing

Susceptibility testing was performed according to EUCAST e.def 7.3.1 standards [32]. Fluconazole (FLZ), voriconazole (VRZ), posaconazole (POS), and amphotericin B (AMB) substances were purchased from Discovery fine Chemicals Ltd. (Bournemouth, UK), micafungin (MFG) was kindly provided by Astellas, and caspofungin (CAS) was provided by Merck Sharp & Dohme Corp (MSD). Sequencing of the ERG11 and MRR1 genes was performed as previously described [33].

Preformed biofilms reduction

Cells were pre-grown on Sabouraud dextrose agar (SDA) for 96 h at 30 °C, and one colony was sub-cultured in 5 mL of YEPD broth overnight at 37 °C in an orbital incubator at 200 rpm. Cells were harvested by centrifugation and resuspended in Phosphate-buffered saline (PBS). Upon counting cells in a Neubauer chamber, the suspensions were adjusted to 1×10^6 cells/mL in both RPMI (2 g/L glucose, pH 7) and YEPD (20 g/L glucose, pH 6.7). One hundred µL of the inoculum was pipetted into each well of a Bioscreen plate (Labsystem, Helsinki, Finland), and the plates were incubated for 24 h at 37 °C to allow biofilm formation. Next, planktonic cells were removed, and the plates were washed twice in PBS leaving just the biofilm in the wells. Two-fold serial dilutions of four antifungal drugs were prepared in RPMI or YEPD ranging from 0.25 to 32 µg/mL for POS, VRZ, and MFG, and from 0.0125 to 16 µg/mL for AMB. Subsequently, 100 µl of each dilution was added to the corresponding wells with biofilm in triplicate, and the plates were incubated again at 37 °C for 24 h. Finally, plates were washed twice with PBS, and reduction of the biofilm metabolic activity was determined by measuring the absorbance at 492 nm with the XTT (2,3-bis-(2-methoxy-4-nitro-5-sulfophenyl)-2H- tetrazolium-5-carboxanilide) colorimetric method [34].

2.4. Morphotype Development and Agar Invasion

Selected *C. parapsilosis* isolates were cultured overnight in YEPD liquid media in an orbital shaker at 220 rpm at 30 °C. Cell density was adjusted to 2×10^2 cells/mL, after which 100 µL was plated onto YEPD agar plates and incubated at 30 °C for ten successive days. Starting after 48 h, the morphotype development of colonies was captured every 24 h over ten days using a stereoscopic binocular loupe (SZM-1, OPTIKA®, Ponteranica, Italy) mounted with a digital camera. Morphotypes and agar invasion were classified according to the references given in Supplementary Figure S1.

For analysis of agar invasion, colonies with different morphotypes were plated onto YEPD agar plates supplemented with 5 mg/mL of phloxine B [25], and morphotype development was followed as described above. Agar invasion was scored from day 4 onwards by scraping selected colonies with an inoculation loop and eventually washing off the cells under running water on the last day. Agar invasion was classified as low (1), low-medium (2), medium (3), medium-high (4), high (5), and finally as very high (6) when cells could not be removed by rinsing (see scoring reference in Supplementary Figure S1).

2.5. Statistical Analyses

For statistical analyses of biofilms and antifungal drug susceptibility, unpaired two-samples Student's *t*-tests were used. All data used were the average of three independent analyses, and *p* values < 0.05 were considered statistically significant.

To detect potential correlations between biofilm formation capacity, colony morphotype, and/or agar invasion capacity, regression analyses were performed, and Pearson's correlation coefficient r was used as a predictor for correlation. All data were analyzed using IMB SPSS 22 statistics software.

3. Results

3.1. Biofilm Formation Capacity Is Independent of Body Site of Isolation

Over the course of two years, we collected 215 *C. parapsilosis* clinical isolates from our routine diagnostics (Figure 2). Isolates were classified according to nine different categories depending on the body site of isolation. *C. parapsilosis* is known to frequently occur in the nape region, reaching up to the ear. Consequently, most isolates stemmed from ear infections; however, a substantial number of isolates from invasive infections at other body sites as well as from indwelling devices such as central venous or urine catheters were included in the study. *C. parapsilosis* was only infrequently isolated from locations of the GI (2,3-bis-(2-methoxy-4-nitro-5-sulfophenyl)-2H- tetrazolium-5-carboxanilide) tract, the oral cavity, or the skin.

Isolates obtained were systematically screened for their capacity to form biofilms in standard biofilm formation tests in polystyrol microtiter plates. No body site, including those isolate groups obtained from plastic materials, could be identified to be significantly associated with elevated numbers of biofilm-forming isolates ($p = 0.371$, Figure 2A). When stratified by quantitative measurement values, we observed a near even distribution across the study group; only a tentative cut-off for low biofilm formation capacity was observed at OD (optical density) measurement values of approximately 0.1 (Figure 2B, intersection of black lines). Microscopical imaging of cells in biofilms from some representative isolates confirmed the already established idea that the capacity to form biofilms is correlated with pseudohyphal development (Supplementary Figure S3) [25–28].

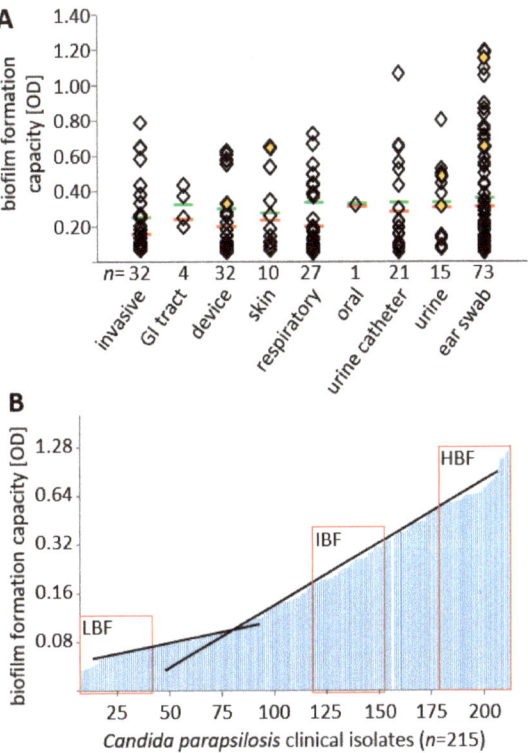

Figure 2. *C. parapsilosis* collection and selection of isolates for downstream experiments. (**A**) Distribution of collection isolates stratified according to site of isolation and biofilm production on polystyrol. Category "invasive" includes, e.g., blood culture, biopsies, or intraoperative swabs. Orange diamonds: six isolates used in pre-formed biofilm experiments, see text. Red and green lines: mean and two-fold mean values. (**B**) Biofilm formation capacity; isolates sorted by value from low to high. Intersection of black lines: approximated cut-off. Red boxes indicate strain selection of representative low (LBF, left box), intermediate (IBF, middle box) and high (HBF, right box) biofilm formers for subsequent experiments.

3.2. Effect of Biofilm Formation on Antifungal Drug Susceptibility

In order to estimate the correlation of the lead phenotype (biofilm formation on polystyrol) with drug susceptibility, we selected 40 isolates each of low (LBF), intermediate (IBF), and high (HBF) biofilm formation capacity (Figure 2B, red boxes) from our collection including two non-adherent control strains (CDC317 and ATCC22019). The strains were tested for susceptibility to selected azoles (FLZ, POS, VRZ), echinocandins (CAS, MFG), and one polyene (AMB) after one (young colonies) and eight days (matured colonies) of growth on phloxine B agar plates.

Four IBF isolates (PEU651, PEU768, PEU941, and PEU950), and reference strain CDC317 showed elevated (minimum inhibitory concentration) MIC (values of 4–16 µg/mL for FLC. To exclude potential biases through resistance mutations (e.g., Y132F [35]), we sequenced the ERG11 and MRR1 genes in these isolates. A non-synonymous ERG11 point mutation was found only in CDC317, which was heterozygous with respect to the Y132F amino acid exchange. Y132F is known to confer resistance to fluconazole [36,37]. MRR1 only contained non-synonymous SNPs (Single nucleotide polymorphisms) in PEU651. Since we could not exclude a potential influence of these mutations, data for PEU651 as well as those of the two reference strains were excluded from the drug susceptibility analysis, leaving a total of 117 isolates in three groups of 39 isolates each.

We did not observe large-scale differences in drug susceptibility between experiments undertaken with young or mature colonies except for CAS (LBF $p = 0.017$ and HBF $p = 0.028$, Figure 3A white vs. gray boxes).

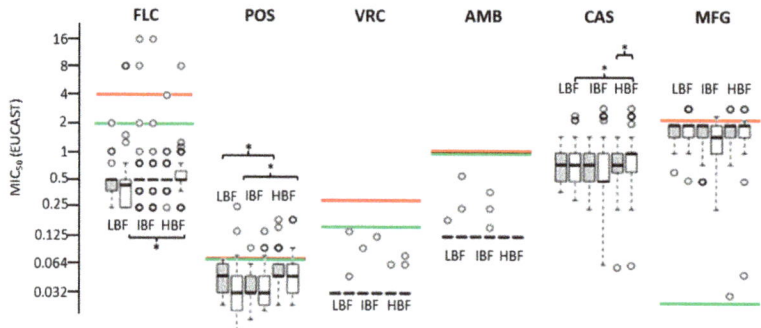

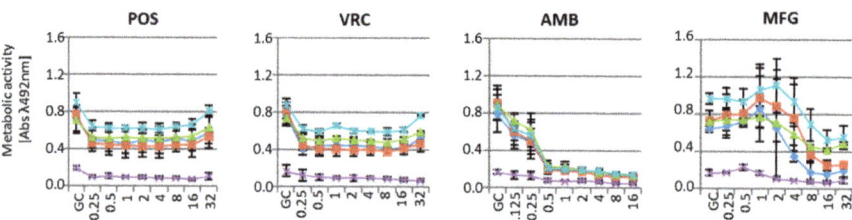

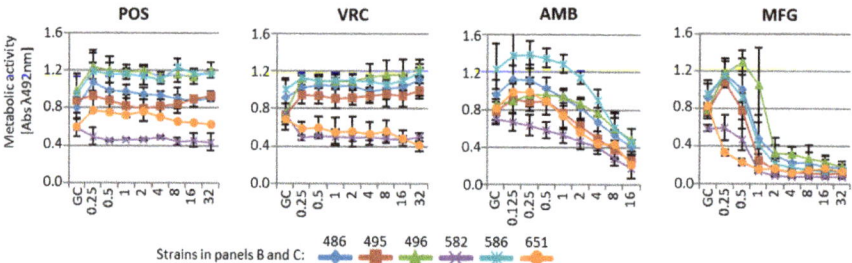

Figure 3. Drug susceptibility. (**A**) Biofilm formation-phenotype dependent susceptibility testing where inoculum was prepared from cells after 1 day of growth on Sabouraud dextrose agar (SDA) (gray boxes) and after 8 days of growth (white boxes) on the same plates, when colonies had fully developed morphotypes. For each substance tested, the values for 1 and 8-day inoculum are depicted for each group (LBF, IBF, and HBF). Red lines: EUCAST clinical breakpoint (R>); green lines, susceptible cut-off (S ≤). *: statistical significance (**B**,**C**) Effect of antifungal drugs on cell viability in pre-formed biofilms of selected biofilm-forming isolates tested in (**B**) RPMI (Roswell Park Memorial Institute)or (**C**) YEPD(yeast extract peptone dextrose) media.

Although statistically significant differences between HBF versus IBF or LBF isolate groups were clearly evident for some antifungal drugs (POS: LBF vs. HBF with young colonies $p = 0.014$, mature colonies $p = 0.072$, CAS: LBF vs. HBF with young colonies $p = 0.015$), the observed mean MIC differences did not result in a major change in classification of either susceptible (S) or resistant (R) according to EUCAST breakpoints. Differences in mean susceptibility values were 1-2 log2-fold decreases for VRZ, POS (mature colonies only), CAS, and MFG in the HBF group, as compared to the LBF group. No apparent differences for either FLZ or AMB were seen.

3.3. Susceptibility of Biofilms to Antifungal Drugs

Next, for six selected intermediate to high biofilm-forming isolates, we analyzed to which degree pre-formed *C. parapsilosis* biofilms resisted antifungal drug treatment in two different media, RPMI and YEPD. RPMI is considered the reference medium for antifungal drug susceptibility testing and, as mentioned above, it was also used for MIC determination according to the EUCAST protocol. Likewise, YEPD is a glucose-rich medium that is widely used in assays with yeasts due to the large amount of peptone and dextrose extremely necessary for yeast growth and biofilm formation. The ability to form biofilms was evaluated using this culture medium. Since both media are widely used in the literature, we decided to test the drug susceptibility of preformed biofilms in both of them, observing that some strains are more prone to form biofilms in one media and not in the other, as well as behaving differently when interacting with antifungal drugs. More specifically, one of the six isolates (PEU651) was not able to form biofilm in RPMI (Figure 3B), whereas another (PEU582) grew only at reduced rates. Both isolates also showed a reduction in biofilm development in YEPD (Figure 3C) but were kept in these assays as the results were qualitatively in agreement with the other strains used.

Antifungal drugs had different quantitative effects when the assay was carried out in RPMI (Figure 3B) or in YEPD (Figure 3C). In YEPD, sub-inhibitory drug concentrations caused increases in metabolic activity, as measured by XTT reduction. This may be a stress-response effect countering drugs at these levels, and it was considered an artifact for the purpose of this study. Higher concentrations of azoles (POS, VRZ) reduced biofilm metabolic activity by only 30–50% as compared to the drug-free control. There was no azole drug concentration in the measurement range (up to 32 µg/mL) that led to a full reduction in biofilm metabolic activity (all $p > 0.05$). In contrast, both MFG and AMB did achieve a strong reduction of metabolic activity, although under different conditions: in RPMI, an AMB concentration of 0.5 µg/mL was sufficient for 70% reduction, while 16 µg/mL were required in YEPD. For MFG, this was the opposite: in YEPD, a clear effect was seen at 2 µg/mL with only residual metabolic activity apparent up to the upper assay boundaries (32 µg/mL).

3.4. Biofilm Formation Capacity on Polystyrol Correlates with Colony Morphotype and Agar Invasiveness

On culture plates, individual *C. parapsilosis* isolates showed specific, stable morphotypes. Only a minority of isolates (18%) were also able to switch between such morphotypes upon re-plating (Figure 1 and scoring reference shown in Supplementary Figure S1).

In a preliminary analysis on a selected subset (Supplementary Figure S2), non-smooth colony morphologies were already apparent at the start of the observation period (20%) and reliably appeared after 72 h of growth. Across the entire collection, agar invasion (Supplementary Figure S1A) and colony morphotype (Supplementary Figures S1B and S2) were therefore scored over a course of four to ten days (Figure 4). Most LBF isolates (90%) showed smooth morphotypes, and only a small proportion (10%), for instance PEU944, developed wrinkled or crepe phenotypes. On day 10, about 20% had developed non-smooth morphotypes as their major morphology (Figure 4A). With increasing biofilm formation capacity, also the frequency of non-smooth colony morphotypes increased. Of the IBF isolates, 20% had developed non-smooth morphotypes at day 4, and 55% had developed non-smooth morphotypes on day 10. HBF isolates mainly, but not exclusively, produced non-smooth phenotypes (66% on day 4, 83% on day 10), which in most cases were already distinguishable at day 2. Some isolates presented two independent stable morphotypes (e.g., PEU525: non-smooth (cr) and smooth (s)), which were distinguishable from day 2 until day 10. Along with the increased formation of non-smooth colony morphotypes in IBF and HBF strains (r = 0.832, *p* < 0.001), also agar invasiveness increased from day 4 to day 10 (r = 0.969, *** *p* < 0.001 (Figure 4B, Table 1).

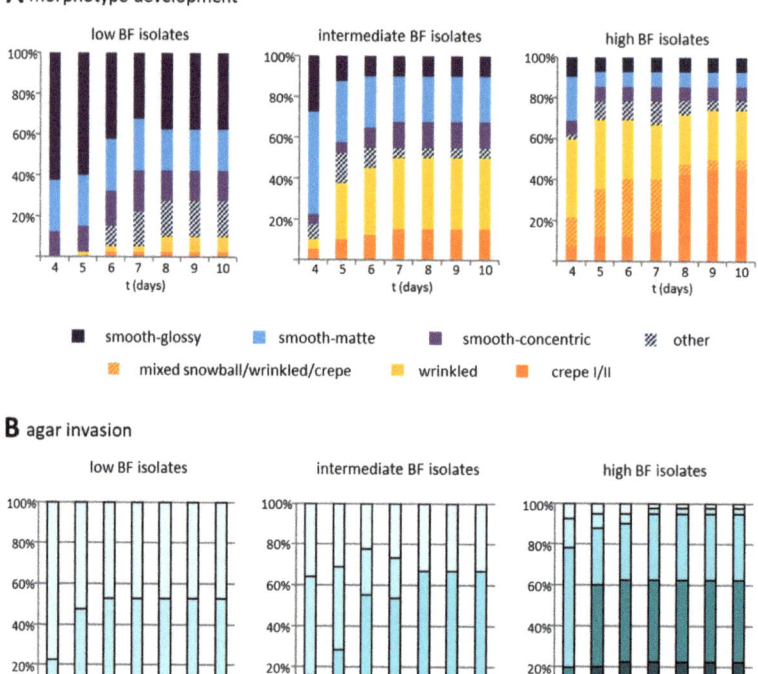

Figure 4. Emergence of colony morphotype over time. (**A**) Development of colony morphotype and (**B**) agar invasiveness scoring the same plates consecutively from 4 days to 10 days after inoculation. Isolates with low biofilm formation capacity (left panels), intermediate biofilm formation capacity (middle panels), and high biofilm formation capacity (right panels) were scored for the most frequent colony morphotype visible. Of note, HBF isolates rated "smooth" still developed minor frequencies of non-smooth colonies. See Supplementary Figure S1 for scoring references.

Table 1. Agar invasiveness and colony morphology.

Morphology [a]	n	Agar Invasion [a]					
		Low	Low-Medium	Medium	Medium-High	High	Very High
smooth	59	34%	27%	5%	32%	2%	0%
wrinkled	22	5%	9%	23%	50%	9%	5%
mixed/infrequent	16	0%	6%	6%	63%	19%	6%
crepe I and II	25	4%	4%	0%	36%	28%	28%

[a] see Supplementary Figure S1 for classification of agar invasion and morphotypes.

4. Discussion

C. parapsilosis is frequently found as a cause of pathologies due to biofilm formation on medical devices in long-term hospitalized patients suffering from endocarditis, peritonitis, arthritis, or general sepsis [22,38–40]. We hypothesized that the capacity to form biofilm might be related to the origin of the clinical specimen, that is, infections at different body sites or fungus growing on medical devices such as indwelling catheters. However, when the 215 clinical isolates in our collection were scored for their biofilm-forming capacity on rich medium (YEPD), a strong inducer of biofilms in *C. parapsilosis* [41], no clear distribution of low (LBF) versus high (HBF) biofilm formation depending on the site of isolation was detected. Nevertheless, a high percentage of catheter-associated isolates belonged to the IBF and HBF groups, which is consistent with the notion that *C. parapsilosis* infections often start from infected indwelling devices [42,43].

Then, we raised the question of whether there might be a possible link between the biofilm-forming capacity of clinical isolates and their drug susceptibility [21,22], which could be useful for decision making about treatment strategies in the clinic. However, tests with the three groups of isolates (LBF, IBF, and HBF), reflecting a wide range—from negligible to high quantities of biomass—of biofilm-formation capacity on polystyrol, and six commonly used azole-, echinocandin-, and polyene antifungal agents did not reveal any such correlation. Observed MIC values were similar to those reported previously by others [44–47], and also, no remarkable differences were observed between inocula prepared from young or matured cells (as found in biofilms). Therefore, we conclude that the drug susceptibility data obtained with the standard EUCAST protocol do not seem to generate predictive information toward the biofilm-formation capacity of clinical isolates.

Nevertheless, fungal cells embedded within biofilms, including those formed by *C. parapsilosis*, are considered to be less susceptible to antifungal compounds [21,22]. This notion was confirmed here by studying the antifungal drug susceptibility of six biofilm-forming strains embedded in preformed biofilms, which showed significantly reduced sensitivity to azoles. This experiment was executed in both YEPD (high glucose) and RPMI (lower glucose) medium. As expected [41], biofilm formation in YEPD was higher than in RPMI, and media-dependent differences in echinocandin and polyene sensitivity were also noted. These observations support earlier reported overall quantitative dependences of biofilm formation and drug susceptibility on glucose levels in the media [41,48,49].

Another important aspect of our study was the question of whether *C. parapsilosis* colony morphotypes might perhaps serve to forecast the biofilm-forming capacity of clinical isolates. We hypothesized that high biofilm formers would show more non-smooth morphotypes and pseudohyphae than poor biofilm formers and have an increased tendency to invade agar [50]. When following colony morphotype development in the three isolate groups (LBF, IBF, and HBF) over a course of ten days, we indeed observed a strong correlation of the HBF group with non-smooth colony morphotypes. In contrast, the appearance of non-smooth colonies occurred only in a minority of the isolates in the LBF group. As surface adherence represents the first step in biofilm formation, our data are supported by studies showing that non-smooth colonies are generally more adherent to plastic than smooth colonies [51].

Interestingly, in most cases, non-smooth morphotypes could already be observed within 48 h of growth, and only little change was observed after 96 h, indicating that prolonged incubation beyond this time point is not needed for morphotype determination. In addition, all the morphotypes appeared stable, as they were reproduced upon repeating the experiment, which is consistent with the idea that switching is not a common or frequent event. Finally, biofilm-forming capacity and the appearance of non-smooth morphotypes and pseudohyphae were positively correlated to agar invasion. However, a large proportion of smooth colony types also displayed medium-strength agar invasion, indicating pseudohyphae formation at least at the base of the colony [52,53].

In summary, our experiments show that there is a strong correlation between colony morphotype and biofilm formation capacity in isolates from clinical samples and that this is not reflected in the results from standard antifungal drug susceptibility testing. Our data are the first to indicate that the observation of non-smooth colony morphotypes of *C. parapsilosis* may help to consider the initiation of anti-biofilm-active therapy. This may include antifungal lock therapy and shifting treatment from azole-based to echinocandin- or polyene-based strategies to eliminate biofilms from catheters [39]. However, due to the inherent ability of some strains to switch between morphotypes [25–28,54], the absence of such colonies should not be taken as an absolute indicator that biofilms do *not* exist in the patient.

Supplementary Materials: The following are available online at https://www.mdpi.com/2309-6 08X/7/1/33/s1, Supplementary Figure S1. Morphological classification of *C. parapsilosis* colony morphotypes. (A) Semi-quantitative classification of agar invasion on phloxine B-containing SDA. (B) Colony morphotypes observed in our isolate collection. In picture pairs, left pictures represent colony morphotype after 10 d incubation, right pictures show agar imprint left on phloxine B agar plates after flushing off colonies with running water. Scale bars = 0.25 cm; Supplementary Figure S2. Colony morphotype development during a ten-day time-lapse experiment. Morphotype development of colonies was followed during ten days of growth on YEPD agar at 30 °C. (A) Five selected low biofilm-forming (LBF) clinical isolates, (B) five intermediate biofilm-forming (IBF) isolates, and (C) five high-biofilm-forming (HBF) isolates. d, derby; cn, concentric; cr, crater; s, smooth; wr, wrinkled; Supplementary Figure S3. Morphology of *C. parapsilosis* cells in biofilms onto polystyrol. Representative strains with low (LBF, row 1), intermediate (IBF, row2) and high (HBF, rows 3 and 4) biofilm formation capacity are shown. Biofilms were let to develop for 24 h in YEPD as described in materials and methods. Unbound cells were removed by washing with PBS. Remaining biofilm cells were observed with a Leica DM1000 microscope mounted with a HC PL 100×/1.32 objective and MC170 HD digital camera.

Author Contributions: Conceptualization, E.G.-M., P.W.J.d.G. and O.B.; Formal analysis, E.G.-M., I.D.-l.-P., J.F.-P. and P.W.J.d.G.; Funding acquisition, U.G., G.Q., P.W.J.d.G. and O.B.; Investigation, E.G.-M., I.D.-l.-P. and J.F.-P.; Methodology, E.G.-M., M.W. and G.Q.; Project administration, O.B.; Resources, U.G. and M.W.; Supervision, G.Q., P.W.J.d.G. and O.B.; Writing–original draft, E.G.-M., M.W., P.W.J.d.G. and O.B.; Writing–review & editing, G.Q. and O.B. All authors have read and agreed to the published version of the manuscript.

Funding: This work was funded in part by grants or scholarships from the ZabaldUz program (Universidad del País Vasco/Euskal Herriko Unibertsitatea) to IDlP, the Consejería de Educación, Universidades e Investigación (GIC15/78 IT-990-16) of Gobierno Vasco-Eusko Jaurlaritza to GQ, the Ministerio de Economía y Competitividad (grants SAF2013-47570-P and SAF2017-86188-P, the latter co-financed by FEDER) of the Spanish government to P.G. and G.Q., and the FP7-PEOPLE-2013-ITN—Marie-Curie Action: "Initial Training Networks": Molecular Mechanisms of Human Fungal Pathogen Host Interaction, ImResFun, MC-ITN-606786, to O.B. and U.G.

Institutional Review Board Statement: Not applicable.

Informed Consent Statement: Not applicable.

Data Availability Statement: The data presented in this study are available upon reasonable request from the corresponding author.

Acknowledgments: Agnieszka Goretzki and Yvonne Laukat are thanked for performing susceptibility testing.

Conflicts of Interest: The authors declare no conflict of interest.

References

1. Weems, J.J., Jr. *Candida parapsilosis*: Epidemiology, pathogenicity, clinical manifestations, and antimicrobial susceptibility. *Clin. Infect. Dis.* **1992**, *14*, 756–766. [CrossRef] [PubMed]
2. Krcmery, V.; Barnes, A.J. Non-*albicans Candida* spp. causing fungaemia: Pathogenicity and antifungal resistance. *J. Hosp. Infect.* **2002**, *50*, 243–260. [CrossRef] [PubMed]
3. Pfaller, M.A.; Diekema, D.J. Role of sentinel surveillance of candidemia: Trends in species distribution and antifungal susceptibility. *J. Clin. Microbiol.* **2002**, *40*, 3551–3557. [CrossRef] [PubMed]
4. Pammi, M.; Holland, L.; Butler, G.; Gacser, A.; Bliss, J.M. *Candida parapsilosis* is a significant neonatal pathogen: A systematic review and meta-analysis. *Pediatr. Infect. Dis. J.* **2013**, *32*, e206–e216. [CrossRef]
5. Trofa, D.; Gacser, A.; Nosanchuk, J.D. *Candida parapsilosis*, an emerging fungal pathogen. *Clin. Microbiol. Rev.* **2008**, *21*, 606–625. [CrossRef]

6. Lindberg, E.; Hammarstrom, H.; Ataollahy, N.; Kondori, N. Species distribution and antifungal drug susceptibilities of yeasts isolated from the blood samples of patients with candidemia. *Sci. Rep.* **2019**, *9*, 3838. [CrossRef]
7. Toth, R.; Nosek, J.; Mora-Montes, H.M.; Gabaldon, T.; Bliss, J.M.; Nosanchuk, J.D.; Turner, S.A.; Butler, G.; Vagvolgyi, C.; Gacser, A. Candida parapsilosis: From Genes to the Bedside. *Clin. Microbiol. Rev.* **2019**, *32*. [CrossRef]
8. Lupetti, A.; Tavanti, A.; Davini, P.; Ghelardi, E.; Corsini, V.; Merusi, I.; Boldrini, A.; Campa, M.; Senesi, S. Horizontal transmission of Candida parapsilosis candidemia in a neonatal intensive care unit. *J. Clin. Microbiol.* **2002**, *40*, 2363–2369. [CrossRef]
9. Gacser, A.; Trofa, D.; Schafer, W.; Nosanchuk, J.D. Targeted gene deletion in Candida parapsilosis demonstrates the role of secreted lipase in virulence. *J. Clin. Investig.* **2007**, *117*, 3049–3058. [CrossRef]
10. Linden, J.R.; De Paepe, M.E.; Laforce-Nesbitt, S.S.; Bliss, J.M. Galectin-3 plays an important role in protection against disseminated candidiasis. *Med. Mycol.* **2013**, *51*, 641–651. [CrossRef]
11. Kuhn, D.M.; Chandra, J.; Mukherjee, P.K.; Ghannoum, M.A. Comparison of biofilms formed by Candida albicans and Candida parapsilosis on bioprosthetic surfaces. *Infect. Immun.* **2002**, *70*, 878–888. [CrossRef] [PubMed]
12. Neji, S.; Hadrich, I.; Trabelsi, H.; Abbes, S.; Cheikhrouhou, F.; Sellami, H.; Makni, F.; Ayadi, A. Virulence factors, antifungal susceptibility and molecular mechanisms of azole resistance among Candida parapsilosis complex isolates recovered from clinical specimens. *J. Biomed. Sci.* **2017**, *24*, 67. [CrossRef] [PubMed]
13. Silva, S.; Henriques, M.; Martins, A.; Oliveira, R.; Williams, D.; Azeredo, J. Biofilms of non-Candida albicans Candida species: Quantification, structure and matrix composition. *Med. Mycol.* **2009**, *47*, 681–689. [CrossRef] [PubMed]
14. Lattif, A.A.; Mukherjee, P.K.; Chandra, J.; Swindell, K.; Lockhart, S.R.; Diekema, D.J.; Pfaller, M.A.; Ghannoum, M.A. Characterization of biofilms formed by Candida parapsilosis, C. metapsilosis, and C. orthopsilosis. *Int. J. Med. Microbiol.* **2010**, *300*, 265–270. [CrossRef] [PubMed]
15. Pannanusorn, S.; Fernandez, V.; Romling, U. Prevalence of biofilm formation in clinical isolates of Candida species causing bloodstream infection. *Mycoses* **2013**, *56*, 264–272. [CrossRef] [PubMed]
16. Kozik, A.; Karkowska-Kuleta, J.; Zajac, D.; Bochenska, O.; Kedracka-Krok, S.; Jankowska, U.; Rapala-Kozik, M. Fibronectin-, vitronectin- and laminin-binding proteins at the cell walls of Candida parapsilosis and Candida tropicalis pathogenic yeasts. *BMC Microbiol.* **2015**, *15*, 197. [CrossRef]
17. Butler, G.; Rasmussen, M.D.; Lin, M.F.; Santos, M.A.; Sakthikumar, S.; Munro, C.A.; Rheinbay, E.; Grabherr, M.; Forche, A.; Reedy, J.L.; et al. Evolution of pathogenicity and sexual reproduction in eight Candida genomes. *Nature* **2009**, *459*, 657–662. [CrossRef]
18. Pryszcz, L.P.; Nemeth, T.; Gacser, A.; Gabaldon, T. Unexpected genomic variability in clinical and environmental strains of the pathogenic yeast Candida parapsilosis. *Genome Biol. Evol.* **2013**, *5*, 2382–2392. [CrossRef]
19. Neale, M.N.; Glass, K.A.; Longley, S.J.; Kim, D.J.; Laforce-Nesbitt, S.S.; Wortzel, J.D.; Shaw, S.K.; Bliss, J.M. Role of the Inducible Adhesin CpAls7 in Binding of Candida parapsilosis to the Extracellular Matrix under Fluid Shear. *Infect. Immun.* **2018**, *86*. [CrossRef]
20. Rossignol, T.; Ding, C.; Guida, A.; d'Enfert, C.; Higgins, D.G.; Butler, G. Correlation between biofilm formation and the hypoxic response in Candida parapsilosis. *Eukaryot. Cell* **2009**, *8*, 550–559. [CrossRef]
21. Katragkou, A.; Chatzimoschou, A.; Simitsopoulou, M.; Dalakiouridou, M.; Diza-Mataftsi, E.; Tsantali, C.; Roilides, E. Differential activities of newer antifungal agents against Candida albicans and Candida parapsilosis biofilms. *Antimicrob. Agents Chemother.* **2008**, *52*, 357–360. [CrossRef] [PubMed]
22. Soldini, S.; Posteraro, B.; Vella, A.; De Carolis, E.; Borghi, E.; Falleni, M.; Losito, A.R.; Maiuro, G.; Trecarichi, E.M.; Sanguinetti, M.; et al. Microbiologic and clinical characteristics of biofilm-forming Candida parapsilosis isolates associated with fungaemia and their impact on mortality. *Clin. Microbiol. Infect.* **2018**, *24*, 771–777. [CrossRef] [PubMed]
23. Soll, D.R. The role of phenotypic switching in the basic biology and pathogenesis of Candida albicans. *J. Oral Microbiol.* **2014**, *6*. [CrossRef] [PubMed]
24. Gómez-Molero, E.; Willis, J.; Dudakova, A.; Gacser, A.; Weig, M.; Groß, U.; Gabaldón, T.; Bader, O. Phenotypic variability in a coinfection with three independent C. parapsilosis lineages. *Front. Microbiol.* **2020**, *11*. [CrossRef] [PubMed]
25. Laffey, S.F.; Butler, G. Phenotype switching affects biofilm formation by Candida parapsilosis. *Microbiology* **2005**, *151*, 1073–1081. [CrossRef] [PubMed]
26. Lott, T.J.; Kuykendall, R.J.; Welbel, S.F.; Pramanik, A.; Lasker, B.A. Genomic heterogeneity in the yeast Candida parapsilosis. *Curr. Genet.* **1993**, *23*, 463–467. [CrossRef] [PubMed]
27. Enger, L.; Joly, S.; Pujol, C.; Simonson, P.; Pfaller, M.; Soll, D.R. Cloning and characterization of a complex DNA fingerprinting probe for Candida parapsilosis. *J. Clin. Microbiol.* **2001**, *39*, 658–669. [CrossRef]
28. Nosek, J.; Holesova, Z.; Kosa, P.; Gacser, A.; Tomaska, L. Biology and genetics of the pathogenic yeast Candida parapsilosis. *Curr. Genet.* **2009**, *55*, 497–509. [CrossRef]
29. Bernhard, M.; Weig, M.; Zautner, A.E.; Gross, U.; Bader, O. Yeast on-target lysis (YOTL), a procedure for making auxiliary mass spectrum data sets for clinical routine identification of yeasts. *J. Clin. Microbiol.* **2014**, *52*, 4163–4167. [CrossRef]
30. Chandra, J.; Kuhn, D.M.; Mukherjee, P.K.; Hoyer, L.L.; McCormick, T.; Ghannoum, M.A. Biofilm formation by the fungal pathogen Candida albicans: Development, architecture, and drug resistance. *J. Bacteriol.* **2001**, *183*, 5385–5394. [CrossRef] [PubMed]
31. Gómez-Molero, E.; de Boer, A.D.; Dekker, H.L.; Moreno-Martínez, A.; Kraneveld, E.A.; Ichsan Chauhan, N.; Weig, M.; de Soet, J.J.; de Koster, C.G.; Bader, O.; et al. Proteomic analysis of hyperadhesive Candida glabrata clinical isolates reveals a core wall proteome and differential incorporation of adhesins. *FEMS Yeast Res.* **2015**, *15*, fov098. [CrossRef] [PubMed]

32. EUCAST. Available online: http://www.eucast.org/fileadmin/src/media/PDFs/EUCAST_files/AFST/Files/EUCAST_E_Def_7_3_1_Yeast_testing__definitive.pdf (accessed on 16 April 2019).
33. Grossman, N.T.; Pham, C.D.; Cleveland, A.A.; Lockhart, S.R. Molecular mechanisms of fluconazole resistance in *Candida parapsilosis* isolates from a U.S. surveillance system. *Antimicrob. Agents Chemother.* **2015**, *59*, 1030–1037. [CrossRef]
34. Ramage, G.; Vande Walle, K.; Wickes, B.L.; Lopez-Ribot, J.L. Standardized method for in vitro antifungal susceptibility testing of *Candida albicans* biofilms. *Antimicrob. Agents Chemother.* **2001**, *45*, 2475–2479. [CrossRef] [PubMed]
35. Arastehfar, A.; Daneshnia, F.; Hilmioglu-Polat, S.; Fang, W.; Yasar, M.; Polat, F.; Yesim Metin, D.; Rigole, P.; Coenye, T.; Ilkit, M.; et al. First report of candidemia clonal outbreak caused by emerging fluconazole-resistant *Candida parapsilosis* isolates harboring Y132F and/or Y132F+K143R in Turkey. *Antimicrob. Agents Chemother.* **2020**. [CrossRef] [PubMed]
36. Souza, A.C.; Fuchs, B.B.; Pinhati, H.M.; Siqueira, R.A.; Hagen, F.; Meis, J.F.; Mylonakis, E.; Colombo, A.L. *Candida parapsilosis* Resistance to Fluconazole: Molecular Mechanisms and *In Vivo* Impact in Infected *Galleria mellonella* Larvae. *Antimicrob. Agents Chemother.* **2015**, *59*, 6581–6587. [CrossRef] [PubMed]
37. Magobo, R.E.; Lockhart, S.R.; Govender, N.P. Fluconazole-resistant *Candida parapsilosis* strains with a Y132F substitution in the *ERG11* gene causing invasive infections in a neonatal unit, South Africa. *Mycoses* **2020**, *63*, 471–477. [CrossRef]
38. Van Asbeck, E.C.; Clemons, K.V.; Stevens, D.A. *Candida parapsilosis*: A review of its epidemiology, pathogenesis, clinical aspects, typing and antimicrobial susceptibility. *Crit. Rev. Microbiol.* **2009**, *35*, 283–309. [CrossRef]
39. Imbert, C.; Rammaert, B. What Could Be the Role of Antifungal Lock-Solutions? From Bench to Bedside. *Pathogens* **2018**, *7*, 6. [CrossRef]
40. Borges, K.R.A.; Pimentel, I.V.; Lucena, L.; Silva, M.; Monteiro, S.G.; Monteiro, C.A.; Nascimento, M.; Bezerra, G.F.B. Adhesion and biofilm formation of *Candida parapsilosis* isolated from vaginal secretions to copper intrauterine devices. *Rev. Inst. Med. Trop. Sao Paulo* **2018**, *60*, e59. [CrossRef]
41. Tan, Y.; Leonhard, M.; Ma, S.; Schneider-Stickler, B. Influence of culture conditions for clinically isolated non-albicans *Candida* biofilm formation. *J. Microbiol. Methods* **2016**, *130*, 123–128. [CrossRef]
42. Silva, S.; Negri, M.; Henriques, M.; Oliveira, R.; Williams, D.W.; Azeredo, J. *Candida glabrata*, *Candida parapsilosis* and *Candida tropicalis*: Biology, epidemiology, pathogenicity and antifungal resistance. *FEMS Microbiol. Rev.* **2012**, *36*, 288–305. [CrossRef] [PubMed]
43. Thomaz, D.Y.; de Almeida, J.N., Jr.; Lima, G.M.E.; Nunes, M.O.; Camargo, C.H.; Grenfell, R.C.; Benard, G.; Del Negro, G.M.B. An Azole-Resistant *Candida parapsilosis* Outbreak: Clonal Persistence in the Intensive Care Unit of a Brazilian Teaching Hospital. *Front. Microbiol.* **2018**, *9*, 2997. [CrossRef] [PubMed]
44. Melo, A.S.; Bizerra, F.C.; Freymuller, E.; Arthington-Skaggs, B.A.; Colombo, A.L. Biofilm production and evaluation of antifungal susceptibility amongst clinical *Candida* spp. isolates, including strains of the *Candida parapsilosis* complex. *Med. Mycol.* **2011**, *49*, 253–262. [CrossRef] [PubMed]
45. Espinel-Ingroff, A.; Barchiesi, F.; Cuenca-Estrella, M.; Pfaller, M.A.; Rinaldi, M.; Rodriguez-Tudela, J.L.; Verweij, P.E. International and multicenter comparison of EUCAST and CLSI M27-A2 broth microdilution methods for testing susceptibilities of *Candida* spp. to fluconazole, itraconazole, posaconazole, and voriconazole. *J. Clin. Microbiol.* **2005**, *43*, 3884–3889. [CrossRef] [PubMed]
46. Modiri, M.; Hashemi, S.J.; Ghazvin, I.R.; Khodavaisy, S.; Ahmadi, A.; Ghaffari, M.; Rezaie, S. Antifungal susceptibility pattern and biofilm-related genes expression in planktonic and biofilm cells of *Candida parapsilosis* species complex. *Curr. Med. Mycol.* **2019**, *5*, 35–42. [CrossRef]
47. Khodavaisy, S.; Badali, H.; Meis, J.F.; Modiri, M.; Mahmoudi, S.; Abtahi, H.; Salehi, M.; Dehghan Manshadi, S.A.; Aala, F.; Agha Kuchak Afshari, S.; et al. Comparative in vitro activities of seven antifungal drugs against clinical isolates of *Candida parapsilosis* complex. *J. Mycol. Med.* **2020**, *30*, 100968. [CrossRef]
48. Rodriguez-Tudela, J.L.; Gomez-Lopez, A.; Arendrup, M.C.; Garcia-Effron, G.; Perlin, D.S.; Lass-Florl, C.; Cuenca-Estrella, M. Comparison of caspofungin MICs by means of EUCAST method EDef 7.1 using two different concentrations of glucose. *Antimicrob. Agents Chemother.* **2010**, *54*, 3056–3057. [CrossRef]
49. Santos, F.; Leite-Andrade, M.C.; Brandao, I.S.; Alves, A.; Buonafina, M.D.S.; Nunes, M.; Araujo-Neto, L.N.; Freitas, M.A.; Brayner, F.A.; Alves, L.C.; et al. Anti-biofilm effect by the combined action of fluconazole and acetylsalicylic acid against species of *Candida parapsilosis* complex. *Infect. Genet. Evol.* **2020**, *84*, 104378. [CrossRef]
50. Pannanusorn, S.; Ramirez-Zavala, B.; Lunsdorf, H.; Agerberth, B.; Morschhauser, J.; Romling, U. Characterization of biofilm formation and the role of *BCR1* in clinical isolates of *Candida parapsilosis*. *Eukaryot. Cell* **2014**, *13*, 438–451. [CrossRef]
51. De Bernardis, F.; Mondello, F.; San Millan, R.; Ponton, J.; Cassone, A. Biotyping and virulence properties of skin isolates of *Candida parapsilosis*. *J. Clin. Microbiol.* **1999**, *37*, 3481–3486. [CrossRef]
52. Rupp, S.; Summers, E.; Lo, H.J.; Madhani, H.; Fink, G. MAP kinase and cAMP filamentation signaling pathways converge on the unusually large promoter of the yeast *FLO11* gene. *EMBO J.* **1999**, *18*, 1257–1269. [CrossRef] [PubMed]
53. Chakraborty, T.; Toth, Z.; Toth, R.; Vagvolgyi, C.; Gacser, A. Iron Metabolism, Pseudohypha Production, and Biofilm Formation through a Multicopper Oxidase in the Human-Pathogenic Fungus *Candida parapsilosis*. *mSphere* **2020**, *5*. [CrossRef] [PubMed]
54. Cassone, A.; De Bernardis, F.; Pontieri, E.; Carruba, G.; Girmenia, C.; Martino, P.; Fernandez-Rodriguez, M.; Quindos, G.; Ponton, J. Biotype diversity of *Candida parapsilosis* and its relationship to the clinical source and experimental pathogenicity. *J. Infect. Dis.* **1995**, *171*, 967–975. [CrossRef] [PubMed]

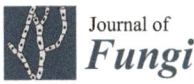

Article

The Membranotropic Peptide *gH625* to Combat Mixed *Candida albicans/Klebsiella pneumoniae* Biofilm: Correlation between In Vitro Anti-Biofilm Activity and In Vivo Antimicrobial Protection

Angela Maione [1], Elisabetta de Alteriis [1], Federica Carraturo [1], Stefania Galdiero [2], Annarita Falanga [3], Marco Guida [1], Anna Di Cosmo [1], Valeria Maselli [1,*] and Emilia Galdiero [1,*]

[1] Department of Biology, University of Naples Federico II, Via Cinthia 26, 80126 Naples, Italy; angela.maione@unina.it (A.M.); dealteri@unina.it (E.d.A.); federica.carraturo@unina.it (F.C.); marco.guida@unina.it (M.G.); dicosmo@unina.it (A.D.C.)

[2] Department of Pharmacy, School of Medicine, University of Naples Federico II, Via Domenico Montesano 49, 80131 Naples, Italy; sgaldier@unina.it

[3] Department of Agricultural Science, University of Naples Federico II, Via dell'Università 100, 80055 Portici, Naples, Italy; annarita.falanga@unina.it

* Correspondence: valeria.maselli@unina.it (V.M.); egaldieri@unina.it (E.G.)

Citation: Maione, A.; de Alteriis, E.; Carraturo, F.; Galdiero, S.; Falanga, A.; Guida, M.; Di Cosmo, A.; Maselli, V.; Galdiero, E. The Membranotropic Peptide *gH625* to Combat Mixed *Candida albicans*/*Klebsiella pneumoniae* Biofilm: Correlation between In Vitro Anti-Biofilm Activity and In Vivo Antimicrobial Protection. *J. Fungi* 2021, 7, 26. https://doi.org/10.3390/jof7010026

Received: 29 October 2020
Accepted: 31 December 2020
Published: 5 January 2021

Publisher's Note: MDPI stays neutral with regard to jurisdictional claims in published maps and institutional affiliations.

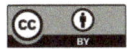

Copyright: © 2021 by the authors. Licensee MDPI, Basel, Switzerland. This article is an open access article distributed under the terms and conditions of the Creative Commons Attribution (CC BY) license (https://creativecommons.org/licenses/by/4.0/).

Abstract: The antibiofilm activity of a gH625 analogue was investigated to determine the in vitro inhibition and eradication of a dual-species biofilm of *Candida albicans* and *Klebsiella pneumoniae*, two leading opportunistic pathogens responsible for several resistant infections. The possibility of effectively exploiting this peptide as an alternative anti-biofilm strategy in vivo was assessed by the investigation of its efficacy on the *Galleria mellonella* larvae model. Results on larvae survival demonstrate a prophylactic efficacy of the peptide towards the infection of each single microorganism but mainly towards the co-infection. The expression of biofilm-related genes in vivo showed a possible synergy in virulence when these two species co-exist in the host, which was effectively prevented by the peptide. These findings provide novel insights into the treatment of medically relevant bacterial–fungal interaction.

Keywords: *Galleria mellonella*; polymicrobial biofilm; experimental method in vivo

1. Introduction

Microorganisms rarely exist as single-species planktonic forms, and the biofilm mode of growth is the most common lifestyle adopted. Biofilms can be defined as biotic and abiotic surface-associated, structured microorganism communities embedded in an extracellular polysaccharide matrix. Living in a biofilm provides protection in a stressful environment where mechanical stress, desiccation, and biocides are frequent threats.

Progress in biofilm research has highlighted that these communities are rarely composed of a single-species microorganism, but mainly exist as complex, diverse, and heterogeneous structures. In fact, multiple species (fungi, bacteria, and viruses) frequently exist together in complex polymicrobial biofilm communities attached to sites where they compete for space and nutrients [1–3]. Moreover, polymicrobial biofilms are likely to influence disease severity by promoting intensified pathogenic phenotypes, including increased resistance to both host defense and antimicrobial therapies. Despite their clinical significance, polymicrobial biofilm infections continue to be largely understudied [4].

Candida albicans and *Klebsiella pneumoniae* are important pathogens causing a wide variety of infections. They possess the ability to co-exist as complex polymicrobial biofilms within the human host [5]. *C. albicans* is the predominant fungus frequently present in hospital infections with significant morbidity and mortality rates; unfortunately, it is difficult to prevent, diagnose and treat. It is an opportunistic pathogen, which is a major cause of invasive fungal disease, principally in immunocompromised individuals, such as patients with organ transplantation and HIV infection or patients undergoing chemotherapy. The superficial mucosal and dermal infections caused by *C. albicans* can be disseminated to bloodstream infections with a mortality rate higher than 40% [6].

Klebsiella pneumoniae, the most common carbapenem-resistant member of the *Enterobacteriaceae* family, has emerged as an important opportunistic pathogen, mostly causing nosocomial infections associated with mortality rates up to 50% [7]. *K. pneumoniae* is responsible of infections both in human gastrointestinal tract and lung environments, and has a high propensity to form mono- and polymicrobial biofilms with consequent treatment difficulties [8].

Mixed biofilms of *Candida* with different bacteria, including *K. pneumoniae*, are present on implanted devices such as intravascular or urinary catheters, as well as in the oral environment [2].

Notwithstanding its clinical importance, information on mixed biofilms of *Candida/Klebsiella* is relatively scarce [9].

The potential use of antimicrobial peptides (AMPs) as a valid alternative to conventional antibiotics has been acknowledged and widely studied. In fact, their fast and strong antimicrobial activity, their antibiofilm action, and their reduced induction of resistance compared to conventional antibiotics make AMPs relevant compounds for controlling infections due to multi-drug resistant microorganisms embedded in a biofilm [10–12]. Among AMPs, there is a particularly relevant class of peptides, known as membranotropic peptides, which, apart from their eventual antimicrobial activity, present a high ability to disrupt the biofilm and thus may have an action both in the inhibition and in the eradication of the biofilm [13].

In this study, we evaluated the anti-biofilm activity of an analogue of the membranotropic peptide gH625, namely gH625-M, on a dual-species *C. albicans*/*K. pneumoniae* biofilm. Peptide gH625-M (HGLASTLTRWAHYNALIRAFGGGKKKK) is derived from gH625 (HGLASTLTRWAHYNALIRAF) and presents a C-terminal lysine sequence conjugated to the gH625 peptide by a glycine linker; the lysine functions to enhance the interaction with the negatively charged surfaces of bacterial biofilms and to enhance solubility. The glycine linker between the gH625 sequence and the lysine residues provides conformational flexibility to the peptide. gH625-M was shown to have activity on polymicrobial biofilms of *Candida tropicalis* and *Serratia marcescens* or *Staphylococcus aureus* [14] and on biofilms derived from *C. albicans* persister cells [15]. Therefore, the peptide was selected as a good candidate to evaluate the antibiofilm activity in vitro on a static biofilm of *C. albicans*/*K. pneumoniae*.

Since in vivo studies are crucial for the evaluation of the antimicrobial activities of new therapeutic agents and their modulatory effects on immune response, the larvae of the wax moth *G. mellonella* were used. In particular, *G. mellonella* is frequently exploited as an alternative to the murine model for studying microbial infections, because it is a simple, cheap and fast method, and implies fewer ethical concerns compared to the use of vertebrate models. As a matter of fact, several other studies have recently used *G. mellonella* to investigate the in vivo activity of antimicrobial agents against pathogenic microorganisms, including bacteria and fungi [16].

Here, we investigated for the first time, the correlation between the susceptibility profile shown by gH625-M in vitro and its antimicrobial efficacy in vivo. Therefore, the infection in the *G. mellonella* larva model was evaluated through the impact of gH625-M on the survival rate and on the immune response (galiomycin) of the larvae [17]. Furthermore, the expression of biofilm related genes of *C. albicans* (*HWP1*, *ALS3*) [18], and *K. pneumoniae* (*luxS*, *mrkA*) in *G. mellonella* larvae was investigated [19,20].

2. Materials and Methods

2.1. Peptide Synthesis

Peptide gH625-M (HGLASTLTRWAHYNALIRAFGGGKKKK) was synthetized by the Fmoc-solid-phase method [21]. Briefly, all amino acids were protected at their amino terminus with the Fmoc (9-fluorenylmethoxycarbonyl) group and coupled to the growing chain after activation of the carboxylic acid group. Consecutive cycles of amino deprotection (30% piperidine in dimethylformamide, for 10 min, twice) and coupling were performed to obtain the desired sequence. In particular, the first coupling was performed with four equivalents (equiv) of amino acid and four equiv DIC (Diisopropyl carbodiimide); while from the second coupling, we used four equiv amino acid, four equiv HATU (O-(7-azabenzotriazol-1-yl)-1,1,3,3-tetramethyluroniumhexafluorophosphate) and eight equiv DIPEA (diisopropylethylamine): the synthesis was performed using a rink amide resin MBHA (4-methyl-benzhydrylamine-resin, 0.44 mmol/g). Side chain deprotection and cleavage of the peptide from the resin was achieved using an acid solution (95% v/v of TFA, trifluoroacetic acid). The peptide was precipitated in cold ethylic ether and the crude peptide was analyzed by HPLC–MS using a gradient of acetonitrile (0.1% TFA) in water (0.1% TFA) from 20 to 80% in 15 min. The purified peptide was obtained with a good yield (approximatively 60%) and its identity was confirmed using a LTQ-XL Thermo Scientific linear ion trap mass spectrometer.

2.2. Microorganisms Culture and Biofilm Formation

Candida albicans ATCC 90028 and *Klebsiella pneumoniae* ATCC 10031 were selected as pathogen representative of fungus and Gram-negative bacteria forming biofilm in hospital environments. *C. albicans* ATCC 90028 was subcultured into Tryptone Soya Broth (TSB) (Oxoid) medium with 1% of glucose and propagated in Sabouraud dextrose agar (1% yeast extract, 1% peptone, 4% glucose, 1% agar) as described previously [14]. *K. pneumoniae* ATCC 10031 was grown in Tryptone Soya Broth (TSB and maintained in Tryptone Soya Agar (TSA) at $-80\ ^\circ$C.

Biofilm formation was carried out on microtiter plates, as previously described [14], with minor modifications. Briefly, for single species biofilms. *C. albicans* and *K. pneumoniae* suspensions were adjusted to 10^6 colony-forming units (CFU) mL^{-1} in fresh TSB with 0.1% glucose and TSB, respectively. In the case of the dual species biofilm, microorganism suspensions were mixed in TSB with 0.1% glucose (1:1). Aliquots (100 µL) of these suspensions (single or mixed) were added to the wells of sterile flat-bottom 96-well microtiter test plates to allow single or mixed biofilm formation and incubated for 24 or 48 h at 37 $^\circ$C. Then, the wells were washed with PBS in order to remove planktonic and sessile cells weakly attached to the surface. Quantification of biofilm biomass was carried out with crystal violet (CV) staining [22].

Experimental conditions were run in triplicate. Results are presented as mean values from at least four independent experiments.

2.3. Minimum Inhibition Concentration (MIC)

The concentration of the peptide that inhibited 80% microbial growth (MIC$_{80}$) was determined by the microdilution method according to Clinical Laboratory Standards Institute guidelines [23]. Briefly, 100 µL of TSB with 1% glucose and TSB containing strain of *C. albicans* or *K. pneumoniae*, respectively (1×10^6 CFU/mL), was introduced into each well of 96-well microplate with different concentrations of gH625-M (2.5 µM–50 µM) and incubated for 24 h at 37 $^\circ$C. The growth of each strain was measured at 590 nm wavelength with a plate reader (SYNERGY H4 BioTek).

2.4. Inhibition and Eradication Biofilm Assays

The inhibition activity of gH625-M on mono- and polymicrobial biofilm formation and the eradication activity against preformed biofilm were evaluated by using sub-MIC concentrations of the peptide ranging from 2.5 to 50 µM.

Briefly, for the inhibition assay, peptide was added together with the standardized inoculum in each well of a 96-well polystyrene microtiter plate and incubated at 37 °C for 24 h. Non-adherent microorganisms were removed by washing twice with 200 µL sterile PBS and adherent cells were fixed by incubation for 1 h at 60 °C and stained for 5 min at room temperature with 100 µL 1% crystal violet solution. Wells were then rinsed with distilled water and dried at 37 °C for 30 min. Biofilms were de-stained by treatment with 100 µL 33% glacial acetic acid for 15 min and OD_{570} measured.

The eradication activity of the peptide was evaluated exposing 24 h mono- and polymicrobial biofilms for additional 24 h to different sub-MIC concentrations of peptide and quantified the biomass by crystal violet assay as previously described. The percentages of inhibition or eradication were calculated as biofilm reduction % = OD_{570} control − OD_{570} sample/OD_{570} control × 100, where OD_{570} control and sample were the biomass formed in the absence and in the presence of the peptide, respectively. All tests were performed in triplicate in three independent experiments.

2.5. Galleria Mellonella Survival Assay

To determinate the in vivo effects of gH625-M, a *G. mellonella* survival assay was performed as described previously [24,25]. In brief, larvae of 250–300 mg each were used for each treatment (20 for each group). They were chosen to have clear color and a lack of spots and/or dark pigments on their cuticle. The experiments were performed in triplicate.

Larvae were cleaned by an alcohol swab prior to injection. Larvae were injected directly into the hemocoel with 10 µL *C. albicans* and/or *K. pneumoniae* suspensions prepared in PBS at a concentration of 1×10^6 CFU/larvae/pathogen (1×10^6 CFU/larvae total for co-infection), using a 50 µL microsyringe via the last left proleg. An aliquot of 10 µL of 50 µM gH625-M was delivered behind the last proleg on the opposite side of the pathogen injection site either 2 h pre-infection (for prevention experiments) or 2 h post-infection (for treatment experiments). One group of untreated larvae served as a blank control group (intact larvae), one group received 10 µL of PBS solution per leg and one group was injected with 10 µL of 50 µM gH625-M in one leg and 10 µL PBS in the other, in order to assess peptide toxicity.

Larvae were then incubated at 35 °C in plastic containers provided with a perforated lid and monitored daily for survival for 4 days. A larva was considered dead when it displayed no response to touch.

2.6. Fungal/Bacterial Burden

Larvae were inoculated with *C. albicans* or *K. pneumoniae* or co-infected with the two, at concentration of 1×10^6 CFU/larvae/pathogen or 1×10^6 CFU/larvae total for co-infection. The peptide was administered before or after infection/co-infection, as described in the previous paragraph. The infected models were incubated at 30 °C, and after 24 h of infection, two larvae were randomly selected and washed in 70% ethanol. Larvae were cut into small pieces using a sterile scalpel and added to falcon tubes containing 1 mL of PBS vortexed and 100 µL of each sample was collected and serially diluted. The dilutions were plated and incubated 48 h at 30 °C and colony forming units (CFU) of *C. albicans* and *K. pneumoniae* were counted on Sabouraud dextrose agar plus 20 µg mL^{-1} cloramphenicol and TSA plus 1 µg mL^{-1} caspofungin, respectively. The experiments were performed in triplicate.

2.7. RNA Extraction and Gene Expression Analysis

Larvae were infected, and RNA was extracted at 4 and 24 h post-treatment.

Therefore, three live larvae from each experimental group (4 and 24 h post-treatment) were snap-frozen in liquid nitrogen and ground to a powder by mortar and pestle in TRIzol (Invitrogen, Paisley, UK). The samples were further homogenized using a TissueLyser II (Qiagen, Valencia, CA, USA) and steal beads of 5 mm diameter (Qiagen, Valencia, CA, USA). RNA was extracted with RNeasy minikit (Qiagen, Valencia, CA, USA), following the manufacturer's protocol. The quality and amount of purified RNA were analyzed spectrophotometrically with Nanodrop2000 (Thermo Scientific Inc., Waltham, MA, USA). 1000 ng of RNA was reverse transcribed with the QuantiTect Reverse Transcription Kit (Qiagen, Valencia, CA, USA), used as described by the manufacturer. Afterwards, Real-Time PCR was performed using the QuantiTect SYBR Green PCR Kit (Qiagen, Valencia, CA, USA) in a final volume of 25 µL, with 100 ng of cDNA, 1 µM of each primer, 12.5 µL of QuantiFast SYBR Green PCR Master Mix (2×). PCR cycling profile consisted of a cycle at 95 °C for 5 min, 40 two-step cycles at 95 °C for 15 s, at 60 °C for 60 s. Quantitative RT-PCR analysis was conducted using the $2^{(-\Delta\Delta C(T))}$ method [26]. RT-PCR was performed in a Rotor-Gene Q cycler (Qiagen, Valencia, CA, USA). All primers used for quantitative PCR (qPCR) studies are shown in Table 1. At the end of each test, a melting curve analysis was done (plate read every 0.5 °C from 55 to 95 °C) to determine the formation of the specific products. Each sample was tested and run in duplicate. No-template controls were included.

Table 1. Primers used in this study.

Primer Name	Primer Sequence (5'-3')	Melting Temperature (°C)	Amplicon Length (bp)
G.mellonella_actin_F	GGACTTGTACGCCAACACAG	60	196
G.mellonella_actin_R	CCACATCTGCTGGAATGTCG	62	
G.mellonella_galiomycin_F	GGTGCGACGAATTACACCTC	62	101
G.mellonella_galiomycin_R	TCGCACCAACAATTGACGTT	55	
K.pneumoniae_16S_F	AGCACAGAGAGCTTG	54	126
K.pneumoniae_16S_R	ACTTTGGTCTTGCGAC	59	
K.pneumoniae_luxS_F	ATCGACATTTCGCCAATGGG	58	157
K.pneumoniae_luxS_R	ACTGGTAGACGTTGAGCTCC	66	
K.pneumoniae_mrkA_F	ACGTCTCTAACTGCCAGGC	64	115
K.pneumoniae_mrkA_R	TAGCCCTGTTGTTTGCTGGT	66	
C.albicans_actin_F	AGCCCAATCCAAAAGAGGTATT	62	153
C.albicans_actin_R	GCTTCGGTCAACAAAACTGG	63	
C.albicans_HWP1_F	CAGCCACTGAAACACCAACT	63	135
C.albicans_HWP1_R	CAGAAGTAACAACAACAACACCAG	63	
C.albicans_ALS3_F	CTAATGCTGCTACGTATAATT	56	201
C.albicans_ALS3_R	CCTGAAATTGACATGTAGCA	58	

mRNA levels in the different treatments were compared by ANCOVA (analysis of covariance). The control and the treatment groups in various assays were compared and analyzed using a Wilcoxon two group test and data with p-values < 0.05 were considered statistically significant [27].

Transcriptional activation is represented by the RNA fold change of the expression; for the *galiomycin* gene evaluation in *G. mellonella* actin was used as housekeeping gene, for the *luxS* and *mrkA* genes in *K. pneumoniae* 16S was used as housekeeping gene, and for *HWP1* and *ALS3* genes in *C. albicans* actin was used as housekeeping gene.

2.8. Scanning Electron Microscopy (SEM)

The 48 h polymicrobial biofilm was formed in multi-well plates as described above. The slides were prepared for scanning electron microscopy (SEM) using a previously published protocol [14]. Briefly, the slides were placed in 3% glutaraldehyde at 4 °C, then washed with PBS and post-fixed in 1% aqueous solution of osmium for 90 min at room temperature. Then, samples were dehydrated in a series of graded alcohols, dried to the critical drying point, and finally coated with gold. Specimens were evaluated with a scanning electron microscope (QUANTA 200 ESEM FEI Europe Company, Eindhoven, The Netherlands).

2.9. Statistical Analysis

Statistical analyses were performed using Microsoft® Excel 2016/XLSTAT©-Pro (version 7.2, Addinsoft, Inc., Brooklyn, NY, USA). Error bars in the graphs represent standard error of the mean (SEM and gene expression analysis) or standard deviations (SD, for biomass in mono- and polymicrobial biofilms, inhibition and eradication biofilm assay, CFU assay).

In the *G. mellonella* model of infection, the survival curves were plotted using Kaplan–Meier method and log-rank test. In all other assays, Tukey test was used to compare the means within the same set of experiments and ANOVA to consider the differences among the groups. A *p*-value of <0.05 was considered statistically significant.

3. Results

Both the examined strains were able to form single- and dual-species biofilm in vitro (Figure 1) under the experimental conditions adopted. In particular, the single biofilm production was weak for both species and moderate for dual species. The biomass of the dual species biofilm was even higher than the sum of the single species biofilm biomass, which likely indicated a synergism between the two species forming the biofilm. The analysis of the SEM images clearly showed the strict interconnection between the two species in the mixed biofilm (Figure 2). The co-existence of *C. albicans* and *K. pneumoniae* was clearly shown in the SEM image (Figure 2) and also confirmed by cell count: $4.1 \times 10^8 \pm 0.2$ (SD) and $4.6 \times 10^8 \pm 0.4$ (SD), respectively.

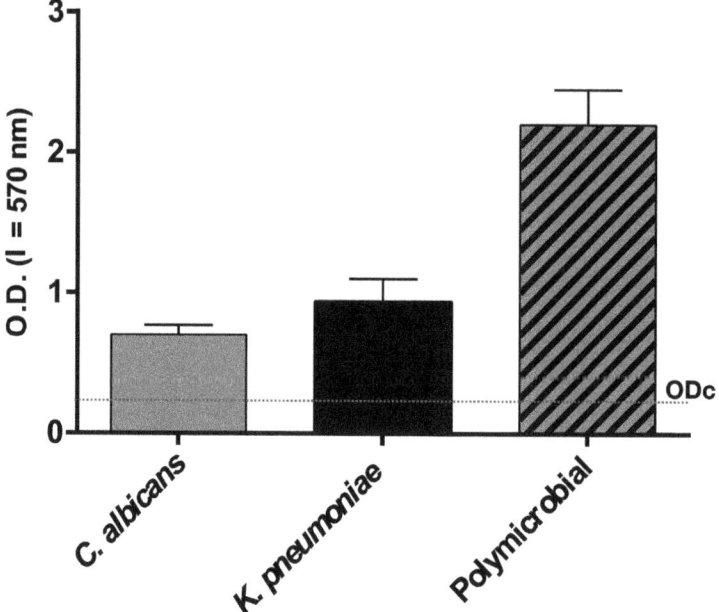

Figure 1. Biomass in mono- (*K. pneumoniae* and *C. albicans*) and polymicrobial biofilms ($n = 3$, mean ± SD) quantified by crystal violet staining and expressed as OD_{570}. The dotted line corresponds to ODc, that is the cut-off value, defined as three standard deviations above the mean OD of the negative control. Negative (OD ≤ ODc), weak (ODc ≤ OD ≤ 2 ODc), moderate (2 ODc < OD ≤ 4 ODc), and strong biofilm production (4 ODc < OD), according to Stepanovich [22].

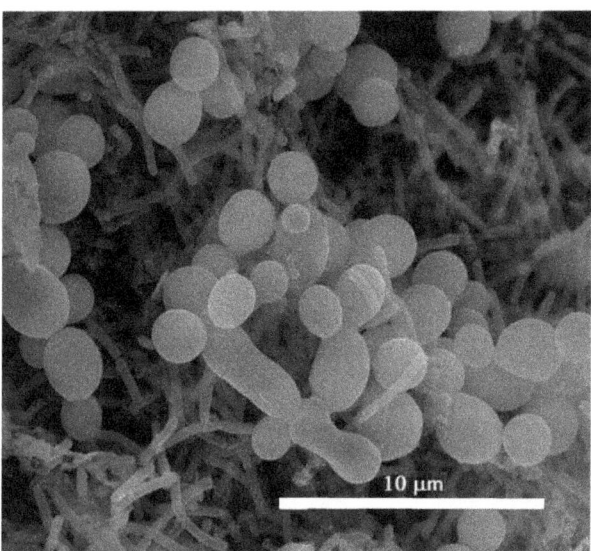

Figure 2. SEM observation of the 48 h dual species biofilm of *C. albicans* and *K. pneumoniae*. Scale bar = 10 μm.

The peptide gH625-M is an analogue of gH625, a peptide, which proved to be very effective in crossing membrane bilayers [15,28]. *In vitro*, gH625-M showed weak anticandidal activity with a MIC_{80} > 50 μM, which was in agreement with our previous studies [15]. Similarly, the MIC_{80} value of *K. pneumoniae* was higher than 50 μM, indicating a relatively scarce antibacterial activity of the peptide.

Interestingly, gH625-M was able to inhibit the formation of the biofilm, as well as to eradicate it (Figure 3A,B). After treatment with sub-MIC doses of gH625-M, the formation of mono- and polymicrobial biofilm was inhibited significantly (Figure 3A).

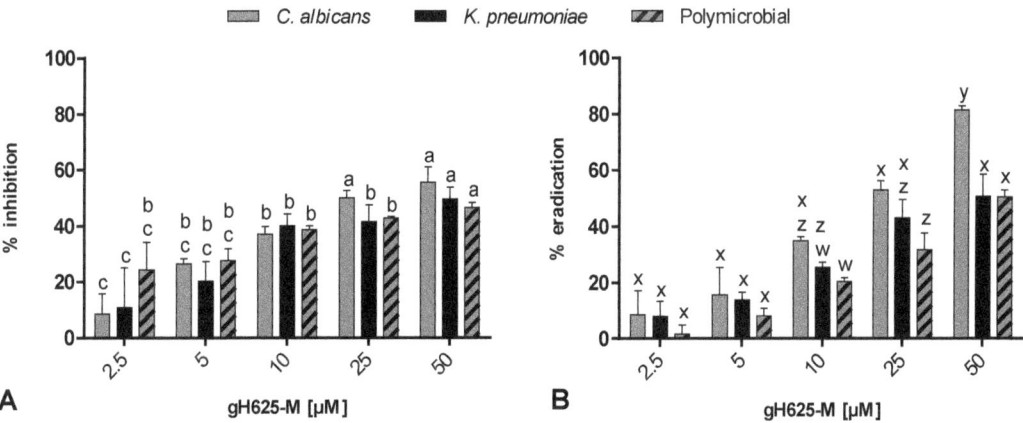

Figure 3. Action of increasing gH625-M concentrations on inhibition (**A**) and eradication (**B**) of mono- and polymicrobial biofilms. Quantification of the residual biofilm biomass was performed by crystal violet staining. Data with different letters (a–c; w–z) are significantly different (Tukey's, $p < 0.05$).

Figure 3B showed the eradication effect of gH625-M on preformed mono- and polymicrobial biofilm (48 h old). At 50 µM, gH625-M reduced the mono-preformed biofilms of *C. albicans* and *K. pneumoniae* of 80% and 50%, respectively, and the mixed biofilm of 50%.

The in vivo antimicrobial activity of gH625-M was evaluated using *G. mellonella* larvae infected with *C. albicans* and *K. pneumoniae* isolates alone or mixed as shown in Figure 4.

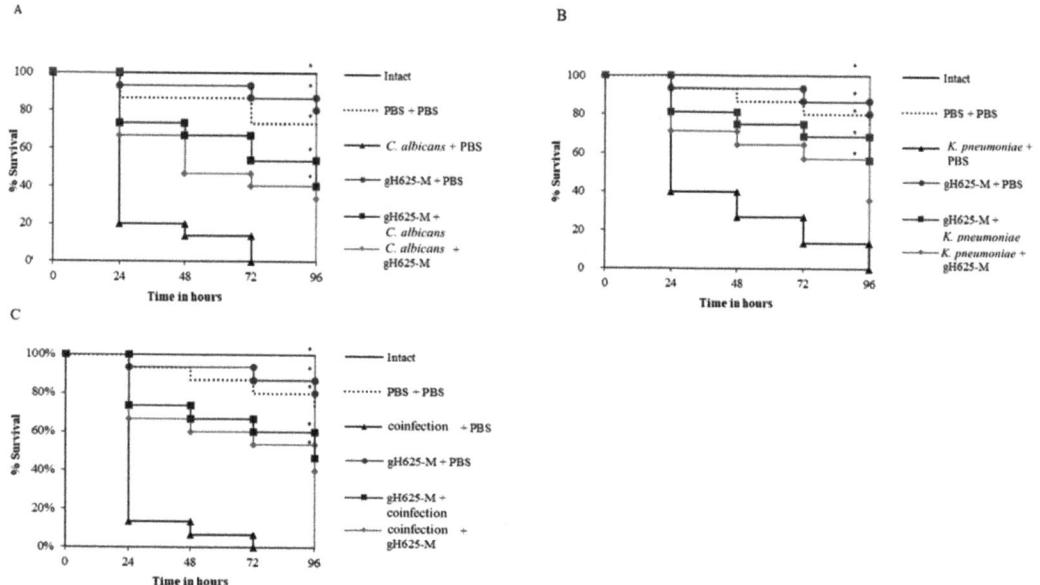

Figure 4. Kaplan–Meier plots of survival curves of *G. mellonella* larvae infected with *C. albicans* (**A**), *K. pneumoniae* (**B**), and co-infected with *C. albicans* + *K. pneumoniae* (**C**). In all panels, survival curves of larvae are shown. All groups were treated with 50 µM gH625-M before or after infection/co-infection are reported. All groups were compared with control (infected or co-infected larvae). In all panels, survival curves of intact larvae, larvae injected with PBS, larvae injected with gH625 alone are reported. * represents *p*-value < 0.001 (log-rank test).

Larval survival assay indicated that groups of larvae injected with PBS alone and gH625-M alone presented about 80% survival up to 96 h of observation with respect to intact larvae, indicating that gH625-M was not toxic for the larvae. Survival of larvae infected with *C. albicans* or *K. pneumoniae* (Figure 4A,B) was only 20% and 40% after 24 h, with 100% mortality observed after at 72 and 96 h, respectively.

To determine whether gH625-M had an effect in vivo, *G. mellonella* larvae were treated with gH625-M at 50 µM before or after the infection with each of the two species (Figure 4A,B) and before or after co-infection with the two (Figure 4C).

Both pre- and post-infection treatments showed significantly higher survival rates. In particular, the survival of larvae treated with gH625-M before infection with *C. albicans* was about 70%, and for *K. pneumoniae* was 80% after 24 h, preserving about 50% and 70% survival respectively at the end of the observation period. Moreover, the survival of the larvae treated with gH625-M after the infection with *C. albicans* or *K. pneumoniae* was significant, resulting in higher than 60% at 24 h, and 40% at 72 h of the experiment for both the microorganisms.

These results indicate that when gH625-M was administered before the infection, it was more effective compared to when administered after infection for both microorganisms. However, the increased survival rate of infected *Galleria* further confirms the significant activity of gH625-M.

In Figure 4C, survival of larvae co-infected with both *C. albicans* and *K. pneumoniae* is reported. Compared to single infection, mortality was enhanced, being 90% and 100% after 24 and 72 h. For co-infections, the administration of gH625-M greatly improved larvae survival both when given before and after the co-infection, with a slightly better prophylactic effect.

To detect the effect of gH625-M on the fungal and bacterial burden of infected larvae, a burden analysis was performed (Figure 5).

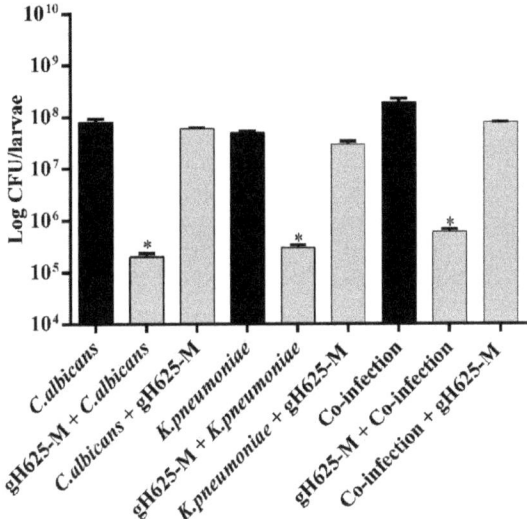

Figure 5. Effect pre- and post-treatment with gH625-M on bacterial/fungal burden in *G. mellonella* infected with *C. albicans* or *K. pneumoniae* and co-infected with *C. albicans* + *K. pneumoniae*. The peptide was administered before or after infection/co-infection. * indicates that the differences vs. larvae injected with microorganisms alone or together is statistically significant (*t*-test; $p < 0.05$). Error bars represent the SD.

There was a significant decrease in the microbial burden for the gH625-M pre-treated groups and only a slight decrease for the gH625-M post-treated groups. These results corroborated the protective action of gH625-M towards infection and co-infection, as already seen in the analysis of survival curves.

The expression of the galiomycin peptide-encoding gene is associated with the immune response of *G. mellonella*. Galiomycin is an antimicrobial peptide playing a major role in innate immunity, showing broad-spectrum microbicidal activity and specificity to *G. mellonella*. To evaluate the insect humoral response after infection with and co-infection each of the two microorganisms and co-infection, as well as the role of gH625-M on infection and co-infection we evaluated the expression of the *galiomycin* peptide-encoding gene.

Figure 6 reports expression levels of *galiomycin* gene in *G. mellonella* larvae after 4 and 24 h after infection with each species, after co-infection with the two species and after treatment with the peptide. Analysis by real-time quantitative PCR showed that the levels of galiomycin were higher in insects infected after 4 h with *C. albicans* alone ($p < 0.05$) and co-infected with *C. albicans* and with *K. pneumoniae* ($p < 0.05$) than those found in insects infected with *K. pneumoniae* alone. Instead, the expression levels of the same gene after 24 h from the infection did not significantly differ among the insects infected with both microorganisms. In this context, it could be reasonable to explore some other markers able to evidence the biofilm-associated damage in infected larvae, or lack thereof in gH625M-treated larvae.

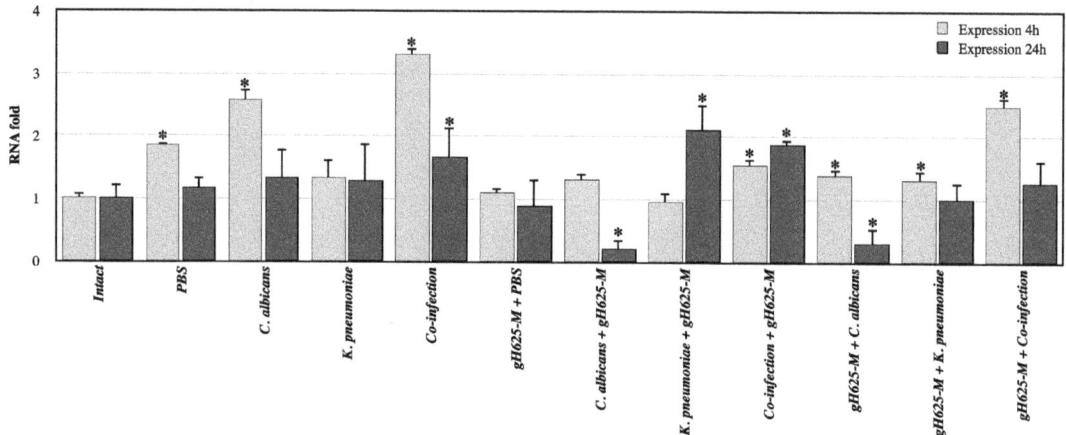

Figure 6. Relative mRNA expression levels of galiomycin gene in *G. mellonella* larvae infected with *C. albicans* and *K. pneumoniae* alone or together and pre-treated or post-treated with gH625-M, at 4 and 24 h, measured using real-time PCR analysis and calculated by the $2^{(-\Delta\Delta C(T))}$ method. Actin gene was used as housekeeping. Each sample was tested and run in duplicate. No-template controls were included. * asterisk indicates that the difference vs. intact larvae expression is statistically significant (Wilcoxon two group test, $p < 0.05$). Error bars represent the SEM.

Analysis of the expression of the selected genes revealed that the use of gH625-M before and after the infection, and the co-infection, significantly affects expression, decreasing the level of *galiomycin* compared to the corresponding intact and not treated samples. Data also show that the treatment with gH625-M produces an inhibition of galiomycin gene expression.

In Figure 7, levels of hyphal-specific and biofilm-related genes in *C. albicans* in the absence and presence of gH625-M at 24 h were quantified by real-time PCR. Hyphal specific gene, *HWP1* was downregulated in all cases showing hyphal structure formation failure. Biofilm-related gene *ALS3* was significantly downregulated in the presence of gH625-M 2 h after infection with *C. albicans* and in polymicrobial treated with gH625-M two hours before the infection. It was upregulated in larvae with only *C. albicans* infection pre-treated and in polymicrobial biofilm untreated or post-treated with gH625-M.

The relative expressions of *luxS* and *mrkA* genes were evaluated in *G. mellonella* infected with *K. pneumoniae* alone or in combination with *C. albicans* (Figure 8). The *luxS* gene encodes the AI-2 proteins of quorum sensing that play an important role in biofilm formation in Gram-negative bacteria such as *K. pneumoniae*, while *mrkA* gene (type 3 fimbriae) is a virulence-related gene detected in *K. pneumoniae*; both have critical roles in biofilm formation and antibiotic resistance.

It is interesting to observe that in co-infections, when the peptide was administered before, both *mrkA* and *luxS* genes were significantly down-regulated compared to untreated co-infections. The effect of pre-treatment was also observed in the case of *K. pneumoniae* infection. In contrast, both *mrkA* and *luxS* genes were upregulated when gH625-M was administered after infection and co-infection.

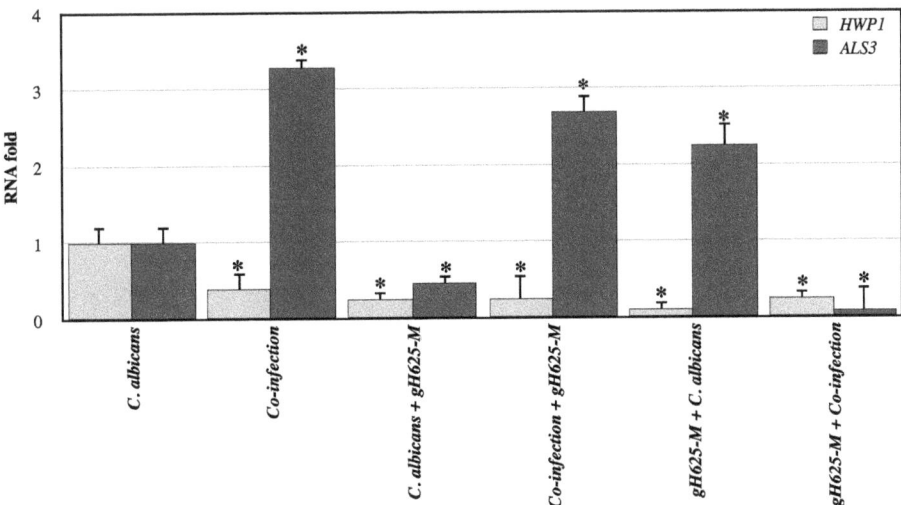

Figure 7. Relative mRNA expression levels of *C. albicans* virulence genes (*HWP1* and *ALS3*) in *G. mellonella* larvae at 24 h, measured using real-time PCR analysis and calculated by the $2^{(-\Delta\Delta C(T))}$ method. Actin gene was used as housekeeping. Each sample was tested and run in duplicate. No-template controls were included. * asterisk indicates that the difference vs. expression of larvae treated with *C. albicans* only is statistically significant (Wilcoxon two group test, $p < 0.05$). Error bars represent the SEM.

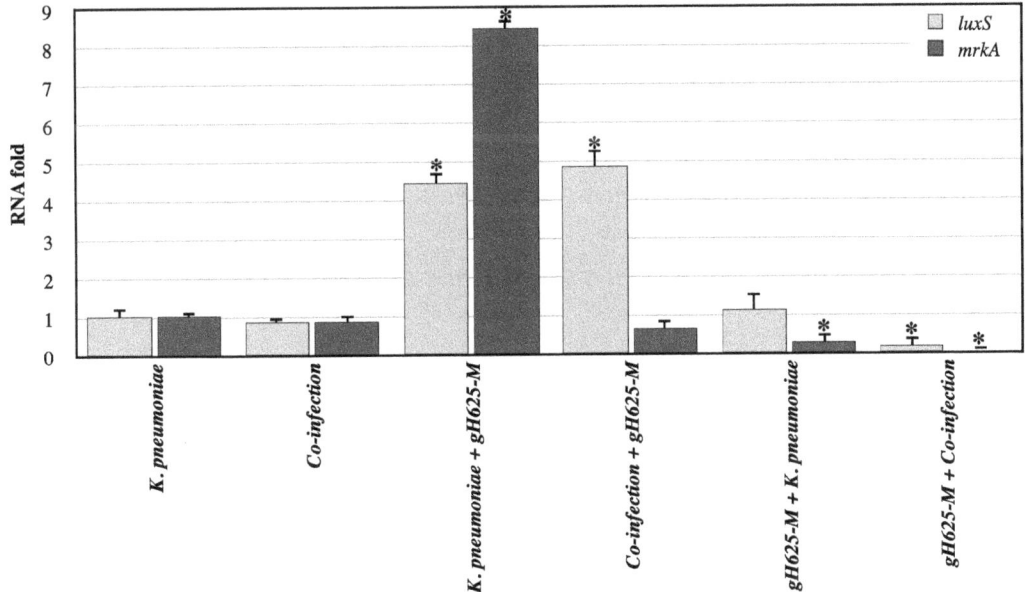

Figure 8. Relative mRNA expression levels of *K. pneumoniae* virulence genes (*luxS* and *mrkA*) in *G. mellonella* larvae at 24 h, measured using real-time PCR analysis and calculated by the $2^{(-\Delta\Delta C(T))}$ method. 16S gene was used as housekeeping. Each sample was tested and run in duplicate. No-template controls were included. * asterisk indicates that the difference vs. expression of larvae treated with *K. pneumoniae* only is statistically significant (Wilcoxon two group test $p < 0.05$). Error bars represent the SEM.

4. Discussion

Infections associated with polymicrobial fungal/bacterial biofilms represent a huge challenge due to intrinsic heterogeneity of these consortia, the low susceptibility to traditional drugs, as well as the high toxicity of many common antifungals. In this context, the development of novel strategies to combat polymicrobial biofilms of pathogen species is of great relevance.

In this paper, we focused our attention on the dual-species biofilms formed by *C. albicans* and *K. pneumoniae*, with *C. albicans* being the most common fungal opportunistic pathogen and *K. pneumoniae* being recognized in the group of 'ESKAPE' (*Enterococcus faecium, Staphylococcus aureus, Klebsiella pneumoniae, Acinetobacter baumannii, Pseudomonas aeruginosa, Enterobacter* spp.) pathogens, which 'escape' from the action of several antibiotics [29].

Previous work has demonstrated that the membranotropic peptide gH625-M was very effective against *C. albicans* biofilm, also when the biofilm was developed from persister cells [15]. In the present paper, we explored the efficacy of the peptide towards the dual-species *Candida/Klebsiella* biofilm, showing its ability of both inhibiting and eradicating in vitro the biofilm at sub-MIC concentrations. The low antimicrobial activity of the peptide used in this work towards *C. albicans* and *K. pneumoniae* was very low and was similar to that of other previously tested membranotropic peptides [14,15]; nevertheless, these characteristics may represent an advantageous property in the prevention of the possible development of resistances in the entire microbial consortium, a feature typical of several compounds proposed as anti-biofilms molecules [11]. The mechanism of action of gH625-M against *C. albicans* monospecies biofilm, as shown by a CSLM analysis previously reported [15], is initially directed towards the esopolymeric matrix of the biofilm and then penetrates across cell membranes, producing a local and temporary destabilization of membranes, which nonetheless has scarce effects on cell viability. The results obtained in the present paper, with the scarce antimicrobial activity (MIC values > 50 uM) exhibited in the case of both fungal (*Candida*) and bacterial (*Klebsiella*) cells, further support the hypothesis that the de-structuring property is presumably at the basis of the inhibiting and eradicating efficacy of the peptide also in the case of the *Candida/Klebsiella* biofilm. Interestingly, the dual-species biofilm is characterized by a strict interconnection established between the two species, thus the ability to disrupt the structure of the biofilm is of even greater relevance.

Candida/Klebsiella biofilm-associated infections have been reported in mammalian hosts; nonetheless, the description of the interactions between *Candida* spp. and *K. pneumoniae* in mixed biofilms has been limited to few observations, derived from in vitro models [9]. Our results show an increase in the total biomass of the polymicrobial biofilm in vitro compared to the sum of the single species biofilm, suggesting a possible synergy between the two species.

In vivo studies are crucial for the evaluation of the efficacy of new therapeutic agents and their modulatory effects on the host immune response, which makes it necessary to evaluate outcomes in animal models. In this study, we used the larvae of the wax moth *G. mellonella* as an in vivo model, for its well-known advantages as an alternative to vertebrate models. Although *G. mellonella* does not replace the vertebrate model, it can be exploited as a screening step between in vitro and in vivo evaluations [16].

One of the main outcomes was derived from the analysis of the survival curves after fungal/bacterial infection in the larvae [30]. Our results clearly show that the killing of *G. mellonella* larvae by infection of the two pathogens together is greater than the sum of killing with each pathogen alone; this pattern suggests a synergistic pathogen–pathogen interaction or a change in host–pathogen interactions that is characterized by increased host susceptibility to one or both of the pathogens.

The analysis of the survival curves in experiments with gH625-M, showed that the peptide functions in vivo both as a prophylactic and therapeutic agent towards both single infections and co-infections, with a higher efficacy in prophylaxis as revealed also with the fungal burden analysis.

The actual interaction established in vivo between the two species examined and the host, as well as the action of the peptide, was further investigated in the larvae model through the analysis of the transcriptional profiles of both biofilm-associated genes and gene associated with the larvae innate immune response. Following infection, the expression of the biofilm-associated genes of the two species examined was enhanced in the larvae, suggesting the occurrence of a biofilm-like interaction in the animal, which was concomitant to the overexpression of the *galiomycin* gene indicating an activation of the larvae immune response, as expected. The reduction in the expression of the *galiomycin* gene following administration of the peptide seems to suggest that gH625-M could have an anti-inflammatory effect which may result in the protection of the infected larvae.

Interestingly, gH625-M treatment before the infection, significantly reduced the biofilm-associated gene expression of *HWP1* and *ALS3* particularly in co-culture, supporting the efficacy of the peptide already observed in vitro. It was previously reported that *HWP1* mutants produce a thin biofilm with less hyphae in vitro, but display serious biofilm defects in vivo, only forming yeast microcolonies, while *ALS3* mutants are able to form hyphae, but exhibit defects in biofilm formation [31,32]. Thus, the observed down-regulation of hyphal specific gene, *HWP1*, could determine a loss of physical scaffolds for yeast cell adhesion and aggregation, producing a decreased biofilm strength, integrity, and maturation. The results obtained confirm previous hypothesis on the ability of gH625-M in regulating the initial adhesion of yeast cells to surfaces, which is essential for all stages of biofilm development.

For *K. pneumoniae*, too, genes involved in biofilm formation and virulence indicated that only the pre-treatment with gH625-M before infection has a significant effect in decreasing gene activity, confirming that this peptide was able to reduce infection and biofilm formation. However, future experiments relative to differential gene expression after 4 h and 12 h, when % of viability is higher than 50%, could clarify the action of these genes involved in *G. mellonella* immune response and biofilm formation in *C. albicans* and *K. pneumoniae*.

The results obtained in this study confirm the importance of developing new strategies for dealing with polymicrobial biofilms and we foresee a novel role for membranotropic peptides such as gH625 for the inhibition of biofilm formation thanks to their physico-chemical properties. It is likely that conformational flexibility and ability to destabilize hydrophobic domains typically present in membrane bilayers makes them able to disrupt the structure of the biofilm (eradication) or interfere with biofilm formation (inhibition). In conclusion, membranotropic peptides represent an appealing strategy to further evaluate for the development of innovative therapies meant to address problems such as biofilm inhibition/eradication and resistance.

Author Contributions: Conceptualization, E.d.A. and E.G.; Data curation, A.F.; Formal analysis, V.M.; Funding acquisition, M.G.; Investigation, A.M.; Project administration, F.C.; Resources, M.G.; Software, A.M.; Supervision, S.G.; Validation, E.d.A. and A.D.C.; Visualization, E.G.; Writing—original draft, V.M.; Writing—review & editing, S.G. and E.G., All authors have read and agreed to the published version of the manuscript.

Funding: This research received no external funding.

Institutional Review Board Statement: Ethical review and approval were not required for this animal species.

Informed Consent Statement: Not applicable.

Data Availability Statement: The data presented in this study are available on request from the corresponding author.

Conflicts of Interest: The authors declare no conflict of interest.

References

1. Lobo, C.I.V.; Rinaldi, T.B.; Christiano, C.M.S.; De Sales Leite, L.; Barbugli, P.A.; Klein, M.I. Dual-species biofilms of *Streptococcus mutans* and *Candida albicans* exhibit more biomass and are mutually beneficial compared with single-species biofilms. *J. Oral Microbiol.* **2019**, *11*, 1581520. [CrossRef]
2. Rodrigues, M.E.; Gomes, F.; Rodrigues, C.F. *Candida* spp./Bacteria Mixed Biofilms. *J. Fungi* **2019**, *6*, 5. [CrossRef]
3. Lohse, M.B.; Gulati, M.; Johnson, A.D.; Nobile, C.J. Development and regulation of single- and multi-species *Candida albicans* biofilms. *Nat. Rev. Microbiol.* **2018**, *16*, 19–31. [CrossRef] [PubMed]
4. Bhardwaj, R.G.; Ellepolla, A.; Drobiova, H.; Karched, M. Biofilm growth and IL-8 & TNF-α-inducing properties of *Candida albicans* in the presence of oral gram-positive and gram-negative bacteria. *BMC Microbiol.* **2020**, *20*, 156. [CrossRef]
5. Welp, A.L.; Bomberger, J.M. Bacterial Community Interactions During Chronic Respiratory Disease. *Front. Cell Infect. Microbiol.* **2020**, *10*, 213. [CrossRef] [PubMed]
6. Zhang, C.; Xue, Z.; Yu, Z.; Wang, H.; Liu, Y.; Li, H.; Wang, L.; Li, C.; Song, L. A tandem-repeat galectin-1 from *Apostichopus japonicus* with broad PAMP recognition pattern and antibacterial activity. *Fish Shellfish. Immunol.* **2020**, *99*, 167–175. [CrossRef] [PubMed]
7. Effah, C.Y.; Sun, T.; Liu, S.; Wu, Y. *Klebsiella pneumoniae*: An increasing threat to public health. *Ann. Clin. Microbiol. Antimicrob.* **2020**, *19*, 1. [CrossRef] [PubMed]
8. Lagrafeuille, R.; Miquel, S.; Balestrino, D.; Vareille-Delarbre, M.; Chain, F.; Langella, P.; Forestier, C. Opposing effect of Lactobacillus on in vitro *Klebsiella pneumoniae* in biofilm and in an in vivo intestinal colonisation model. *Benef. Microbes* **2018**, *9*, 87–100. [CrossRef]
9. Fox, E.P.; Cowley, E.S.; Nobile, C.J.; Hartooni, N.; Newman, D.K.; Johnson, A.D. Anaerobic bacteria grow within *Candida albicans* biofilms and induce biofilm formation in suspension cultures. *Curr. Biol.* **2014**, *24*, 2411–2416. [CrossRef]
10. Magana, M.; Pushpanathan, M.; Santos, A.L.; Leanse, L.; Fernandez, M.; Ioannidis, A.; Giulianotti, M.A.; Apidianakis, Y.; Bradfute, S.; Ferguson, A.L.; et al. The value of antimicrobial peptides in the age of resistance. *Lancet Infect. Dis.* **2020**, *20*, e216–e230. [CrossRef]
11. Kovács, R.; Majoros, L. Fungal Quorum-Sensing Molecules: A Review of Their Antifungal Effect against *Candida* Biofilms. *J. Fungi* **2020**, *6*, 99. [CrossRef] [PubMed]
12. Batoni, G.; Maisetta, G.; Esin, S. Antimicrobial peptides and their interaction with biofilms of medically relevant bacteria. *Biochim. Biophys. Acta* **2016**, *1858*, 1044–1060. [CrossRef] [PubMed]
13. Falanga, A.; Galdiero, M.; Galdiero, S. Membranotropic Cell Penetrating Peptides: The Outstanding Journey. *Int. J. Mol. Sci.* **2015**, *16*, 25323–25337. [CrossRef] [PubMed]
14. de Alteriis, E.; Lombardi, L.; Falanga, A.; Napolano, M.; Galdiero, S.; Siciliano, A.; Carotenuto, R.; Guida, M.; Galdiero, E. Polymicrobial antibiofilm activity of the membranotropic peptide gH625 and its analogue. *Microb. Pathog.* **2018**, *125*, 189–195. [CrossRef] [PubMed]
15. Galdiero, E.; de Alteriis, E.; De Natale, A.; D'Alterio, A.; Siciliano, A.; Guida, M.; Lombardi, L.; Falanga, A.; Galdiero, S. Eradication of *Candida albicans* persister cell biofilm by the membranotropic peptide gH625. *Sci. Rep.* **2020**, *10*, 5780. [CrossRef]
16. Campos-Silva, R.; Brust, F.R.; Trentin, D.S.; Macedo, A.J. Alternative method in *Galleria mellonella* larvae to study biofilm infection and treatment. *Microb. Pathog.* **2019**, *137*, 103756. [CrossRef]
17. Rossoni, R.D.; Fuchs, B.B.; de Barros, P.P.; Velloso, M.D.; Jorge, A.O.; Junqueira, J.C.; Mylonakis, E. *Lactobacillus paracasei* modulates the immune system of *Galleria mellonella* and protects against *Candida albicans* infection. *PLoS ONE* **2017**, *12*, e0173332. [CrossRef]
18. Priya, A.; Pandian, S.K. Piperine Impedes Biofilm Formation and Hyphal Morphogenesis of *Candida albicans*. *Front. Microbiol.* **2020**, *11*, 756. [CrossRef]
19. Chen, L.; Wilksch, J.J.; Liu, H.; Zhang, X.; Torres, V.V.L.; Bi, W.; Mandela, E.; Cao, J.; Li, J.; Lithgow, T.; et al. Investigation of LuxS-mediated quorum sensing in *Klebsiella pneumoniae*. *J. Med. Microbiol.* **2020**, *69*, 402–413. [CrossRef]
20. Wang, Y.M.; Dong, W.L.; Odah, K.A.; Kong, L.C.; Ma, H.X. Transcriptome Analysis Reveals AI-2 Relevant Genes of Multi-Drug Resistant *Klebsiella pneumoniae* in Response to Eugenol at Sub-MIC. *Front. Microbiol.* **2019**, *10*, 1159. [CrossRef]
21. Galdiero, S.; Capasso, D.; Vitiello, M.; D'Isanto, M.; Pedone, C.; Galdiero, M. Role of surface-exposed loops of *Haemophilus influenzae* protein P2 in the mitogen-activated protein kinase cascade. *Infect. Immun.* **2003**, *71*, 2798–2809. [CrossRef] [PubMed]
22. Stepanović, S.; Vuković, D.; Hola, V.; Di Bonaventura, G.; Djukić, S.; Cirković, I.; Ruzicka, F. Quantification of biofilm in microtiter plates: Overview of testing conditions and practical recommendations for assessment of biofilm production by staphylococci. *APMIS* **2007**, *115*, 891–899. [CrossRef]
23. CLSI. *Methods for Dilution Antimicrobial Susceptibility Tests for Bacteria That Grow Aerobically*; Approved Standards; Clinical and Laboratory Standards Institute: Wayne, PA, USA, 2006; p. 6.
24. Gu, W.; Yu, Q.; Yu, C.; Sun, S. In vivo activity of fluconazole/tetracycline combinations in *Galleria mellonella* with resistant *Candida albicans* infection. *J. Glob. Antimicrob. Resist.* **2018**, *13*, 74–80. [CrossRef] [PubMed]
25. Gu, W.; Guo, D.; Zhang, L.; Xu, D.; Sun, S. The Synergistic Effect of Azoles and Fluoxetine against Resistant *Candida albicans* Strains Is Attributed to Attenuating Fungal Virulence. *Antimicrob. Agents Chemother.* **2016**, *60*, 6179–6188. [CrossRef] [PubMed]
26. Livak, K.J.; Schmittgen, T.D. Analysis of Relative Gene Expression Data Using Real-Time Quantitative PCR and the 2-ΔΔCT Method. *Methods* **2001**, *25*, 402–408. [CrossRef] [PubMed]
27. Yuan, J.S.; Reed, A.; Chen, F.; Stewart, C.N. Statistical analysis of real-time PCR data. *BMC Bioinform.* **2006**, *7*, 85. [CrossRef]

28. Falanga, A.; Valiante, S.; Galdiero, E.; Franci, G.; Scudiero, O.; Morelli, G.; Galdiero, S. Dimerization in tailoring uptake efficacy of the HSV-1 derived membranotropic peptide gH625. *Sci. Rep.* **2017**, *7*, 9434. [CrossRef] [PubMed]
29. Ribeiro, S.M.; Cardoso, M.H.; Cândido Ede, S.; Franco, O.L. Understanding, preventing and eradicating *Klebsiella pneumoniae* biofilms. *Future Microbiol.* **2016**, *11*, 527–538. [CrossRef]
30. Peleg, A.Y.; Hogan, D.A.; Mylonakis, E. Medically important bacterial-fungal interactions. *Nat. Rev. Microbiol.* **2010**, *8*, 340–349. [CrossRef]
31. Nobile, C.J.; Andes, D.R.; Nett, J.E.; Smith, F.J.; Yue, F.; Phan, Q.T.; Edwards, J.E.; Filler, S.G.; Mitchell, A.P. Critical role of Bcr1-dependent adhesins in *C. albicans* biofilm formation in vitro and in vivo. *PLoS Pathog.* **2006**, *2*, e63. [CrossRef]
32. Nobile, C.J.; Mitchell, A.P. Genetics and genomics of *Candida albicans* biofilm formation. *Cell. Microbiol.* **2006**, *8*, 1382–1391. [CrossRef] [PubMed]

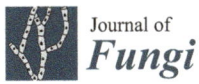

Article

A Screen for Small Molecules to Target *Candida albicans* Biofilms

Matthew B. Lohse [1,2], Craig L. Ennis [3,4], Nairi Hartooni [1,†], Alexander D. Johnson [1,5,*] and Clarissa J. Nobile [4,6,*]

1. Department of Microbiology and Immunology, University of California—San Francisco, San Francisco, CA 94158, USA; matthew.lohse@ucsf.edu (M.B.L.); Nairi.Hartooni@ucsf.edu (N.H.)
2. Department of Biology, BioSynesis, Inc., San Francisco, CA 94114, USA
3. Quantitative and Systems Biology Graduate Program, University of California—Merced, Merced, CA 95343, USA; cennis@ucmerced.edu
4. Department of Molecular and Cell Biology, School of Natural Sciences, University of California—Merced, Merced, CA 95343, USA
5. Department of Biochemistry and Biophysics, University of California—San Francisco, San Francisco, CA 94158, USA
6. Health Sciences Research Institute, University of California—Merced, Merced, CA 95343, USA
* Correspondence: ajohnson@cgl.ucsf.edu (A.D.J.); cnobile@ucmerced.edu (C.J.N.)
† Current Address: Tetrad Graduate Program, University of California—San Francisco, San Francisco, CA 94158, USA.

Abstract: The human fungal pathogen *Candida albicans* can form biofilms on biotic and abiotic surfaces, which are inherently resistant to antifungal drugs. We screened the Chembridge Small Molecule Diversity library containing 30,000 "drug-like" small molecules and identified 45 compounds that inhibited biofilm formation. These 45 compounds were then tested for their abilities to disrupt mature biofilms and for combinatorial interactions with fluconazole, amphotericin B, and caspofungin, the three antifungal drugs most commonly prescribed to treat *Candida* infections. In the end, we identified one compound that moderately disrupted biofilm formation on its own and four compounds that moderately inhibited biofilm formation and/or moderately disrupted mature biofilms only in combination with either caspofungin or fluconazole. No combinatorial interactions were observed between the compounds and amphotericin B. As members of a diversity library, the identified compounds contain "drug-like" chemical backbones, thus even seemingly "weak hits" could represent promising chemical starting points for the development and the optimization of new classes of therapeutics designed to target *Candida* biofilms.

Keywords: high-throughput screens; biofilms; biofilm inhibition; biofilm disruption; *Candida albicans*; antimicrobial resistance; therapeutics; Chembridge Small Molecule Diversity library

Citation: Lohse, M.B.; Ennis, C.L.; Hartooni, N.; Johnson, A.D.; Nobile, C.J. A Screen for Small Molecules to Target *Candida albicans* Biofilms. *J. Fungi* 2021, 7, 9. https://dx.doi.org/10.3390/jof7010009

Received: 30 October 2020
Accepted: 23 December 2020
Published: 27 December 2020

Publisher's Note: MDPI stays neutral with regard to jurisdictional claims in published maps and institutional affiliations.

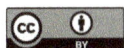

Copyright: © 2020 by the authors. Licensee MDPI, Basel, Switzerland. This article is an open access article distributed under the terms and conditions of the Creative Commons Attribution (CC BY) license (https://creativecommons.org/licenses/by/4.0/).

1. Introduction

Candida albicans is a normal commensal of the human microbiota that asymptomatically colonizes the skin, the mouth, and the gastrointestinal tract of healthy humans [1–4]. *C. albicans* is also one of the most common fungal pathogens of humans, typically causing superficial mucosal infections in healthy individuals [1,5–11]. When a host's immune system is compromised (e.g., in patients with AIDS), *C. albicans* can give rise to disseminated bloodstream infections with mortality rates exceeding 40% [1,12–15].

A notable virulence trait of *C. albicans* is its ability to form biofilms, multilayered, structured communities of cells that can grow on biotic and abiotic surfaces, such as mucosal surfaces and implanted medical devices (e.g., catheters, dentures, and heart valves) [1,2,10,16–21]. These biofilms are often resistant to antifungal drugs at concentrations that are normally effective against planktonic (free-floating) cells [20–25]. The drug-resistant nature of *C. albicans* biofilms frequently makes removal of biofilm-infected medical devices the only effective option to mitigate a biofilm-based infection, which can be especially problematic if patients are already critically ill or when device removal requires surgical procedures (e.g., heart valve or prosthetic replacement) [20,26,27]. Since there are no biofilm-specific therapeutics available on the market today and only three major classes of antifungal drugs used to treat fungal infections in humans, the development of new therapeutics effective against *C. albicans* biofilms is an important and unmet medical need.

The search for new antibiofilm therapeutics has encompassed a wide range of approaches, many of which focus on compounds that have combinatorial effects with known antifungal drugs rather than (or in addition to) compounds that affect *Candida* biofilms by themselves [28–43]. One approach has focused on screening libraries of existing drugs and/or pharmacologically active compounds that would make promising candidates for repurposing [38–40,43,44]. A second approach has focused on targeted classes of compounds (e.g., compounds with known effects on signaling pathways [28,29], compounds with known effects on cell–cell communication [34], and secreted aspartyl protease inhibitors [42]) that influence specific aspects of *Candida* biology. In addition, compounds that might affect *Candida* that are produced by other organisms (e.g., antimicrobial peptides [35] and chemicals produced by plants [36,37]) are also included in this targeted approach. A third approach has focused on screening large, chemically diverse compound libraries to identify pharmacophores that inhibit and/or disrupt biofilms through novel mechanisms [41,45]. Examples of this third approach taken to identify compounds with effects against *C. albicans* biofilms include a screen of a 20,000 compound Chembridge NOVACore library [45] and a screen of a 120,000 compound National Institutes of Health Molecular Libraries Small Molecule Repository library [41]. Here, we report a screen of a 30,000 compound Chembridge Small Molecule Diversity library (a library which, we note, has few compounds that overlap with the NOVACore library from the same commercial vendor) for the ability of the compounds to inhibit biofilm formation and/or disrupt mature biofilms by themselves or in combination with the known antifungal drugs fluconazole, amphotericin B, and caspofungin.

2. Materials and Methods

2.1. Media and Strains

Media were prepared in accordance with previously reported biofilm protocols [46,47]. Yeast extract peptone dextrose (YEPD) liquid media contains 2% Bacto^{TM} peptone (Difco #211677 (Becton, Dickinson and Company, Franklin Lakes, NJ, USA)), 2% dextrose, and 1% yeast extract (Difco #212750 (Becton, Dickinson and Company, Franklin Lakes, NJ, USA)). YEPD plates also contain 2% agar. Biofilm assays were performed in Roswell Park Memorial Institute (RPMI)-1640 media (containing L-glutamine and lacking sodium biocarbonate, MP Biomedicals #0910601 (MP Biomedicals, Santa Ana, CA, USA)) supplemented with 34.5 g/L 3-(*N*-morpholino)propanesulfonic acid (MOPS) (Sigma #M3183 (Sigma Aldrich, St. Louis, MO, USA)) and adjusted to pH 7.0 with sodium hydroxide before sterilizing using a 0.22 µm filter. All biofilm assays used the previously reported SC5314-derived strain SN425, a commonly used prototrophic **a**/α *C. albicans* standard strain, which was created by introducing *HIS1*, *LEU2*, and *ARG4* markers back into the SN152 **a**/α *his1 leu2 arg4* strain [48]. Cells were recovered from glycerol stocks for two days at 30 °C on yeast extract peptone dextrose (YEPD) plates. Overnight cultures for assays were grown approximately 16 h at 30 °C in YEPD media.

2.2. Reagents

The Chembridge Small Molecule Diversity library, which consists of 30,000 "drug-like" compounds, including diverse and target-directed compounds, was obtained by the University of California – San Francisco's (UCSF's) Small Molecule Discovery Center (SMDC) from commercial vendors and proprietary sources. Stocks of candidate compounds (as well as the three positive control compounds (PC12, 2-[(1,5-dimethyl-1*H*-pyrazol-4-yl)methyl]-7-(4-isopropylbenzyl)-2,7-diazaspiro[4.5]decane, Chembridge Catalog #17159859; PC26, 7-(4-isopropylbenzyl)-2-(tetrahydro-2*H*-thiopyran-4-yl)-2,7-diazaspiro[4.5]decan-6-one, Chembridge Catalog #80527891; PC27, 7-(4-isopropylbenzyl)-2-[(2-methyl-5-pyrimidinyl)methyl]-

2,7-diazaspiro[4.5]decan-6-one, Chembridge Catalog #61894700) from the Chembridge NOVACore library that were hits from another high-throughput biofilm screen of a different Chembridge compound library [45]) were obtained directly from Chembridge (http://www.hit2lead.com/index.asp) for follow-up testing. Working stocks of the compounds were made at 20 mM in dimethyl sulfoxide (DMSO).

2.3. Biofilm Assays

The adherence inhibition, the sustained inhibition, and the disruption optical density biofilm assays followed previously reported 384-well format standard protocols [46,47,49,50]. In brief, for the biofilm inhibition assays, compounds were added during the 90 min adherence step (for the adherence and the sustained inhibition optical density biofilm assays) and/or at the 24 h growth step (for the sustained inhibition optical density biofilm assay). For the disruption optical density biofilm assay, a biofilm was grown for 24 h, after which the biofilm was incubated for an additional 24 h in the presence of the compound of interest. At the end of each assay, the media were removed from each well, and the OD_{600} of each well was measured using a Tecan Infinite M1000 Pro or a Tecan M200 plate reader (Tecan Group Ltd., Männedorf, Switzerland), taking the average of five reads per well.

The high-throughput adherence inhibition optical density biofilm assay screen of the Chembridge Small Molecule Diversity library was robotically conducted at UCSF's SMDC. Compounds were included at a final concentration of 10 µM per well in 384-well plates in the high-throughput adherence inhibition optical density biofilm assay. Compounds were included at a final concentration of 40 µM per well in 384-well plates in the sustained inhibition optical density biofilm and the disruption optical density biofilm assays. Candidate compounds were tested at 12.5 µM in the combination sustained inhibition optical density biofilm and the disruption optical density biofilm assays. In line with previously reported studies [42,43], the combination sustained inhibition optical density biofilm assays used 1 µg/mL amphotericin B, 0.125 µg/mL caspofungin, or 256 µg/mL fluconazole. The combination disruption optical density biofilm assays used 2 µg/mL amphotericin B, 0.5 µg/mL caspofungin, or 256 µg/mL fluconazole. These amphotericin B, caspofungin, and fluconazole concentrations were chosen to be close to but below the effective concentrations (as measured by OD_{600}) in the respective assays in order to leave a dynamic range for observing any combinatorial interactions. The sensitivity of SN425 to the antifungal drugs amphotericin B, caspofungin, and fluconazole in the sustained inhibition optical density biofilm and the disruption optical density biofilm assays is included in File S3.

2.4. Candidate Compound Selection

Candidate compounds based on the results of the adherence inhibition optical density biofilm assay high throughput screen of the 30,000 compound Chembridge Small Molecule Diversity library were selected as follows. Separate lists of candidate compounds were developed for those compounds with an absorbance at least two standard deviations below that of the DMSO only controls and for those compounds with a B-score of less than −4 [51,52]. Other factors were also included in our selection criteria prioritizations, such as the selection of compounds with most favorable chemistries for optimizations as well as the selection of compounds that are available for purchase from Chembridge (http://www.hit2lead.com/index.asp) (some compounds became unavailable for commercial purchase during this study). In total, we selected 64 compounds, 28 from the standard deviation list and 36 from the B-score list. Nineteen of these compounds were on both lists for a total of 45 candidate compounds (File S2). We selected three additional compounds available from Chembridge (PC12, Chembridge Catalog #17159859; PC26, Chembridge Catalog #80527891; PC27, Chembridge Catalog #61894700) that were not in the Chembridge Small Molecule Diversity library but were previously reported by Pierce and colleagues to inhibit biofilm formation in a screen of a different Chembridge libraries (the Chembridge NOVACore library) [45] to serve as positive controls. Data from our adherence inhibition optical density biofilm assay screen of the 30,000 compound Chembridge Small Molecule Diversity library can be found in File S1. A list of the 45 selected candidate compounds can be found in File S2.

2.5. Statistical Analysis and "Hit" Calling for the Biofilm Assays

Statistical analyses and "hit" calling for the Biofilm Assays followed previously reported protocols [42,43]. For the stand-alone sustained inhibition and disruption optical density biofilm assays, individual repeats of candidate compounds (and controls) were performed in groups of eight wells. Between two and four repeats (16–32 total wells) were performed for each candidate compound. Each plate had seven sets of control wells (56 total wells) containing equivalent volumes of DMSO to the experimental wells spread throughout the plate to reduce positional effects. For each experimental set of eight wells, significance was evaluated relative to all of the control wells from the same plate using Welch's t-tests (two-tailed, assuming unequal variance). In order to correct for the multiple comparisons performed, we then applied the Bonferroni correction with $\alpha = 0.05$. All of the comparisons for a given type of assay (e.g., all of the stand-alone sustained inhibition optical density biofilm assays) were pooled for the multiple comparisons correction step, giving a number of hypotheses, m, of 146 for the sustained inhibition optical density biofilm assay and of 105 for the disruption optical density biofilm assay (for final thresholds of 3.42×10^{-4} and 4.76×10^{-4}, respectively). We then determined whether each experimental repeat (1) had an average absorbance less than the average of the control wells and (2) was significant after the multiple comparisons correction. To be considered a validated "hit", a compound had to satisfy both of these criteria.

For the combination sustained inhibition and disruption optical density biofilm assays, compounds (and controls) were again tested in groups of eight wells, and two distinct groups of controls were included on each plate. The first set of controls were wells where the candidate compound but no known antifungal drug was included. The second set of controls were wells where the antifungal drug but no candidate compound was included. In both cases, we used the same concentration of candidate compound or antifungal drug as was used in the experimental wells. Controls were included for all candidate compounds and antifungal drugs being tested on a given plate. In general, a single set of eight wells was included for each experimental or control condition on a given plate. Statistical analysis was performed using Welch's t-test and the Bonferroni correction as described above with the following modifications. Each experimental condition was compared to both the relevant antifungal drug control and the relevant candidate control (e.g., a compound CB01 plus caspofungin experiment was compared to the CB01 only control and the caspofungin only control from the same plate). All of the same comparisons for a given assay (e.g., all of the antifungal drug comparisons for the combination sustained inhibition optical density biofilm assay) were pooled for the multiple comparisons correction step, giving a number of hypotheses, m, of 144 for both the antifungal drug and the candidate compound comparisons in both the sustained inhibition and the disruption optical density biofilm assays (for a final threshold of 3.47×10^{-4}). To be considered a validated combination hit, a given experimental condition had to have (1) an average absorbance less than the averages of both sets of relevant control wells and (2) remain significant after the multiple comparisons correction for both sets of comparisons.

Data and statistics for the stand-alone and the combination biofilm assays are compiled in File S3. The chemical properties of the "hit" compounds (including molecular weights, polar surface area, logP, logSW, the number of rotatable bonds, and the numbers of H-bond acceptors and donors) that were available at the ChemBridge Online Chemical Store (www.hit2lead.com) are also included in File S3.

3. Results

The Chembridge Small Molecule Diversity library of 30,000 "drug-like" compounds covering a wide range of chemical scaffolds, diverse chemical backbones, chemotypes, and pharmacophores was robotically screened for compounds that inhibit *C. albicans* biofilm formation. This screen used the adherence inhibition optical density biofilm assay [46,47] (Figure 1a), where the compound of interest was added during the 90 min initial step of biofilm formation and then washed out (along with unadhered cells). The biofilm was then allowed to develop for 24 h in the absence of the compound. In total, 45 candidate compounds were then selected for further evaluation in secondary assays (Figure 1b, Files S1 and S2).

The 45 candidate Chembridge compounds (as well as the three positive control Chembridge compounds previously reported to inhibit biofilm formation that were not present in the 30,000 compound Small Molecule Diversity library [45]) were then evaluated for antibiofilm activity in the sustained inhibition optical density biofilm assay and the disruption optical density biofilm assay [46,47]. In the sustained inhibition optical density biofilm Assay, the compounds were added to the media during both the 90 min adherence step and the 24 h growth step of biofilm formation (Figure 1a). In the disruption optical density biofilm assay, a biofilm was grown for 24 h, after which the biofilm was incubated for an additional 24 h in the presence of the compound (Figure 1a). Other than the three positive controls (PC12, 2-[(1,5-dimethyl-1H-pyrazol-4-yl)methyl]-7-(4-isopropylbenzyl)-2,7-diazaspiro[4.5]decane, Chembridge Catalog #17159859; PC26, 7-(4-isopropylbenzyl)-2-(tetrahydro-2H-thiopyran-4-yl)-2,7-diazaspiro[4.5]decan-6-one, Chembridge Catalog #80527891; PC27, 7-(4-isopropylbenzyl)-2-[(2-methyl-5-pyrimidinyl)methyl]-2,7-diazaspiro[4.5]decan-6-one, Chembridge Catalog #61894700) [45], none of the compounds tested inhibited biofilm formation throughout the duration of biofilm development (Figure 1c and Figure S1a). We do not fully understand why some compounds showed significant inhibition in the adherence inhibition optical density biofilm assay but not in the sustained inhibition optical density biofilm assay, but these different assays may be sensitive to different compound parameters such as solubility, stability, and pH dependence. Given the lack of a biofilm inhibition phenotype in the sustained inhibition optical density biofilm assay, we were surprised to find that one of the 45 compounds (CB17, 1-[2-(2-methylphenoxy)-3-pyridinyl]-*N*-(3-pyridinylmethyl)methanamine, Chembridge Catalog #80338143) disrupted mature *C. albicans* biofilms on its own at the same concentration (Figure 1d,e and Figure S1b). See File S3 for names and chemical properties of this compound.

Given the previous reports suggesting antibiofilm synergies between known antifungal drugs and certain drug classes, we next tested our initial 45 candidate compounds for their abilities to inhibit biofilm formation (using the sustained inhibition optical density biofilm assay and/or to disrupt mature biofilms (using the disruption optical density biofilm assay) when combined with sub-inhibitory concentrations of amphotericin B, caspofungin, or fluconazole (Figure 2 and Figures S2 and S3). Three compounds disrupted mature biofilms in the presence of caspofungin (CB14, 2,2′-({[2-(ethylsulfonyl)-1-(3-phenylpropyl)-1H-imidazol-5-yl]methyl}imino)diethanol, Chembridge Catalog #10068182; CB36, *N*-[2-({2-[3-(1-azocanyl)-2-hydroxypropoxy]-4-methoxybenzyl}amino)ethyl]acetamide, Chembridge Catalog #29059737; CB40, 1-{3-[5-(1,3-benzodioxol-5-yl)-1,3,4-oxadiazol-2-yl]propanoyl}-4-(2-ethoxyphenyl)piperazine, Chembridge Catalog #35558198) (Figure 2a and Figure S2a). One of these compounds (CB36) also inhibited biofilm formation in the presence of caspofungin (Figure 2b and Figure S3a). In addition, a fourth compound (CB06, *N*-(2,3-dihydro-1,4-benzodioxin-6-yl)-1-[3-(1H-pyrazol-4-yl)propanoyl]-3-piperidinamine, Chembridge Catalog #22164746) inhibited biofilm formation in the presence of fluconazole (Figure 2c and Figure S3b). As noted above, none of these compounds had effects on biofilms on their own in this assay. Chemical properties of these compounds can be found in File S3. We also note that the positive control compounds PC12, PC26, and PC27 all disrupted mature biofilms in the presence of caspofungin, PC12 disrupted mature biofilms in the presence of fluconazole, and PC26 inhibited biofilm formation in the presence of fluconazole (Figure 2 and Figures S2 and S3).

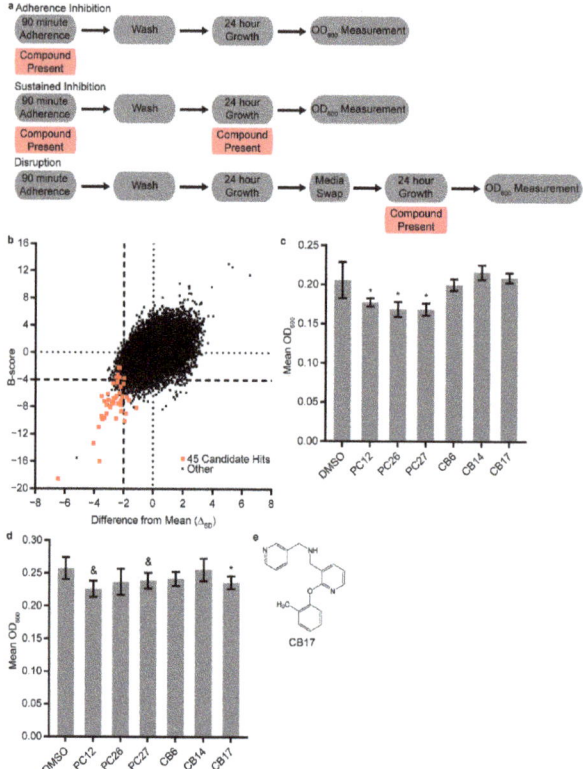

Figure 1. Screen of the Chembridge 30,000 "drug-like" member library for compounds with the ability to inhibit *C. albicans* biofilm formation. (**a**) Overview of the adherence inhibition, the sustained inhibition, and the disruption optical density biofilm assays. (**b**) Comparisons of the differences from the mean (in units of standard deviation, x-axis) and the B-score (y-axis) for the entire library screened at a concentration of 10 µM in the adherence inhibition optical density biofilm assay. The 45 candidate hits that were pursued further are indicated in red, and all other compounds are indicated in black. (**c,d**) Statistically significant hits, positive controls, and additional selected candidates from the (**c**) stand-alone sustained inhibition optical density biofilm assay and the (**d**) stand-alone disruption optical density biofilm assay; compounds were included at concentrations of 40 µM. In both panels, the mean OD_{600} readings with standard deviations are shown. Significant differences from the DMSO solvent control, as determined by Welch's *t*-test (two-tailed, assuming unequal variance) with the Bonferroni correction, are indicated for $\alpha = 0.05$ (*) or mixed results (&). In the cases of PC12 (2-[(1,5-dimethyl-1*H*-pyrazol-4-yl)methyl]-7-(4-isopropylbenzyl)-2,7-diazaspiro[4.5]decane, Chembridge Catalog #17159859) and PC27 (7-(4-isopropylbenzyl)-2-[(2-methyl-5-pyrimidinyl)methyl]-2,7-diazaspiro[4.5]decan-6-one, Chembridge Catalog #61894700) in the disruption optical density biofilm assay, only one of the two repeats performed met the significance threshold. Data within a chart were taken from the same plate. (**e**) Structure of compound CB17 (1-[2-(2-methylphenoxy)-3-pyridinyl]-*N*-(3-pyridinylmethyl)methanamine, Chembridge Catalog #80338143) disrupted mature *C. albicans* biofilms on its own at a concentration of 40 µM.

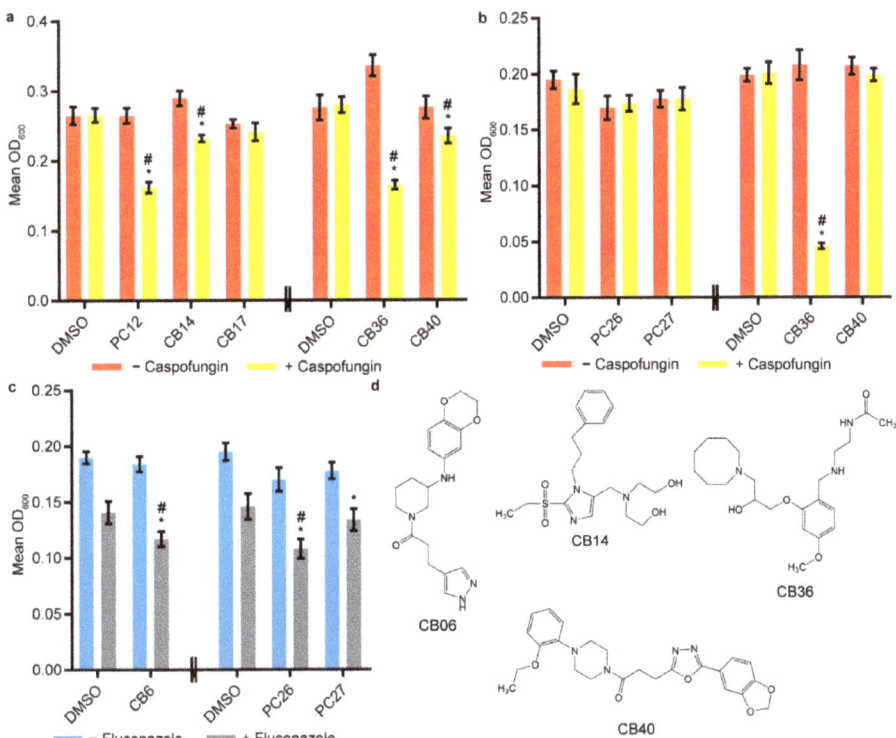

Figure 2. Combination screening of candidate compounds with the antifungal drugs caspofungin and fluconazole. (**a**) combination disruption optical density biofilm assay and (**b**) combination sustained inhibition optical density biofilm assay with caspofungin. For each compound, wells with caspofungin (+ caspofungin) are indicated in yellow, and wells without caspofungin (− caspofungin) are indicated in red. (**c**) Combination sustained inhibition optical density biofilm assay with fluconazole. For each compound, wells with fluconazole (+ fluconazole) are indicated in grey and wells without fluconazole − fluconazole) are indicated in blue. Mean OD_{600} readings with standard deviations are shown, significant differences from the compound without antifungal drug controls (e.g., PC12, − caspofungin), as determined by Welch's *t*-test (two-tailed, assuming unequal variance) with the Bonferroni correction, are indicated for $\alpha = 0.05$ (*). Significant differences from the antifungal drug without compound control (e.g., DMSO, + caspofungin), determined by the same statistical analysis, are indicated for $\alpha = 0.05$ (#). Data from different plates are separated by two vertical lines on the *x*-axis, and DMSO solvent controls are shown for each plate. Candidate compounds were included at concentrations of 12.5 μM in each of these assays. (**d**) Structures of compounds CB06 (*N*-(2,3-dihydro-1,4-benzodioxin-6-yl)-1-[3-(1*H*-pyrazol-4-yl)propanoyl]-3-piperidinamine, Chembridge Catalog #22164746), CB14 (2,2′-({[2-(ethylsulfonyl)-1-(3-phenylpropyl)-1*H*-imidazol-5-yl]methyl}imino)diethanol, Chembridge Catalog #10068182), CB36 (*N*-[2-({2-[3-(1-azocanyl)-2-hydroxypropoxy]-4-methoxybenzyl}amino)ethyl]acetamide, Chembridge Catalog #29059737), and CB40 (1-{3-[5-(1,3-benzodioxol-5-yl)-1,3,4-oxadiazol-2-yl]propanoyl}-4-(2-ethoxyphenyl)piperazine, Chembridge Catalog #35558198) inhibited and/or disrupted *C. albicans* biofilms in combination with at least one of the known antifungal drugs tested.

4. Discussion

Starting from an initial screen of a 30,000 compound diversity library and following standard high-throughput screening procedures for hit identification [53], we identified four compounds capable of inhibiting biofilm formation and/or disrupting mature biofilms in combination with caspofungin or fluconazole and a fifth compound capable of disrupting mature *C. albicans* biofilms on its own. As members of a diversity library, the identified compounds contain "drug-like" chemical backbones that represent promising chemical starting points for the development and the optimization of new classes of therapeutics designed to target *Candida* biofilms. For example, all compounds within this library have low molecular weights, low polar surface areas, and are predicted to be soluble and capable of crossing membranes. Given the distinct structures of our specific individual and combination hits, these compounds are likely to display broad ranges of biological activities and should provide multiple amenable opportunities for structural elaboration. Thus, even seemingly "weak" hits have the potential to become potent hits upon chemical optimizations [53–55]. Therefore, even compounds we identified with relatively minor yet significant antibiofilm effects on their own (e.g., CB17) have promise. In addition, our combination results indicate potent effects for certain compounds (e.g., CB06, CB14, CB36, CB40) in combination with fluconazole and caspofungin, suggesting that these compounds are a priority for future chemical optimizations.

In addition to identifying several promising antibiofilm compounds, our results illustrate the degree to which the experimental setup for biofilm formation can affect compound efficacy. One example is our identification of several compounds with efficacy in combination with known antifungal drugs, where the combined effect is dependent on the assay conditions. A second example is our identification of compounds that disrupt mature biofilms but that do not inhibit biofilm formation (either on their own or in combination with known antifungal drugs). Given these findings, drug efficacy testing that focuses solely on one aspect of biofilm formation (e.g., inhibition of initial biofilm formation) may overlook promising compounds that may be broadly effective against mature biofilms, and vice versa. Thus, multiple testing parameters of compounds against different stages of biofilm formation are useful in identifying the most promising compounds for therapeutic development.

Supplementary Materials: The following are available online at https://www.mdpi.com/2309-608X/7/1/9/s1. File S1, Screen of the Chembridge 30,000 "drug-like" member library for compounds with the ability to inhibit *C. albicans* biofilm formation in the adherence inhibition optical density biofilm assay. Differences from the mean (in units of standard deviation) and the B-score for the entire library screened at a concentration of 10 μM are provided. File S2, Identities of the 45 candidate compounds selected based on the initial adherence inhibition optical density biofilm assay as well as the three positive controls. Differences from the mean (in units of standard deviation) and the B-score are indicated for these compounds. File S3, Compiled data and statistics from the stand-alone and combination sustained inhibition and disruption optical density biofilm assays. For each compound, the average OD_{600}, average OD_{600} of relevant control(s), and value(s) for Welch's *t*-test versus the relevant control(s) are provided. Whether the average OD_{600} was below the average OD_{600} of the relevant control(s) and whether the difference from the relevant control(s) remains significant following the Bonferroni Correction ($\alpha = 0.05$) are indicated. The chemical properties of the "hit" compounds (including molecular weights, polar surface area, logP, logSW, the number of rotatable bonds, and the numbers of H-bond acceptors and donors) that were available at the ChemBridge Online Chemical Store (www.hit2lead.com) are also included. Figure S1, Additional results from the (**a**) stand-alone sustained inhibition and the (**b**) stand-alone disruption optical density biofilm assays. Mean OD_{600} readings with standard deviations are shown, significant differences from the DMSO solvent control, as determined by Welch's *t*-test (two-tailed, assuming unequal variance) with the Bonferroni Correction, are indicated for $\alpha=0.05$ (*) or mixed results (&). In the cases of CB36 and CB40 in the sustained inhibition optical density biofilm assay, only one of the two repeats performed met the significance threshold. In the case of CB40 in the disruption optical density biofilm assay, only two of the four repeats performed met the significance threshold. Data within a chart are all taken from the same plate on the same day. Figure S2, Additional results from the disruption optical density biofilm assay combination screening of candidate compounds with the antifungal agents caspofungin, fluconazole, and amphotericin B. Combination disruption biofilm assays with (**a**) caspofungin, (**b**) fluconazole, and (**c**) amphotericin B. In panel **a**, wells with caspofungin (+ caspofungin) are indicated in yellow and wells without caspofungin (− caspofungin) are indicated in red. In panel **b**, wells with fluconazole (+ fluconazole) are indicated in grey and wells without fluconazole (−fluconazole) are indicated in blue. In panel **c**, wells with amphotericin B (+ amphotericin B) are indicated in orange and wells without amphotericin B (− amphotericin B) are indicated in green. Mean OD_{600} readings with standard deviations are shown, significant differences from the compound without antifungal agent controls (e.g., CB6, − caspofungin), as determined by Welch's t-test (two-tailed, assuming unequal variance) with the Bonferroni Correction, are indicated for $\alpha = 0.05$ (*). Significant differences from the antifungal agent without compound control (e.g., DMSO, + caspofungin), determined by the same statistical testing, are indicated for $\alpha = 0.05$ (#). Candidate compounds were included at a concentration of 12.5 µM. Data from different plates are separated by two vertical lines on the x-axis, DMSO solvent controls are shown for each plate. Figure S3, Additional results from the sustained inhibition optical density biofilm assay combination screening of candidate compounds with the antifungal agents caspofungin, fluconazole, and amphotericin B. Combination sustained inhibition assays with (**a**) caspofungin, (**b**) fluconazole, and (**c**) amphotericin B. In panel **a**, wells with caspofungin (+ caspofungin) are indicated in yellow and wells without caspofungin (− caspofungin) are indicated in red. In panel **b**, wells with fluconazole (+ fluconazole) are indicated in grey and wells without fluconazole (− fluconazole) are indicated in blue. In panel **c**, wells with amphotericin B (+ amphotericin B) are indicated in orange and wells without amphotericin B (− amphotericin B) are indicated in green. Mean OD_{600} readings with standard deviations are shown, significant differences from the compound without antifungal agent controls (e.g., CB6, − caspofungin), as determined by Welch's t-test (two-tailed, assuming unequal variance) with the Bonferroni Correction, are indicated for $\alpha=0.05$ (*). Significant differences from the antifungal agent without compound control (e.g. DMSO, + caspofungin), determined by the same statistical tests, are indicated for $\alpha=0.05$ (#). Candidate compounds were included at a concentration of 12.5 µM. Data from different plates are separated by two vertical lines on the x-axis, DMSO solvent controls are shown for each plate.

Author Contributions: Conceptualization, A.D.J. and C.J.N.; data curation, M.B.L. and C.L.E.; formal analysis, M.B.L. and C.L.E.; funding acquisition, A.D.J. and C.J.N.; investigation, M.B.L., C.L.E. and N.H.; methodology, M.B.L., C.L.E. and N.H.; project administration, C.J.N.; resources, A.D.J. and C.J.N.; supervision, C.J.N.; writing—original draft, M.B.L. and C.J.N.; writing—reviewing and editing, M.B.L, C.L.E., N.H., A.D.J., and C.J.N. All authors have read and agreed to the published version of the manuscript.

Funding: This work was supported by National Institutes of Health (NIH) grants R43AI131710 (to M.B.L.), R01AI083311 (to A.D.J.), R35GM124594 (to C.J.N.), and R41AI112038 (to C.J.N.). C.L.E. was supported by NIH fellowship F31DE028488. This work was also supported by the Kamangar family in the form of an endowed chair (to C.J.N.). The content is the sole responsibility of the authors and does not represent the views of the NIH. The NIH had no role in study design, data collection and interpretation, or the decision to submit the work for publication.

Acknowledgments: We thank the staff at UCSF's Small Molecule Discovery Center, especially Kenny Ang, for assistance with the high-throughput screens.

Conflicts of Interest: The authors declare the following competing interests. Clarissa J. Nobile and Alexander D. Johnson are cofounders of BioSynesis, Inc., a company developing inhibitors and diagnostics of *C. albicans* biofilms. Matthew Lohse was formerly an employee and currently is a consultant for BioSynesis, Inc.

References

1. Douglas, L.J. *Candida* biofilms and their role in infection. *Trends Microbiol.* **2003**, *11*, 30–36. [CrossRef]
2. Lohse, M.B.; Gulati, M.; Johnson, A.D.; Nobile, C.J. Development and regulation of single- and multi-species *Candida albicans* biofilms. *Nat. Rev. Microbiol.* **2018**, *16*, 19–31. [CrossRef] [PubMed]
3. Gulati, M.; Nobile, C.J. *Candida albicans* biofilms: Development, regulation, and molecular mechanisms. *Microbes Infect.* **2016**, *18*, 310–321. [CrossRef] [PubMed]
4. Nobile, C.J.; Johnson, A.D. *Candida albicans* Biofilms and Human Disease. *Annu. Rev. Microbiol.* **2015**, *69*, 71–92. [CrossRef]
5. Kullberg, B.J.; Oude Lashof, A.M.L. Epidemiology of opportunistic invasive mycoses. *Eur. J. Med. Res.* **2002**, *7*, 183–191.
6. Kim, J.; Sudbery, P. *Candida albicans*, a major human fungal pathogen. *J. Microbiol.* **2011**, *49*, 171–177. [CrossRef]
7. Achkar, J.M.; Fries, B.C. *Candida* infections of the genitourinary tract. *Clin. Microbiol. Rev.* **2010**, *23*, 253–273. [CrossRef]
8. Ganguly, S.; Mitchell, A.P. Mucosal biofilms of *Candida albicans*. *Curr. Opin. Microbiol.* **2011**, *14*, 380–385. [CrossRef]
9. Kennedy, M.J.; Volz, P.A. Ecology of *Candida albicans* gut colonization: Inhibition of *Candida* adhesion, colonization, and dissemination from the gastrointestinal tract by bacterial antagonism. *Infect. Immun.* **1985**, *49*, 654–663. [CrossRef]
10. Kumamoto, C.A. *Candida* biofilms. *Curr. Opin. Microbiol.* **2002**, *5*, 608–611. [CrossRef]
11. Kumamoto, C.A. Inflammation and gastrointestinal *Candida* colonization. *Curr. Opin. Microbiol.* **2011**, *14*, 386–391. [CrossRef] [PubMed]
12. Calderone, R.A.; Fonzi, W.A. Virulence factors of *Candida albicans*. *Trends Microbiol.* **2001**, *9*, 327–335. [CrossRef]

13. Pappas, P.G.; Rex, J.H.; Sobel, J.D.; Filler, S.G.; Dismukes, W.E.; Walsh, T.J.; Edwards, J.E. Guidelines for treatment of candidiasis. *Clin. Infect. Dis.* **2004**, *38*, 161–189. [CrossRef] [PubMed]
14. Wenzel, R.P. Nosocomial candidemia: Risk factors and attributable mortality. *Clin. Infect. Dis.* **1995**, *20*, 1531–1534. [CrossRef]
15. López-Ribot, J.L. *Candida albicans* biofilms: More than filamentation. *Curr. Biol.* **2005**, *15*, R453–R455. [CrossRef]
16. Ramage, G.; Mowat, E.; Jones, B.; Williams, C.; Lopez-Ribot, J. Our current understanding of fungal biofilms. *Crit. Rev. Microbiol.* **2009**, *35*, 340–355. [CrossRef]
17. Douglas, L.J. Medical importance of biofilms in *Candida* infections. *Rev. Iberoam. Micol.* **2002**, *19*, 139–143.
18. Fox, E.P.; Nobile, C.J. A sticky situation: Untangling the transcriptional network controlling biofilm development in *Candida albicans*. *Transcription* **2012**, *3*, 315–322. [CrossRef]
19. Chandra, J.; Kuhn, D.M.; Mukherjee, P.K.; Hoyer, L.L.; McCormick, T.; Ghannoum, M.A. Biofilm formation by the fungal pathogen *Candida albicans*: Development, architecture, and drug resistance. *J. Bacteriol.* **2001**, *183*, 5385–5394. [CrossRef]
20. Kojic, E.M.; Darouiche, R.O. *Candida* infections of medical devices. *Clin. Microbiol. Rev.* **2004**, *17*, 255–267. [CrossRef]
21. Ramage, G.; Martínez, J.P.; López-Ribot, J.L. *Candida* biofilms on implanted biomaterials: A clinically significant problem. *FEMS Yeast Res.* **2006**, *6*, 979–986. [CrossRef] [PubMed]
22. Tumbarello, M.; Posteraro, B.; Trecarichi, E.M.; Fiori, B.; Rossi, M.; Porta, R.; de Gaetano Donati, K.; La Sorda, M.; Spanu, T.; Fadda, G.; et al. Biofilm production by *Candida* species and inadequate antifungal therapy as predictors of mortality for patients with candidemia. *J. Clin. Microbiol.* **2007**, *45*, 1843–1850. [CrossRef] [PubMed]
23. Lebeaux, D.; Ghigo, J.M.; Beloin, C. Biofilm-Related Infections: Bridging the Gap between Clinical Management and Fundamental Aspects of Recalcitrance toward Antibiotics. *Microbiol. Mol. Biol. Rev.* **2014**, *78*, 510–543. [CrossRef] [PubMed]
24. Donlan, R.M. Biofilm formation: A clinically relevant microbiological process. *Clin. Infect. Dis.* **2001**, *33*, 1387–1392. [CrossRef]
25. Tumbarello, M.; Fiori, B.; Trecarichi, E.M.; Posteraro, P.; Losito, A.R.; De Luca, A.; Sanguinetti, M.; Fadda, G.; Cauda, R.; Posteraro, B. Risk factors and outcomes of candidemia caused by biofilm-forming isolates in a tertiary care hospital. *PLoS ONE* **2012**, *7*, e33705. [CrossRef]
26. Andes, D.R.; Safdar, N.; Baddley, J.W.; Playford, G.; Reboli, A.C.; Rex, J.H.; Sobel, J.D.; Pappas, P.G.; Kullberg, B.J. Impact of treatment strategy on outcomes in patients with candidemia and other forms of invasive candidiasis: A patient-level quantitative review of randomized trials. *Clin. Infect. Dis.* **2012**, *54*, 1110–1122. [CrossRef]
27. Fox, E.P.; Singh-Babak, S.D.; Hartooni, N.; Nobile, C.J. Biofilms and Antifungal Resistance. In *Antifungals: From Genomics to Resistance and the Development of Novel Agents*; Caister Academic Press: Poole, UK, 2015; pp. 71–90.
28. Shinde, R.B.; Chauhan, N.M.; Raut, J.S.; Karuppayil, S.M. Sensitization of *Candida albicans* biofilms to various antifungal drugs by cyclosporine A. *Ann. Clin. Microbiol. Antimicrob.* **2012**, *11*, 27. [CrossRef]
29. Bink, A.; Kuchaříková, S.; Neirinck, B.; Vleugels, J.; Van Dijck, P.; Cammue, B.P.A.; Thevissen, K. The Nonsteroidal Antiinflammatory Drug Diclofenac Potentiates the In Vivo Activity of Caspofungin Against *Candida albicans* Biofilms. *J. Infect. Dis.* **2012**, *206*, 1790–1797. [CrossRef]
30. Barchiesi, F.; Spreghini, E.; Maracci, M.; Fothergill, A.W.; Baldassarri, I.; Rinaldi, M.G.; Scalise, G. In Vitro Activities of Voriconazole in Combination with Three Other Antifungal Agents against *Candida glabrata*. *Antimicrob. Agents Chemother.* **2004**, *48*, 3317–3322. [CrossRef]
31. Chatzimoschou, A.; Katragkou, A.; Simitsopoulou, M.; Antachopoulos, C.; Georgiadou, E.; Walsh, T.J.; Roilides, E. Activities of Triazole-Echinocandin Combinations against *Candida* Species in Biofilms and as Planktonic Cells. *Antimicrob. Agents Chemother.* **2011**, *55*, 1968–1974. [CrossRef]
32. Uppuluri, P.; Nett, J.; Heitman, J.; Andes, D. Synergistic Effect of Calcineurin Inhibitors and Fluconazole against *Candida albicans* Biofilms. *Antimicrob. Agents Chemother.* **2008**, *52*, 1127–1132. [CrossRef] [PubMed]
33. Bachmann, S.P.; Ramage, G.; VandeWalle, K.; Patterson, T.F.; Wickes, B.L.; López-Ribot, J.L. Antifungal Combinations against *Candida albicans* Biofilms In Vitro. *Antimicrob. Agents Chemother.* **2003**, *47*, 3657–3659. [CrossRef] [PubMed]
34. Katragkou, A.; McCarthy, M.; Alexander, E.L.; Antachopoulos, C.; Meletiadis, J.; Jabra-Rizk, M.A.; Petraitis, V.; Roilides, E.; Walsh, T.J. In vitro interactions between farnesol and fluconazole, amphotericin B or micafungin against *Candida albicans* biofilms. *J. Antimicrob. Chemother.* **2015**, *70*, 470–478. [CrossRef] [PubMed]
35. Troskie, A.M.; Rautenbach, M.; Delattin, N.; Vosloo, J.A.; Dathe, M.; Cammue, B.P.A.; Thevissen, K. Synergistic Activity of the Tyrocidines, Antimicrobial Cyclodecapeptides from *Bacillus aneurinolyticus*, with Amphotericin B and Caspofungin against *Candida albicans* Biofilms. *Antimicrob. Agents Chemother.* **2014**, *58*, 3697–3707. [CrossRef] [PubMed]
36. Wei, G.; Xu, X.; Wu, C.D. In vitro synergism between berberine and miconazole against planktonic and biofilm *Candida* cultures. *Arch. Oral Biol.* **2011**, *56*, 565–572. [CrossRef] [PubMed]
37. Khan, M.S.A.; Ahmad, I. Antibiofilm activity of certain phytocompounds and their synergy with fluconazole against *Candida albicans* biofilms. *J. Antimicrob. Chemother.* **2012**, *67*, 618–621. [CrossRef] [PubMed]
38. Kaneko, Y.; Fukazawa, H.; Ohno, H.; Miyazaki, Y. Combinatory effect of fluconazole and FDA-approved drugs against *Candida albicans*. *J. Infect. Chemother.* **2013**, *19*, 1141–1145. [CrossRef]
39. De Cremer, K.; Lanckacker, E.; Cools, T.L.; Bax, M.; De Brucker, K.; Cos, P.; Cammue, B.P.A.; Thevissen, K. Artemisinins, New Miconazole Potentiators Resulting in Increased Activity against *Candida albicans* Biofilms. *Antimicrob. Agents Chemother.* **2015**, *59*, 421–426. [CrossRef]

40. Delattin, N.; De Brucker, K.; Vandamme, K.; Meert, E.; Marchand, A.; Chaltin, P.; Cammue, B.P.A.; Thevissen, K. Repurposing as a means to increase the activity of amphotericin B and caspofungin against *Candida albicans* biofilms. *J. Antimicrob. Chemother.* **2014**, *69*, 1035–1044. [CrossRef]
41. LaFleur, M.D.; Lucumi, E.; Napper, A.D.; Diamond, S.L.; Lewis, K. Novel high-throughput screen against *Candida albicans* identifies antifungal potentiators and agents effective against biofilms. *J. Antimicrob. Chemother.* **2011**, *66*, 820–826. [CrossRef]
42. Lohse, M.B.; Gulati, M.; Craik, C.S.; Johnson, A.D.; Nobile, C.J. Combination of Antifungal Drugs and Protease Inhibitors Prevent *Candida albicans* Biofilm Formation and Disrupt Mature Biofilms. *Front. Microbiol.* **2020**, *11*, 1027. [CrossRef] [PubMed]
43. Nobile, C.J.; Ennis, C.L.; Hartooni, N.; Johnson, A.D.; Lohse, M.B. A Selective Serotonin Reuptake Inhibitor, a Proton Pump Inhibitor, and Two Calcium Channel Blockers Inhibit *Candida albicans* Biofilms. *Microorganisms* **2020**, *8*, 756. [CrossRef] [PubMed]
44. Watamoto, T.; Egusa, H.; Sawase, T.; Yatani, H. Screening of Pharmacologically Active Small Molecule Compounds Identifies Antifungal Agents Against *Candida* Biofilms. *Front. Microbiol.* **2015**, *6*, 1453. [CrossRef] [PubMed]
45. Pierce, C.G.; Chaturvedi, A.K.; Lazzell, A.L.; Powell, A.T.; Saville, S.P.; McHardy, S.F.; Lopez-Ribot, J.L. A novel small molecule inhibitor of *Candida albicans* biofilm formation, filamentation and virulence with low potential for the development of resistance. *NPJ Biofilms Microbiomes* **2015**, *1*, 15012. [CrossRef]
46. Gulati, M.; Lohse, M.B.; Ennis, C.L.; Gonzalez, R.E.; Perry, A.M.; Bapat, P.; Arevalo, A.V.; Rodriguez, D.L.; Nobile, C.J. In Vitro Culturing and Screening of *Candida albicans* Biofilms. *Curr. Protoc. Microbiol.* **2018**, *50*, e60. [CrossRef]
47. Lohse, M.B.; Gulati, M.; Arevalo, A.V.; Fishburn, A.; Johnson, A.D.; Nobile, C.J. Assessment and optimizations of *Candida albicans* in vitro biofilm assays. *Antimicrob. Agents Chemother.* **2017**, *61*. [CrossRef]
48. Noble, S.M.; French, S.; Kohn, L.A.; Chen, V.; Johnson, A.D. Systematic screens of a *Candida albicans* homozygous deletion library decouple morphogenetic switching and pathogenicity. *Nat. Genet.* **2010**, *42*, 590–598. [CrossRef]
49. Fox, E.P.; Bui, C.K.; Nett, J.E.; Hartooni, N.; Mui, M.C.; Andes, D.R.; Nobile, C.J.; Johnson, A.D. An expanded regulatory network temporally controls *Candida albicans* biofilm formation. *Mol. Microbiol.* **2015**, *96*, 1226–1239. [CrossRef]
50. Nobile, C.J.; Fox, E.P.; Hartooni, N.; Mitchell, K.F.; Hnisz, D.; Andes, D.R.; Kuchler, K.; Johnson, A.D. A histone deacetylase complex mediates biofilm dispersal and drug resistance in *Candida albicans*. *MBio* **2014**, *5*, e01201–e01214. [CrossRef]
51. Brideau, C.; Gunter, B.; Pikounis, B.; Liaw, A. Improved statistical methods for hit selection in high-throughput screening. *J. Biomol. Screen.* **2003**, *8*, 634–647. [CrossRef]
52. Malo, N.; Hanley, J.A.; Cerquozzi, S.; Pelletier, J.; Nadon, R. Statistical practice in high-throughput screening data analysis. *Nat. Biotechnol.* **2006**, *24*, 167–175. [CrossRef] [PubMed]
53. Dandapani, S.; Rosse, G.; Southall, N.; Salvino, J.M.; Thomas, C.J. Selecting, Acquiring, and Using Small Molecule Libraries for High-Throughput Screening. *Curr. Protoc. Chem. Biol.* **2012**, *4*, 177–191. [CrossRef] [PubMed]
54. Huggins, D.J.; Venkitaraman, A.R.; Spring, D.R. Rational methods for the selection of diverse screening compounds. *ACS Chem. Biol.* **2011**, *6*, 208–217. [CrossRef] [PubMed]
55. Galloway, W.R.J.D.; Isidro-Llobet, A.; Spring, D.R. Diversity-oriented synthesis as a tool for the discovery of novel biologically active small molecules. *Nat. Commun.* **2010**, *1*, 80. [CrossRef]

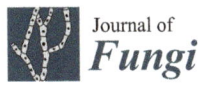

Article

Gene Expression Analysis of Non-Clinical Strain of *Aspergillus fumigatus* (LMB-35Aa): Does Biofilm Affect Virulence?

Teresa D. Rebaza, Yvette Ludeña, Ilanit Samolski and Gretty K. Villena *

Laboratorio de Micología y Biotecnología "Marcel Gutiérrez—Correa", Universidad Nacional Agraria La Molina, 15026 Lima, Peru; damarisrebaza@gmail.com (T.D.R.); yludena@lamolina.edu.pe (Y.L.); isamolski@lamolina.edu.pe (I.S.)
* Correspondence: gkvch@lamolina.edu.pe

Received: 13 November 2020; Accepted: 16 December 2020; Published: 18 December 2020

Abstract: *Aspergillus fumigatus* LMB-35Aa, a saprophytic fungus, was used for cellulase production through biofilms cultures. Since biofilms usually favor virulence in clinical strains, the expression of the related genes of the LMB 35-Aa strain was analyzed by qPCR from the biomass of planktonic cultures and biofilms developed on polyester cloth and polystyrene microplates. For this, virulence-related genes reported for the clinical strain Af293 were searched in *A. fumigatus* LMB 35-Aa genome, and 15 genes were identified including those for the synthesis of cell wall components, hydrophobins, invasins, efflux transporters, mycotoxins and regulators. When compared with planktonic cultures at 37 °C, invasin gene *calA* was upregulated in both types of biofilm and efflux transporter genes *mdr4* and *atrF* were predominantly upregulated in biofilms on polystyrene, while *aspHs* and *ftmA* were upregulated only in biofilms formed on polyester. Regarding the transcription regulators, *laeA* was downregulated in biofilms, and *medA* did not show a significant change. The effect of temperature was also evaluated by comparing the biofilms grown on polyester at 37 vs. 28 °C. Non-significant changes at the expression level were found for most genes evaluated, except for *atrF*, *gliZ* and *medA*, which were significantly downregulated at 37 °C. According to these results, virulence appears to depend on the interaction of several factors in addition to biofilms and growth temperature.

Keywords: *Aspergillus fumigatus*; biofilms; gene expression; virulence

1. Introduction

Filamentous fungi are widely distributed in nature due to their saprophytic condition and their capability to grow in several substrates and surfaces. Additionally, fungi are biotechnologically important due to their ability to produce enzymes, organic acids, and diverse secondary metabolites. Fungi of industrial use are generally recognized as safe and in this sense, it is important to assess the expression of the pathogenicity or virulence genes under different growth and culture conditions.

The *Aspergillus* group, mainly *A. niger*, is widely used in biotechnology [1]. *A. fumigatus* is gaining interest because of its plant polysaccharide modifying and degrading enzymes [2–4]. Particularly, the production of neutral and alkaline endoglucanases, which are in high demand for the textile biofinishing process [5], has been reported for this fungus [6]. However, *A. fumigatus* has also been widely recognized as an opportunistic pathogen which is responsible for many reactions from allergies to invasive pulmonary aspergillosis [7,8].

In clinical strains, certain genes have been reported as key factors for the virulence and pathogenicity of *A. fumigatus*, and their expression is also related to the formation of biofilms in affected tissues.

Although virulence may depend on the isolation origin of strains (environmental or clinical), there is not a specific group of genes in *A. fumigatus* that determines the virulence level. Virulence factors do not include essential genes for normal growth but are associated with some biological processes mainly involved in cell wall structure, thermotolerance, response to stress, signaling, toxin synthesis, nutrition and survival in the host [7,9–11].

On the other hand, biofilm formation is a natural form of growth in fungi, on both biotic and abiotic surfaces, which confer them survival advantages related to metabolic performance and stress resistance. Fungal biofilms have gained much industrial importance, however, at the same time, they can be considered as a virulence factor for opportunistic fungi. Differential gene expression occurs in biofilm as compared with planktonic growth. Some genes expressed in biofilms encode transcription and translation factors, regulators, and those involved in ribosomal protein synthesis and protein turnover, multi-drug resistance transporter genes, enzymes for extracellular matrix synthesis, extracellular enzymes as well as genes for adherence and secondary metabolism (toxins) [12,13].

In this research, *A. fumigatus* LMB-35Aa, an alkaline cellulase producing strain isolated from soil [14], was successfully cultured as a biofilm to improve their cellulase productivity, as has been previously reported for other *Aspergillus* species [15,16]. Nevertheless, considering the saprophytic condition of this strain and its genetic divergence from clinical isolates [17], it was also important to assess the expression of the main genes involved in the pathogenicity and virulence in biofilms.

Multispecies fungal biofilms have great potential for cellulose conversion [18]. However, the industrial production of cellulases, as well as mixed and single species biofilms should be considered. In this study, the reason for using the single biofilms of *A. fumigatus* LMB-35Aa was related to our interest in producing neutral alkaline endoglucanases for use in the textile industry.

Complementarily and according to the systems biology approach, molecular tools are useful to assess bioprocess optimization in industrial biotechnology [19], but most scientific reports are focused on the transcriptomic analysis of clinical strains [7,20], so that information is still incipient for industrial biofilms [3].

2. Materials and Methods

2.1. Fungal Strain

A. fumigatus LMB-35Aa [14] was used throughout this study. The strain was maintained on potato dextrose agar (PDA). For inoculum preparation, before each experiment, the strain was grown in flasks with PDA during 72 h at 37 °C. Then, the spores were washed with 0.1% (*v/v*) Tween 80 solution and diluted until obtaining a concentration of 10^6 spores/mL which was used as inoculum.

2.2. Culture Medium and Growth Conditions

Cellulase production medium was used as reported before [21], except that the carbon source was replaced by 0.5% (*w/v*) carboxymethyl cellulose (CMC).

For biofilms' cultures on polyester support, flasks containing a pre-weighed 3.1 × 3.1 cm piece of cloth and 70 mL of distilled water were used. Each flask was inoculated with a 3% (*v/v*) of spore suspension and incubated with agitation (175 rpm) at 28 or 37 °C (according to the experiment) for 15 min to allow the attachment of spores. The unbound spores were washed twice with sterile distilled water in agitation at the same conditions. Finally, polyester cloths were transferred to 250 mL sterile flasks containing 70 mL of cellulase production medium. Inoculated flasks were incubated at 28/37 °C in a shaker bath at 175 rpm for 72 h.

For the biofilm cultures on polystyrene, flat-bottom 12-well polystyrene microtiter plates were used as a surface for biofilm formation [22]. Each well containing 3 mL of cellulase production medium was inoculated with 90 µL of spore suspension and then incubated without agitation at 37 °C for 15 min. After that, the medium was removed by pipetting and the plate wells were washed three times with distilled water. Finally, each well was refilled with 3 mL of cellulase production medium and microplates were incubated at 37 °C without agitation for 72 h.

For submerged culture, 250 mL flasks containing 70 mL of cellulase production medium were inoculated with 3% (v/v) of spore suspension and incubated at 28 or 37 °C for 72 h in a shaker bath at 175 rpm.

In all cases, for biomass harvesting, biofilms and free mycelium were washed three times with distilled water and maintained at −80 °C until RNA extraction.

2.3. Qualitative Endoglucanase Activity Assay

Qualitative assays of enzymatic activity were performed at different pH's from 4.8 to 9.4 according Vega et al. (2012) with certain modifications [6]. Briefly, 100 µL of culture supernatants of *A. fumigatus* LMB-35Aa biofilms, developed on polyester cloth during 72 h in cellulase production medium, were incorporated into wells of 0.6 cm in diameter, equidistantly distributed in glass plates containing screening medium (1.5% agar and 0.3% CMC in the corresponding buffer). The plates were incubated at 50 °C for 24 h. After the incubation time, a 0.5% Congo Red solution was added on the medium for 15 min at room temperature and then washed with 1 M NaCl. Staining and washings were carried out in an orbital shaker at 50 rpm. The development of a clear zone (halo) around the wells was considered as a positive result of endoglucanase activity. Acetate buffer 50 mM (pH 4.8), borax buffer 50 mM (pH 7.6), and glycine buffer 50 mM (pH 8.4 and pH 9.4) were used correspondingly.

2.4. Quantitative Endoglucanase Activity

Quantitative assays of enzymatic activity were performed in 96-well microplates using 3,5-dinitrosalicylic acid (DNS) reagent according to the method described by Xiao et al. (2005) [23] with certain modifications. Briefly, a 30 µL aliquot of diluted culture supernatant was added into each microwell containing 30 µL of 1% CMC as a substrate prepared in 50 mM of the corresponding buffer (pH 4.8, 7.6, 8.4 or 9.4; see Section 2.3). After 30 min of incubation at 50 °C, 90 µL of DNS reagent was added into each well and incubated at 95 °C for 5 min. Following the color development, a 100 µL aliquot of each sample was transferred to a flat-bottom 96-well microplate and the absorbance was measured at 540 nm in a RT-2100C microplate reader (Rayto). An enzyme blank and substrate blank were also included in each assay. The concentration of glucose released by the secreted enzymes was determined by interpolating from a standard curve constructed with known concentrations of glucose. One enzyme unit (U) was defined as the amount of enzyme required to release 1 µmol of reducing sugar equivalents per minute under the defined assay conditions.

2.5. Extracellular Protein Determination

Soluble extracellular protein concentration was determined at 550 nm by Lowry's colorimetric method using the Folin–Ciocalteu reagent with bovine serum albumin (BSA) as the protein standard [24].

2.6. Confocal Scanning Laser Microscopy (CSLM)

For the microscopy analysis, biofilm cultures on polyester cloth were developed as described above in Section 2.2. After 72 h of growth, the biofilms were washed three times with distilled water and then placed in 50 mM phosphate buffer (pH 7.4). Fluorescein isothiocyanate (FITC) and Concanavalin A (ConA) were used to stain the fungal hyphae and extracellular matrices, respectively. For that, stocks solutions of each dye were prepared in 10 mM phosphate buffer (pH 7.4) and mixed to a final concentration of 10 µg/mL (FITC) and 50 µg/mL (ConA). Biofilms were stained with 15 µL of this mix for 30 min in the dark at room temperature [25]. Finally, the biofilms were washed with 10 mM phosphate buffer four times and a FLUOVIEW FV1200 confocal scanning laser microscope (Olympus Life Science) was used for the image analysis and acquisition. FITC was excited/monitored at 458/488 nm and ConA was excited/monitored at 490/515 nm.

2.7. RNA Extraction and cDNA Synthesis

Total RNA isolation was carried out using RNA Miniprep kit (Zymo Research®, Irvine, CA, USA) after grinding the biomass with liquid nitrogen. The quality and quantity of all RNA samples were analyzed in a NanoDropTM 2000c spectrophotometer (Thermo Scientific®, Waltham, MA, USA) and by agarose gel electrophoresis. In all cases, cDNA was synthesized from 2 µg of total RNA in a 25 µL final volume using a reverse transcription mix containing 200 U of M-MLV RT (Promega®, Madison, WI, USA)), 0.5 mM dNTP mix, 0.5 µg of Oligo(dT)15 and 25 U of RNAse inhibitor. Reaction tubes were incubated at 42 °C for 60 min and stored at −20 °C until required for qPCR analysis.

2.8. Identification of Virulence Genes in A. fumigatus LMB-35Aa Genome

A. fumigatus Af293 clinical strain was used as a reference [26] for the screening of virulence genes in *A. fumigatus* LMB-35Aa genome, which included those encoding synthesis of cell wall components, hydrophobins, invasins, efflux transporters, mycotoxins and regulators.

The selection of virulence genes from the clinical strain *A. fumigatus* Af293 and nucleic sequence alignment was done using BLAST (Basic Local Alignment and Search Tool) to find the corresponding genes in *A. fumigatus* LMB-35Aa genome (Accession PRJNA298653) [14] with a sequence similarity higher than 98%. Table S1 indicates the location of the corresponding genes in the *A. fumigatus* LMB-35Aa genome, including the scaffold number and length (bp).

2.9. Primers Design

Primer Quest SM software (Integrated DNA Technologies, Inc.) was used to the design primers from the *A. fumigatus* LMB-35Aa genome sequence available in GenBank (PRJNA298653). The primers used in this study are listed in Table S2.

2.10. Gene Expression Analysis by qPCR

Gene expression was analyzed by quantitative real-time polymerase chain reaction (qPCR) with KAPA SYBR Fast kit (KAPA Biosystems®, Wilmington, MA, USA) according to the manufacturer's protocol. qPCR was performed in a CFX96 Real Time PCR Detection System (Bio-Rad®, Hercules, CA, USA). Each reaction well with a final volume of 10 µL contained 1 µL of cDNA template and 0.3 µM of each forward and reverse primer (10 mM). The amplification process included an activation step at 95 °C for 3 min followed by 40 cycles at 95 °C for 3 s and 60 °C for 20 s (annealing and extension). After that, a melting curve analysis was included at 60–95 °C to confirm the specific amplification, according to the melting temperature (Tm) expected for each amplicon. Each reaction was carried out in triplicate and each plate included non-target controls. Two independent biological replicates were analyzed. After amplification, the cycle threshold (Ct) number was recorded for the reference and target genes. The amplification efficiency of each pair of primers was validated experimentally from the slope of the log-linear range of the calibration curve constructed with the serial dilutions of target cDNA.

The relative gene expression was calculated according to Hellemans et al. (2007) [27], which constitutes a modified Delta-Delta Ct method by considering the amplification efficiency of target genes and multiple reference genes for the improved normalization of relative quantities. β-Tubulin (*btub*) (F: 5′-TTCACTGCTATGTTCCGTCG-3′; R: 5′-TCGTTCATGTTGCTCTCGG-3′) [28] and elongation factor (*tef1*) (F:5′CCATGTGTGTCGAGTCCTTC-3′, R:5′-GAACGTACAGCAACAGTCTGG-3′) were used as reference genes.

3. Results

3.1. Influence of pH and Temperature on A. fumigatus LMB-35Aa Endoglucanase Activity of Biofilms Formed on Polyester

Endoglucanase production was compared at 28 and 37 °C until 120 h of growth and maximum enzymatic title was obtained at 72 h at both temperatures (Teresa D. Rebaza and Gretty K. Villena. Universidad Nacional Agraria La Molina, Lima, Perú. Diploma Thesis, 2019). At this point, the qualitative and quantitative endoglucanase activity (Figure 1) of the biofilms grown at 37 °C was higher at pH 7.6. At least a two-fold increase in the specific activity (units of enzyme/g of secreted protein) was obtained at 37 °C at pH 7.6 so that this temperature could be used for subsequent assays.

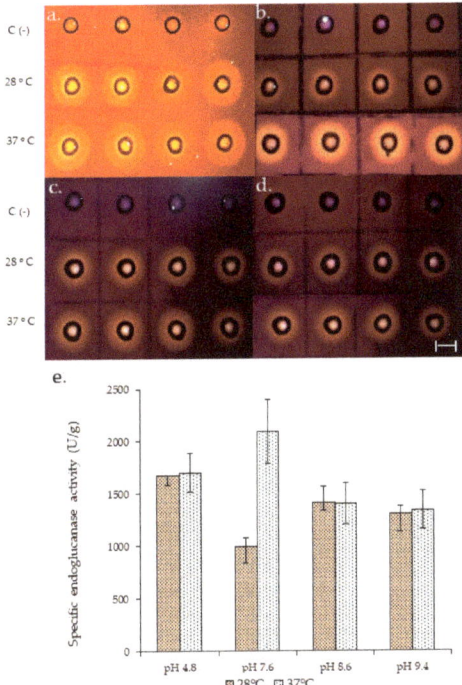

Figure 1. Endoglucanase activity (EG) of *A. fumigatus* LMB-35Aa biofilms developed on polyester cloth at 72 h of growth and 28 or 37 °C. The upper panel shows a qualitative assay for EG at (**a**) pH 4.8; (**b**) 7.6; (**c**) 8.6 and (**d**) 9.4. C (-) represents the negative control for the assay. Specific EG activity (**e**) was calculated by quantitative assay. Specific activity = EG (U/L)/soluble secreted protein (g/L). Scale bar represents 1 cm.

3.2. Influence of Biofilm Formation on A. fumigatus LMB-35Aa Virulence-Related Gene Expression

As better conditions for endoglucanase production and activity, 37 °C and pH 7.6, respectively, could also be favorable for pathogenesis and virulence, a gene expression analysis was performed to evaluate if, in addition, biofilm formation affects the expression of virulence-related genes. For that, 15 virulence-related genes described for the clinical strain *A. fumigatus* Af293, including genes for the synthesis of cell wall components, hydrophobins, invasins, efflux transporters, mycotoxins and regulators, were selected after searching for them in the *A. fumigatus* LMB-35Aa genome. Virulence-related genes found in the genome are described in Table 1.

Table 1. Selected virulence-related genes found in the genome of the saprophytic strain LMB-35Aa, considering the clinical strain *A. fumigatus* Af293 as a reference.

Gene	Gene Function	Role Associated with Virulence	Reference
rho1	β-(1,3) glucan biosynthesis regulation	Regulation of cell wall composition and oxidative alkaline stress	[29]
ags1	α-(1-3) glucan biosynthesis	Conidia adhesion capacity and survival; late phagocytosis	[30,31]
agd3	Deacetylation of galactosaminogalactan (GAG)	Induces biofilms formation	[32,33]
glfA	Galactofuranose biosynthesis	Conidia germination and growth inside macrophages; resistance to antifungal drugs	[34,35]
rodB	Hydrophobin	Upregulation in biofilm conditions and in vivo	[36]
calA	Invasin	Invasion of epithelial and endothelial host cells through endocytosis induction	[37]
mdr4	ABC multidrug transporter	Azole resistance (clinical isolates)	[38]
atrF	ABC multidrug transporter	Azole resistance (environmental isolates)	[39]
gliZ	Gliotoxin biosynthesis regulation	Induces apoptosis and cytotoxicity	[40]
aspf1	Ribotoxin	Cytotoxicity, cell surface allergen	[41]
aspHs	Hemolysin biosynthesis	Hemolysis and cytotoxicity	[42]
ftmA	Fumitremorgins biosynthesis (tremorgenic toxins)	Cytotoxicity	[43]
laeA	Secondary metabolism master regulation	Induces gliotoxin and other secondary metabolites production and cytotoxicity of host cells	[44,45]
rtfA	Developmental and secondary metabolism regulation	Oxidative stress response, protease activity, adhesion capacity	[46]
medA	Developmental regulation	Regulates conidiogenesis, adherence to host cells and biofilm formation, damage of epithelial cells and stimulation of cytokine production	[47,48]

For the gene expression analysis, two biofilm models (Figure 2a,c) and two growth temperatures were evaluated and compared with planktonic cultures. Biofilms were morphologically evaluated by CLSM and in both cases, a typical mycelium organization and extracellular matrix were observed (Figure 2b,d).

When comparing the expression of virulence-related genes (Figure 3a,b), a similar expression pattern was observed in both biofilm models with the exception of fumitremorgin biosynthesis *ftmA* gene, which was upregulated in the biofilms formed on the polyester cloth and downregulated in the biofilms formed on polystyrene, with respect to the planktonic cultures.

On the other hand, a differential gene expression was observed when the biofilms were compared with planktonic cultures. According to Figure 3a, all the genes involved in the cell wall structure (*rho1*, *ags1*, *agd3* and *glfA*) showed a lower expression level in biofilms, a pattern which was especially significant in the case of biofilms developed on polystyrene. This pattern was also observed in the case of the hydrophobin *rodB* gene. Conversely, invasin gene *calA* was significantly upregulated in both types of biofilms. With respect to ABC efflux transporters, genes *mdr4* and *atrF* were predominantly upregulated in biofilm formed on polystyrene.

In the opposite way, Figure 3b shows that the *aspHs* gene, which encodes for hemolysin, and *ftmA*, involved in mycotoxin biosynthesis, were upregulated only in biofilms on polyester, while *gliZ* and *aspF1* genes, encoding proteins involved in secondary metabolism, exhibited a significant downregulation in biofilms formed on polystyrene.

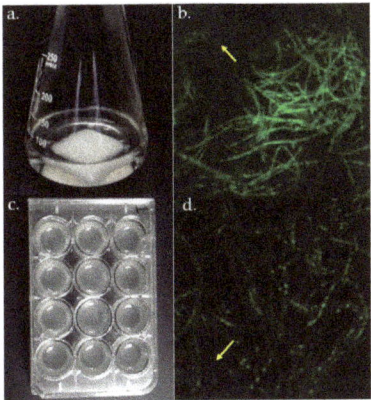

Figure 2. Biofilm models of *A. fumigatus* LMB-35Aa grown on (**a**) polyester and (**c**) polystyrene. Biofilm structure was analyzed by CSLM at 72 h of growth. Average projections of stained biofilms 40× images on (**b**) polyester and (**d**) polystyrene are shown. Green fluorescence depicts fungal viable cells; arrows indicate regions with the extracellular matrices of biofilms.

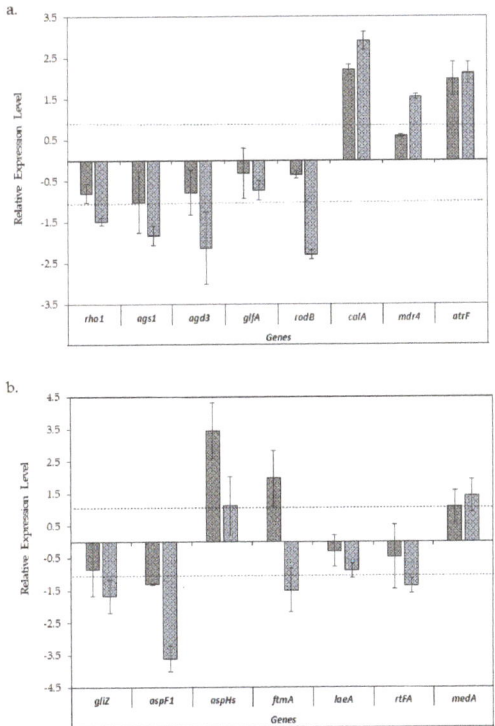

Figure 3. Relative expression ±S.D. of the virulence-related genes of A. fumigatus LMB-35Aa between the biofilms developed on polyester (grey bars) and polystyrene (blue bars) vs. planktonic cultures: (**a**) analysis of genes of the cell wall structure, hydrophobin, invasin and efflux transporters; and (**b**) the genes involved in mycotoxin biosynthesis, adhesion, and secondary metabolism. Gene expression levels were normalized using β-tub and tef1 as reference genes. The relative expression level is represented as a $\log_2$ fold change; dotted lines indicates $\log_2$ fold change thresholds of −1 and 1.

With respect to *medA*, involved in cell adhesion and biofilm formation, it had a slightly higher level of expression in the biofilms formed on polystyrene as compared with those formed on polyester, although in both cases these were not significant. Finally, with regard to regulator genes, *rtfA* was downregulated and the *laeA* gene, encoding for a secondary metabolism regulator, did not show any significant change when *A. fumigatus* formed biofilms.

3.3. Effect of Temperature on A. fumigatus LMB-35Aa Virulence-Related Genes Expression

Given that polyester supports are more suitable for fungal biofilm formation at an industrial level [13] and considering that a greater number of virulence-related genes were upregulated in the biofilms developed on this support, an additional experiment was carried out to evaluate if the temperature could affect the observed gene expression patterns.

Figure 4 shows that the expression levels of analyzed genes involved in cell wall structure did not show any significant change when the biofilms grew at 28 or 37 °C, with the exception of *glfA* and *calA*, which showed a slightly higher level of expression at 37 °C. With regard to the analyzed efflux transporters genes, *atrF* was significantly downregulated at 37 °C compared to 28 °C, while *mdr4* did not show any significant change in any condition. Most of the analyzed genes involved in mycotoxins biosynthesis and regulation did not show notable changes in their expression levels when the biofilms were formed at 28 or 37 °C, except for the *gliZ* gene, involved in gliotoxin biosynthesis, which was significantly downregulated at 37 °C.

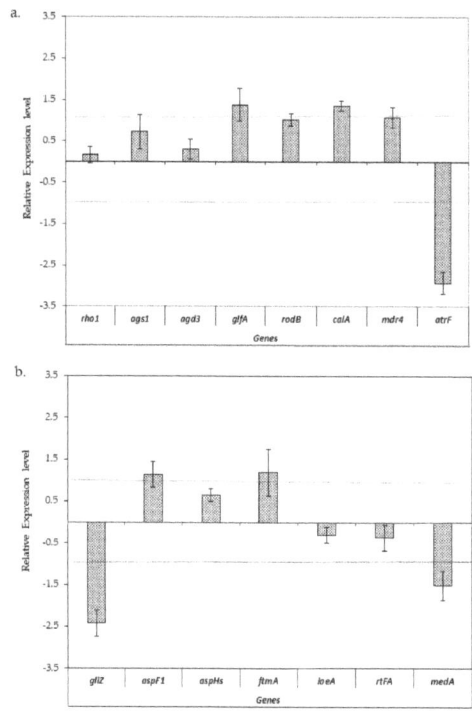

Figure 4. Relative expression ±S.D. of the virulence-related genes of *A. fumigatus* LMB-35Aa biofilms formed on polyester at 37 vs. 28 °C: (**a**) analysis of genes of the cell wall structure, hydrophobin, invasin and efflux transporters; and (**b**) the genes involved in mycotoxin biosynthesis, adhesion and secondary metabolism. Gene expression levels were normalized using β-*tub* and *tef1* as the reference genes. The relative expression level is represented as a $\log_2$ fold change; dotted lines indicates $\log_2$ fold change thresholds of −1 and 1.

4. Discussion

A. fumigatus is gaining great interest as an enzymes producer for biotechnological applications including lignocellulose conversion to added value products [2,4,49–52]. In this case, strain LMB-35Aa was selected as a neutral alkaline endoglucanase producer and grown as biofilms on polyester cloth in order to improve its enzymatic productivity.

Despite its saprophytic condition and not even being grouped with clinical strains, the expression of genes related to virulence in biofilms of *A fumigatus* LMB-35Aa were analyzed. Some particular genetic characteristics of this strain, related to secondary metabolism (SM) cluster variants include the lack of a 54 kb region (five genes from telomere-proximal fumigaclavine C cluster) in the chromosome 2, and a large inversion in the SM gene cluster 14 that contains a transcription factor, an oxidoreductase, and a hypothetical protein [17].

For *A. fumigatus*, biofilm formation is one of the most determining virulence factors [53,54]. In that sense, the strain LMB-35Aa has a good capacity to adhere to abiotic surfaces and form biofilms on polyester and polystyrene supports with a typical structure including an extracellular matrix, as it was also reported for different *Aspergillus* biofilms [13]. Several fungal constituents may be involved in the formation of biofilm in host cells. Associated with this, biofilms formed by the strain LMB-35Aa could be expected to express virulence-related genes, including cell wall components, invasins, and efflux transporters, among others [55].

The cell wall is mainly composed of polysaccharides like β-glucans and galactomannans and some genes like *rho1*, *ags1*, *agd3* and *glfA*, which are involved in the biosynthesis of β-glucans, α-glucans, galactosaminogalactans and galactomannans, respectively, which can also have an impact on virulence, increasing resistance to antifungals and concentrating the extracellular enzymes produced during growth, which are necessary aspects for colonization and tissue infection. Moreover, *rho1* might be required for *A. fumigatus* pathogenicity and internalization into lung epithelial host cells [29]. Gene *ags1* contributes significantly with at least 50% of the cell wall α-1,3-glucan content, however, it is not a determinant for virulence [56], while *agd3* encodes for a deacetylase of galactosaminogalactan, which is an important virulence factor, and induces adherence and biofilms formation [33]. In addition, a Δ*glfA* mutant of *A. fumigatus* produced slower growth and attenuated virulence since a diminished content of glucofuranose causes the thinning of the cell wall and an increased susceptibility to drugs [34]. Interestingly, none of these genes were upregulated in biofilms of LMB-35Aa, probably due to the time of growth (72 h) being much later than the first stages of biofilm formation. Probably, for the same reason, the *medA* gene, involved in biofilm formation and adherence [47,48], was slightly expressed.

By the other hand, gene *rodB*, encoding a Class I hydrophobin in *A. fumigatus*, was downregulated in biofilms, contrarily to the high expression found in a cellophane biofilm model developed by Valsecchi et al. (2018), although, at the same time, they found that the corresponding protein RodB analyzed by Western blots was present in the conidium cell wall but not in the hyphae of planktonic or biofilm cultures [36]. This means that the high gene expression does not always correlate with high protein production. Here, we found that the *rodB* gene was upregulated in our planktonic cultures (pellets) since sporulation occurred early inside the pellet.

Another important virulence gene, *calA*, was upregulated in both biofilm models, especially in biofilms on polystyrene. CalA is dispensable for adherence, but it is important as invasin and induces the host cell endocytosis of pathogenic *A. fumigatus* [37].

Drug efflux transporter genes *cmdr4* and *atrF*, which contribute to itraconazole resistance [57] and are induced by the presence of that drug [58], were also upregulated in biofilms. Even this being a typical resistance for clinical strains, it has also been reported as an environmental route of resistance development [59]. Most of the genes involved in mycotoxin biosynthesis were downregulated in biofilms, except *ftmA*, for the biofilms grown on polyester. In the same way, *aspHs*, a virulence factor which encodes for hemolysin, was slightly overexpressed. This gene has been proposed as a specific target for *A. fumigatus* detection by qPCR for in vivo infections [60]. Thus, it could be related to biofilm formation.

It was remarked that transcription factors are important for fungal pathogenicity because of their role in regulating the transcription of virulence-related pathways [61]. In this case, *medA* was poorly expressed. Additionally, *laeA* was downregulated and correlated with *gliZ* downregulation since LaeA is a transcriptional regulator of secondary metabolite gene clusters including gliotoxin [46].

Gene expression could be also influenced by growth temperature as reported by Sueiro-Olivares et al. (2015) [62] when analyzing the transcriptomes of *A. fumigatus* during the early steps of conidia germination after being grown at 24 and 37 °C. Between the 1249 differentially expressed genes, *gliZ* was upregulated at 37 °C.

Unexpectedly, in our case, when comparing the gene expression patterns of biofilms grown at 37 vs. 28 °C, only a slight but not significant expression of virulence-related genes was observed at 37 °C. However, the fact that some virulence factors such as *gliZ*, *atrF* and *medA* were repressed at this temperature is even more relevant.

This highlights that virulence is a multifactorial condition with many determinants acting together. For industrial purposes, even when *A. fumigatus* biofilm formation slightly induces the level of expression of virulence-related genes, it is not enough to attribute to it a leading role in the virulence for non-clinical strains. Perhaps, together with the influence of the temperature of growth, another signaling mechanism related with host interaction could be explored to discard the potential pathogenicity of the strain LMB-35Aa during biofilm formation.

5. Conclusions

Biofilm formation in the non-clinical *A. fumigatus* LMB-35Aa strain could lightly induce the upregulation of some virulence-related genes, including *calA*, *mdr4*, *atrF*, *aspHs* and *ftmA*, but also the influence of temperature was evident, especially for the downregulation of *gliZ*, *atrF* and *medA* at 37 °C. Further research using an in vivo biofilm model could contribute to a better understanding of the complex virulence phenomena.

Supplementary Materials: The following are available online at http://www.mdpi.com/2309-608X/6/4/376/s1, Table S1: Virulence-related genes identified in *A. fumigatus* LMB-35Aa genome, considering the clinical strain *A. fumigatus* Af293 as reference, Table S2: Primer sequences for gene expression analysis through qPCR for main virulence-related genes found in *A. fumigatus* LMB-35Aa genome.

Author Contributions: G.K.V. conceived the research and designed the experiments. T.D.R. performed the experiments. Y.L. and I.S. supervised the experiments. G.K.V. provide the resources. All authors analyzed the data. T.D.R. and Y.L. wrote the original draft. I.S. and G.K.V. wrote and revised the paper. G.K.V. got funding. All authors have read and agreed to the published version of the manuscript.

Funding: This research was funded by Consejo Nacional de Ciencia, Tecnología e Innovación Tecnológica de Perú (grants N° 177-2015-CONCYTEC-FONDECYT-DE and N° 181-2015-FONDECYT-DE).

Acknowledgments: The authors wish to thank Mary Pasmiño for her technical assistance.

Conflicts of Interest: The authors declare no conflict of interest. The funders had no role in the design of the study; in the collection, analyses, or interpretation of data; in the writing of the manuscript, or in the decision to publish the results.

References

1. Cairns, T.C.; Nai, C.; Meyer, V. How a fungus shapes biotechnology: 100 years of *Aspergillus niger* research. *Fungal Biol. Biotechnol.* **2018**, *5*, 13. [CrossRef] [PubMed]
2. Adav, S.S.; Ravindran, A.; Sze, S.K. Quantitative proteomic study of *Aspergillus fumigatus* secretome revealed deamidation of secretory enzymes. *J. Proteom.* **2015**, *119*, 154–168. [CrossRef] [PubMed]
3. Sun, W.; Liu, L.; Yu, Y.; Yu, B.; Liang, C.; Ying, H.; Liu, D.; Chen, Y. Biofilm-related, time-series transcriptome and genome sequencing in xylanase-producing *Aspergillus niger* SJ1. *ACS Omega* **2020**, *5*, 19737–19746. [CrossRef]
4. De Gouvêa, P.F.; Bernardi, A.V.; Gerolamo, L.E.; de Souza Santos, E.; Riaño-Pachón, D.M.; Uyemura, S.A.; Dinamarco, T.M. Transcriptome and secretome analysis of *Aspergillus fumigatus* in the presence of sugarcane bagasse. *BMC Genom.* **2018**, *19*, 232. [CrossRef] [PubMed]

5. Behera, B.C.; Sethi, B.K.; Mishra, R.R.; Dutta, S.K.; Thatoi, H.N. Microbial cellulases—Diversity & biotechnology with reference to mangrove environment: A review. *J. Genet. Eng. Biotechnol.* **2017**, *15*, 197–210. [PubMed]
6. Vega, K.; Villena, G.K.; Sarmiento, V.H.; Ludeña, Y.; Vera, N.; Gutiérrez-Correa, M. Production of alkaline cellulase by fungi isolated from an undisturbed rain forest of Peru. *Biotechnol. Res. Int.* **2012**, *2012*, 934325. [CrossRef] [PubMed]
7. Puértolas-Balint, F.; Rossen, J.W.A.; Oliveira dos Santos, C.; Chlebowicz, M.M.A.; Raangs, E.C.; van Putten, M.L.; Sola-Campoy, P.J.; Han, L.; Schmidt, M.; García-Cobos, S. Revealing the virulence potential of clinical and environmental *Aspergillus fumigatus* isolates using whole-genome sequencing. *Front. Microbiol.* **2019**, *10*, 1970. [CrossRef]
8. Latgé, J.P.; Chamilos, G. *Aspergillus fumigatus* and aspergillosis in 2019. *Clin. Microbiol. Rev.* **2019**, *33*, e00140-18. [CrossRef]
9. Abad, A.; Fernández-Molina, J.V.; Bikandi, J.; Ramírez, A.; Margareto, J.; Sendino, J.; Hernando, F.L.; Pontón, J.; Garaizar, J.; Rementeria, A. What makes *Aspergillus fumigatus* a successful pathogen? Genes and molecules involved in invasive aspergillosis. *Rev. Iberoam. Micol.* **2010**, *27*, 155–182. [CrossRef]
10. Szalewski, D.A.; Hinrichs, V.S.; Zinniel, D.K.; Barletta, R.G. The pathogenicity of *Aspergillus fumigatus*, drug resistance, and nanoparticle delivery. *Can. J. Microbiol.* **2018**, *64*, 439–453. [CrossRef]
11. Sugui, J.A.; Kwon-Chung, K.J.; Juvvadi, P.R.; Latgé, J.P.; Steinbach, W.J. *Aspergillus fumigatus* and related species. *Cold Spring Harb. Perspect. Med.* **2014**, *5*, a019786. [CrossRef] [PubMed]
12. Fanning, S.; Mitchell, A.P. Fungal biofilms. *PLoS Pathog.* **2012**, *8*, e1002585. [CrossRef] [PubMed]
13. Ramage, G.; Rajendran, R.; Gutierrez-Correa, M.; Jones, B.; Williams, C. *Aspergillus* biofilms: Clinical and industrial significance. *FEMS Microbiol. Lett.* **2011**, *324*, 89–97. [CrossRef] [PubMed]
14. Paul, S.; Zhang, A.; Ludeña, Y.; Villena, G.K.; Yu, F.; Sherman, D.H.; Gutiérrez-Correa, M. Insights from the genome of a high alkaline cellulase producing *Aspergillus fumigatus* strain obtained from Peruvian Amazon rainforest. *J. Biotechnol.* **2017**, *251*, 53–58. [CrossRef]
15. Villena, G.K.; Gutiérrez-Correa, M. Morphological patterns of *Aspergillus niger* biofilms and pellets related to lignocellulolytic enzyme productivities. *Lett. Appl. Microbiol.* **2007**, *45*, 231–237. [CrossRef]
16. Gamarra, N.N.; Villena, G.K.; Gutiérrez-Correa, M. Cellulase production by *Aspergillus niger* in biofilm, solid-state, and submerged fermentations. *Appl. Microbiol. Biotechnol.* **2010**, *87*, 545–551. [CrossRef]
17. Lind, A.L.; Wisecaver, J.H.; Lameiras, C.; Wiemann, P.; Palmer, J.M.; Keller, N.P.; Rodrigues, F.; Goldman, G.H.; Rokas, A. Drivers of genetic diversity in secondary metabolic gene clusters within a fungal species. *PLoS Biol.* **2017**, *15*, e2003583. [CrossRef]
18. Brethauer, S.; Shahab, R.L.; Studer, M.H. Impacts of biofilms on the conversion of cellulose. *Appl. Microbiol. Biotechnol.* **2020**, *104*, 5201–5212. [CrossRef]
19. Knuf, C.; Nielsen, J. Aspergilli: Systems biology and industrial applications. *Biotechnol. J.* **2012**, *7*, 1147–1155. [CrossRef]
20. Muszkieta, L.; Beauvais, A.; Pähtz, V.; Gibbons, J.G.; Anton Leberre, V.; Beau, R.; Shibuya, K.; Rokas, A.; Francois, J.M.; Kniemeyer, O.; et al. Investigation of *Aspergillus fumigatus* biofilm formation by various "omics" approaches. *Front. Microbiol.* **2013**, *4*, 13. [CrossRef]
21. Villena, G.K.; Gutiérrez-Correa, M. Production of cellulase by *Aspergillus niger* biofilms developed on polyester cloth. *Lett. Appl. Microbiol.* **2006**, *43*, 262–268. [CrossRef] [PubMed]
22. Silva-Dias, A.; Miranda, I.M.; Branco, J.; Monteiro-Soares, M.; Pina-Vaz, C.; Rodrigues, A.G. Adhesion, biofilm formation, cell surface hydrophobicity, and antifungal planktonic susceptibility: Relationship among *Candida* spp. *Front. Microbiol.* **2015**, *6*, 205. [CrossRef] [PubMed]
23. Xiao, Z.; Storms, R.; Tsang, A. Microplate-based carboxymethylcellulose assay for endoglucanase activity. *Anal. Biochem.* **2005**, *342*, 176. [CrossRef] [PubMed]
24. Lowry, O.H.; Rosebrough, N.J.; Farr, A.L.; Randall, R.J. Protein measurement with the Folin phenol reagent. *J. Biol. Chem.* **1951**, *193*, 265–275. [PubMed]
25. Strathmann, M.; Wingender, J.; Flemming, H.C. Application of fluorescently labelled lectins for the visualization and biochemical characterization of polysaccharides in biofilms of *Pseudomonas aeruginosa*. *J. Microbiol. Methods* **2002**, *50*, 237–248. [CrossRef]

26. Nierman, W.C.; Pain, A.; Anderson, M.J.; Wortman, J.R.; Kim, H.S.; Arroyo, J.; Berriman, M.; Abe, K.; Archer, D.B.; Bermejo, C.; et al. Genomic sequence of the pathogenic and allergenic filamentous fungus *Aspergillus fumigatus*. *Nature* **2005**, *438*, 1151–1156. [CrossRef]
27. Hellemans, J.; Mortier, G.; De Paepe, A.; Speleman, F.; Vandesompele, J. QBase relative quantification framework and software for management and automated analysis of real-time quantitative PCR data. *Genome Biol.* **2007**, *8*, 1–14. [CrossRef]
28. Gravelat, F.N.; Doedt, T.; Chiang, L.Y.; Liu, H.; Filler, S.G.; Patterson, T.F.; Sheppard, D.C. In vivo analysis of *Aspergillus fumigatus* developmental gene expression determined by real-time reverse transcription-PCR. *Infect. Immun.* **2008**, *76*, 3632–3639. [CrossRef]
29. Zhang, X.; Jia, X.; Tian, S.; Zhang, C.; Lu, Z.; Chen, Y.; Chen, F.; Li, Z.; Su, X.; Han, X.; et al. Role of the small GTPase Rho1 in cell wall integrity, stress response, and pathogenesis of *Aspergillus fumigatus*. *Fungal Genet. Biol.* **2018**, *120*, 30–41. [CrossRef]
30. Beauvais, A.; Maubon, D.; Park, S.; Morelle, W.; Tanguy, M.; Huerre, M.; Perlin, D.S.; Latgé, J.P. Two α-(1-3) glucan synthases with different functions in *Aspergillus fumigatus*. *Appl. Environ. Microbiol.* **2005**, *71*, 1531–1538. [CrossRef]
31. Beauvais, A.; Bozza, S.; Kniemeyer, O.; Formosa, C.; Balloy, V.; Henry, C.; Roberson, R.W.; Dague, E.; Chignard, M.; Brakhage, A.A.; et al. Deletion of the α-(1,3)-glucan synthase genes induces a restructuring of the conidial cell wall responsible for the avirulence of *Aspergillus fumigatus*. *PLoS Pathog.* **2013**, *9*, e1003716. [CrossRef]
32. Lee, M.J.; Geller, A.M.; Bamford, N.C.; Liu, H.; Gravelat, F.N.; Snarr, B.D.; Le Mauff, F.; Chabot, J.; Ralph, B.; Ostapska, H.; et al. Deacetylation of fungal exopolysaccharide mediates adhesion and biofilm formation. *MBio* **2016**, *7*, e00252-16. [CrossRef] [PubMed]
33. Bamford, N.C.; Le Mauff, F.; Van Loon, J.C.; Ostapska, H.; Snarr, B.D.; Zhang, Y.; Kitova, E.N.; Klassen, J.S.; Codée, J.D.C.; Sheppard, D.C.; et al. Structural and biochemical characterization of the exopolysaccharide deacetylase Agd3 required for *Aspergillus fumigatus* biofilm formation. *Nat. Commun.* **2020**, *11*, 2450. [CrossRef] [PubMed]
34. Schmalhorst, P.S.; Krappmann, S.; Vervecken, W.; Rohde, M.; Müller, M.; Braus, G.H.; Contreras, R.; Braun, A.; Bakker, H.; Routier, F.H. Contribution of galactofuranose to the virulence of the opportunistic pathogen *Aspergillus fumigatus*. *Eukaryot. Cell* **2008**, *7*, 1268–1277. [CrossRef]
35. Koch, B.E.V.; Hajdamowicz, N.H.; Lagendijk, E.; Ram, A.F.J.; Meijer, A.H. *Aspergillus fumigatus* establishes infection in zebrafish by germination of phagocytized conidia, while *Aspergillus niger* relies on extracellular germination. *Sci. Rep.* **2019**, *9*, 12791. [CrossRef]
36. Valsecchi, I.; Dupres, V.; Stephen-Victor, E.; Guijarro, J.I.; Gibbons, J.; Beau, R.; Bayry, J.; Coppee, J.Y.; Lafont, F.; Latgé, J.P.; et al. Role of hydrophobins in *Aspergillus fumigatus*. *J. Fungi* **2018**, *4*, 2. [CrossRef]
37. Liu, H.; Lee, M.J.; Solis, N.V.; Phan, Q.T.; Swidergall, M.; Ralph, B.; Ibrahim, A.S.; Sheppard, D.C.; Filler, S.G. *Aspergillus fumigatus* CalA binds to integrin α5β1 and mediates host cell invasion. *Nat. Microbiol.* **2016**, *2*, 16211. [CrossRef]
38. Rajendran, R.; Mowat, E.; McCulloch, E.; Lappin, D.F.; Jones, B.; Lang, S.; Majithiya, J.B.; Warn, P.; Williams, C.; Ramage, G. Azole resistance of *Aspergillus fumigatus* biofilms is partly associated with efflux pump activity. *Antimicrob. Agents Chemother.* **2011**, *55*, 2092–2097. [CrossRef]
39. Meneau, I.; Coste, A.T.; Sanglard, D. Identification of *Aspergillus fumigatus* multidrug transporter genes and their potential involvement in antifungal resistance. *Med. Mycol.* **2016**, *54*, 616–627. [CrossRef]
40. Bok, J.W.; Chung, D.; Balajee, S.A.; Marr, K.A.; Andes, D.; Nielsen, K.F.; Frisvad, J.C.; Kirby, K.A.; Keller, N.P. GliZ, a transcriptional regulator of gliotoxin biosynthesis, contributes to *Aspergillus fumigatus* virulence. *Infect. Immun.* **2006**, *74*, 6761–6768. [CrossRef]
41. Liu, H.; Xu, W.; Solis, N.V.; Woolford, C.; Mitchell, A.P.; Filler, S.G. Functional convergence of *gliP* and *aspf1* in *Aspergillus fumigatus* pathogenicity. *Virulence* **2018**, *9*, 1062–1073. [CrossRef]
42. Zarrin, M.; Ganj, F. Study of hemolysin gene "*aspHS*" and its phenotype in *Aspergillus fumigatus*. *Open Access Maced. J. Med. Sci.* **2019**, *7*, 2399–2403. [CrossRef]
43. Maiya, S.; Grundmann, A.; Li, S.M.; Turner, G. The fumitremorgin gene cluster of *Aspergillus fumigatus*: Identification of a gene encoding brevianamide F synthetase. *ChemBioChem* **2006**, *7*, 1062–1069. [CrossRef]
44. Bok, J.W.; Balajee, S.A.; Marr, K.A.; Andes, D.; Nielsen, K.F.; Frisvad, J.C.; Keller, N.P. LaeA, a regulator of morphogenetic fungal virulence factors. *Eukaryot. Cell* **2005**, *4*, 1574–1582. [CrossRef] [PubMed]

45. Perrin, R.M.; Fedorova, N.D.; Bok, J.W.; Cramer, R.A.; Wortman, J.R.; Kim, H.S.; Nierman, W.C.; Keller, N.P. Transcriptional regulation of chemical diversity in *Aspergillus fumigatus* by LaeA. *PLoS Pathog.* **2007**, *3*, e50. [CrossRef] [PubMed]
46. Myers, R.R.; Smith, T.D.; Elsawa, S.F.; Puel, O.; Tadrist, S.; Calvo, A.M. RtfA controls development, secondary metabolism, and virulence in *Aspergillus fumigatus*. *PLoS ONE* **2017**, *12*, e0176702. [CrossRef] [PubMed]
47. Gravelat, F.N.; Ejzykowicz, D.E.; Chiang, L.Y.; Chabot, J.C.; Urb, M.; Macdonald, K.D.; al-Bader, N.; Filler, S.G.; Sheppard, D.C. *Aspergillus fumigatus* MedA governs adherence, host cell interactions and virulence. *Cell. Microbiol.* **2010**, *12*, 473–488. [CrossRef] [PubMed]
48. Al Abdallah, Q.; Choe, S.I.; Campoli, P.; Baptista, S.; Gravelat, F.N.; Lee, M.J.; Sheppard, D.C. A conserved C-terminal domain of the *Aspergillus fumigatus* developmental regulator MedA is required for nuclear localization, adhesion and virulence. *PLoS ONE* **2012**, *7*, e49959. [CrossRef] [PubMed]
49. Okonji, R.E.; Itakorode, B.O.; Ovumedia, J.O.; Adedeji, O.S. Purification and biochemical characterization of pectinase produced by *Aspergillus fumigatus* isolated from soil of decomposing plant materials. *J. Appl. Biol. Biotech.* **2019**, *7*, 1–8.
50. De Oliveira Júnior, S.D.; de Araújo Padilha, C.E.; de Asevedo, E.A.; de Macedo, G.R.; dos Santos, E.S. Recovery and purification of cellulolytic enzymes from *Aspergillus fumigatus* CCT 7873 using an aqueous two-phase micellar system. *Ann. Microbiol.* **2020**, *70*, 1–12. [CrossRef]
51. Jin, X.; Song, J.; Liu, G.Q. Bioethanol production from rice straw through an enzymatic route mediated by enzymes developed in-house from *Aspergillus fumigatus*. *Energy* **2020**, *190*, 116395. [CrossRef]
52. Mohapatra, S.; Padhy, S.; Mohapatra, P.K.D.; Thatoi, H.N. Enhanced reducing sugar production by saccharification of lignocellulosic biomass, *Pennisetum* species through cellulase from a newly isolated *Aspergillus fumigatus*. *Bioresour. Technol.* **2018**, *253*, 262–272. [CrossRef] [PubMed]
53. Raksha, G.S.; Urhekar, A.D. Virulence factors detection in *Aspergillus* isolates from clinical and environmental samples. *J. Clin. Diagn. Res.* **2017**, *11*, DC13–DC18.
54. Kernien, J.F.; Snarr, B.D.; Sheppard, D.C.; Nett, J.E. The interface between fungal biofilms and innate immunity. *Front. Immunol.* **2018**, *8*, 1968. [CrossRef]
55. Kaur, S.; Singh, S. Biofilm formation by *Aspergillus fumigatus*. *Med. Mycol.* **2014**, *52*, 2–9. [PubMed]
56. Yoshimi, A.; Miyazawa, K.; Abe, K. Cell wall structure and biogenesis in *Aspergillus* species. *Biosci. Biotechnol. Biochem.* **2016**, *80*, 1700–1711. [CrossRef]
57. Nascimento, A.M.; Goldman, G.H.; Park, S.; Marras, S.A.; Delmas, G.; Oza, U.; Lolans, K.; Dudley, M.N.; Mann, P.A.; Perlin, D.S. Multiple resistance mechanisms among *Aspergillus fumigatus* mutants with high-level resistance to itraconazole. *Antimicrob. Agents Chemother.* **2003**, *47*, 1719–1726. [CrossRef]
58. Slaven, J.W.; Anderson, M.J.; Sanglard, D.; Dixon, G.K.; Bille, J.; Roberts, I.S.; Denning, D.W. Increased expression of a novel *Aspergillus fumigatus* ABC transporter gene, *atrF*, in the presence of itraconazole in an itraconazole resistant clinical isolate. *Fungal Genet. Biol.* **2002**, *36*, 199–206.
59. Berger, S.; El Chazli, Y.; Babu, A.F.; Coste, A.T. Azole resistance in *Aspergillus fumigatus*: A consequence of antifungal use in agriculture? *Front. Microbiol.* **2017**, *8*, 1024. [CrossRef]
60. Abad-Diaz-De-Cerio, A.; Fernandez-Molina, J.V.; Ramirez-Garcia, A.; Sendino, J.; Hernando, F.L.; Pemán, J.; Garaizar, J.; Rementeria, A. The *aspHS* gene as a new target for detecting *Aspergillus fumigatus* during infections by quantitative real-time PCR. *Med. Mycol.* **2013**, *51*, 545–554. [CrossRef]
61. Bultman, K.M.; Kowalski, C.H.; Cramer, R.A. *Aspergillus fumigatus* virulence through the lens of transcription factors. *Med. Mycol.* **2017**, *55*, 24–38. [CrossRef] [PubMed]
62. Sueiro-Olivares, M.; Fernandez-Molina, J.V.; Abad-Diaz-de-Cerio, A.; Gorospe, E.; Pascual, E.; Guruceaga, X.; Ramirez-Garcia, A.; Garaizar, J.; Hernando, F.L.; Margareto, J.; et al. *Aspergillus fumigatus* transcriptome response to a higher temperature during the earliest steps of germination monitored using a new customized expression microarray. *Microbiology* **2015**, *161*, 490–502. [CrossRef] [PubMed]

Publisher's Note: MDPI stays neutral with regard to jurisdictional claims in published maps and institutional affiliations.

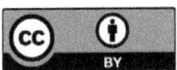

© 2020 by the authors. Licensee MDPI, Basel, Switzerland. This article is an open access article distributed under the terms and conditions of the Creative Commons Attribution (CC BY) license (http://creativecommons.org/licenses/by/4.0/).

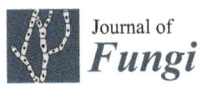

Article

Susceptibility of the *Candida haemulonii* Complex to Echinocandins: Focus on Both Planktonic and Biofilm Life Styles and a Literature Review

Lívia S. Ramos [1], Laura N. Silva [1], Marta H. Branquinha [1] and André L. S. Santos [1,2,*]

[1] Laboratório de Estudos Avançados de Microrganismos Emergentes e Resistentes (LEAMER), Departamento de Microbiologia Geral, Instituto de Microbiologia Paulo de Góes (IMPG), Universidade Federal do Rio de Janeiro (UFRJ), Rio de Janeiro 21941-901, Brazil; liviaramos2@yahoo.com.br (L.S.R.); lauransilva@gmail.com (L.N.S.); mbranquinha@micro.ufrj.br (M.H.B.)

[2] Programa de Pós-Graduação em Bioquímica (PPGBq), Instituto de Química (IQ), Universidade Federal do Rio de Janeiro (UFRJ), Rio de Janeiro 21941-909, Brazil

* Correspondence: andre@micro.ufrj.br; Tel.: +55-21-3938-0366

Received: 20 August 2020; Accepted: 30 September 2020; Published: 1 October 2020

Abstract: *Candida haemulonii* complex (*C. haemulonii*, *C. duobushaemulonii* and *C. haemulonii* var. *vulnera*) is well-known for its resistance profile to different available antifungal drugs. Although echinocandins are the most effective class of antifungal compounds against the *C. haemulonii* species complex, clinical isolates resistant to caspofungin, micafungin and anidulafungin have already been reported. In this work, we present a literature review regarding the effects of echinocandins on this emergent fungal complex. Published data has revealed that micafungin and anidulafungin were more effective than caspofungin against the species forming the *C. haemulonii* complex. Subsequently, we investigated the susceptibilities of both planktonic and biofilm forms of 12 Brazilian clinical isolates of the *C. haemulonii* complex towards caspofungin and micafungin (anidulafungin was unavailable). The planktonic cells of all the fungal isolates were susceptible to both of the test echinocandins. Interestingly, echinocandins caused a significant reduction in the biofilm metabolic activity (viability) of almost all fungal isolates (11/12, 91.7%). Generally, the biofilm biomasses were also affected (reduction range 20–60%) upon exposure to caspofungin and micafungin. This is the first report of the anti-biofilm action of echinocandins against the multidrug-resistant opportunistic pathogens comprising the *C. haemulonii* complex, and unveils the therapeutic potential of these compounds.

Keywords: *Candida haemulonii* complex; planktonic growth; biofilm formation; echinocandins; caspofungin; micafungin

1. Introduction

The members of the *Candida haemulonii* species complex (*C. haemulonii*, *C. duobushaemulonii* and *C. haemulonii* var. *vulnera*) are well-known for their (multi)drug-resistance towards several antifungal agents available in clinical practice. Resistance of the *C. haemulonii* complex to azoles (e.g., fluconazole, itraconazole and voriconazole) and polyenes (e.g., amphotericin B) has been documented extensively [1–7]. On the other hand, susceptibility to prescribed echinocandins (anidulafungin, caspofungin and micafungin) is commonly observed [7–11], although there have been some reports of clinical isolates being resistant to these compounds [5,12].

Echinocandins are the newest class of antifungal agents to be used in clinical practice, exhibiting fungicidal activity against yeasts as well as having a good safety profile [8]. In this sense, the guidelines of the Centers for Disease Control and Prevention (CDC, USA) strongly recommend that echinocandins should be the first choice for the treatment of candidemia in both neutropenic and non-neutropenic patients [9]. The mechanism of action of the echinocandins involves the noncompetitive inhibition of the enzyme β-(1,3)-D-glucan synthase, which is involved in the synthesis of the polysaccharide glucan, resulting in the loss of cell wall integrity and severe stress in the fungal wall [8].

The three clinically available echinocandins usually exhibit both in vitro and in vivo fungicidal activity against a variety of *Candida* species, including those that are intrinsically resistant to azoles or amphotericin B (e.g., *C. krusei*, *C. glabrata* and *C. lusitaniae*), and also emerging species (e.g., *C. famata* and *C. rugosa*) [10]. Additionally, the antifungal activity of echinocandins against *Candida* biofilms represents an aspect that should be highlighted, since microbial biofilm is considered a resistance structure that precludes efficient antimicrobial treatment [10]. For instance, both caspofungin and micafungin, at concentrations attainable in clinical treatments, were able to kill fungal cells in preformed biofilms of either *C. albicans* or *C. parapsilosis* [11]. Therapeutic concentrations of caspofungin and micafungin were active against the biofilms formed by isolates of *C. albicans* and *C. glabrata* recovered from cases of bloodstream infections, but not against *C. tropicalis*, demonstrating that species-specific differences can influence the outcome [12]. Corroborating these findings, caspofungin was also shown to be effective in the treatment and prevention of *C. albicans* biofilms in an in vivo murine model of central venous catheter-associated candidiasis [13].

Considering the aforementioned aspects, the aim of the present study was to evaluate the antifungal susceptibility of both planktonic- and biofilm-forming cells from 12 Brazilian clinical isolates comprising the *C. haemulonii* complex towards caspofungin and micafungin. Furthermore, we have performed a literature review concerning the susceptibility of the *C. haemulonii* species complex towards echinocandins in order to present a comprehensive summary of this field.

2. Materials and Methods

2.1. Microorganisms and Growth Conditions

Twelve clinical fungal isolates, previously identified by molecular methods [6], belonging to the *C. haemulonii* species complex were used in the present study: five isolates of *C. haemulonii* (LIPCh2 recovered from the sole of the foot, GenBank accession number KJ476194; LIPCh3 from a toe nail, KJ476195; LIPCh4 from a finger nail, KJ476196; LIPCh7 from a toe nail, KJ476199; LIPCh12 from blood, KJ476204), four isolates of *C. duobushaemulonii* (LIPCh1 from finger nail, KJ476193; LIPCh6 from a toe nail, KJ476198; LIPCh8 from blood, KJ476200 and LIPCh10 from bronchoalveolar lavage, KJ476202) and three isolates of *C. haemulonii* var. *vulnera* (LIPCh5 from a toe nail, KJ476197; LIPCh9 from urine, KJ476201 and LIPCh11 from blood, KJ476203) [6]. In all experiments, Sabouraud dextrose medium was used to culture the fungal isolates at 37 °C for 48 h under constant agitation (200 rpm). Yeasts were counted in a Neubauer chamber.

2.2. Determination of Minimal Inhibitory Concentration (MIC)

Antifungal susceptibility testing, using the planktonic cells of *C. haemulonii* species complex, against caspofungin and micafungin (Sigma-Aldrich, St. Louis, MO, USA) was performed according to the broth microdilution technique standardized in the M27-Ed4 protocol [14] and interpreted according to the M27-S3 document published by the Clinical and Laboratory Standards Institute (CLSI) [15]. *C. krusei* (ATCC 6258) and *C. parapsilosis* (ATCC 22019) were used as quality control isolates in each test as directed by the CLSI. The clinical breakpoints to echinocandins are detailed below.

2.3. Echinocandins' Breakpoints

Until now, there have been no established breakpoints for echinocandins (or any other antifungal class) regarding the species belonging to the *C. haemulonii* complex. To overcome this problem, researchers working with this fungal complex, as well as "newly identified" *Candida* species, have generally been using a comparative perspective in order to interpret and discuss antifungal susceptibilities. Results are normally presented as CLSI breakpoints which have been established for the *Candida* genus (CLSI document M27S3 [15]) in order to have a minimum (even if not precise) parameter to interpret this kind of experiment. Alternatively, a possible option is to compare the MIC values of *C. haemulonii* complex with the breakpoints established for non-*albicans Candida* species (e.g., *C. glabrata*, *C. tropicalis*, *C. krusei*, *C. parapsilosis* and *C. guilliermondii*) as recently suggested by the CLSI (document M27S4 [16] and protocol M60 [17]). However, this approach varies depending on the particular *Candida* species, since each presents its own breakpoint for each of the echinocandin drugs used. Moreover, the CDC (USA) recently published on its website (https://www.cdc.gov/fungal/candida-auris/c-auris-antifungal.html) a proposal of echinocandins' breakpoints for *C. auris*, a phylogenetically related species to the *C. haemulonii* complex, as follows: resistant breakpoint for caspofungin is ≥2 mg/L and for micafungin and anidulafungin, ≥4 mg/L. After contemplating these various viewpoints, we chose to use, herein, the breakpoints available for *Candida* spp. in the CLSI document M27-S3 [15], which considers as susceptible the strains having MIC values ≤2 mg/L and non-susceptible those with MIC values >2 mg/L for the three clinically available echinocandins; a MIC summary table was prepared.

2.4. Effects of Echinocandins on the Biofilm Formed by the C. haemulonii Species Complex

Fungal suspensions in Sabouraud broth (200 μL containing 10^6 yeast cells) were transferred into each well of a flat-bottom 96-well polystyrene microtiter plate and incubated without agitation at 37 °C for 48 h, which has been shown to be the best incubation time for biofilm formation by species belonging to the *C. haemulonii* complex [18]. Afterwards, the biofilm supernatant fluids were carefully removed, washed once with sterile phosphate-buffered saline (PBS; 10 mM NaH_2PO_4, 10 mM Na_2HPO_4, 150 mM NaCl, pH 7.2) and then 200 μL of Roswell Park Memorial Institute Medium (RPMI) 1640 medium containing different concentrations of echinocandins (range 0.25–8 mg/L) were added to each well. RPMI 1640 medium without echinocandins was used as a positive control and medium-only blanks were used as the negative control. The biofilms were then incubated at 37 °C for an additional 48 h. Afterwards, the supernatant fluids were carefully removed and the wells were washed twice with PBS to remove any non-adherent cells. Finally, two classic biofilm parameters (biomass and metabolic activity/viability) were measured as described below. The results were expressed as percentage of reduction of both viability and biomass. The minimal biofilm eradication concentration (MBEC) was achieved, considering the lowest concentration of each echinocandin capable of causing a 50% reduction in the biofilm viability [19].

2.4.1. Viability Assay

The viability of the fungal cells forming the biofilm was determined using a colorimetric assay that measures the metabolic reduction of 2,3-bis(2-methoxy-4-nitro-5-sulfophenyl)-5-[(phenylamino)carbonyl]-2H-tetrazolium hydroxide (XTT; Sigma-Aldrich) to a water-soluble brown formazan product [20,21]. A XTT/menadione solution was prepared as follows: 2 mg of XTT was dissolved in 10 mL of pre-warmed PBS solution supplemented with 100 μL of a menadione stock solution (made by dissolving 55 mg of menadione in 100 mL of acetone). The XTT/menadione solution (200 μL) was added to all wells containing the biofilms (see Section 2.4 above) and incubated in the dark at 37 °C for 3 h. One hundred microliters of the supernatant from each well were then transferred to a new microplate and the colorimetric readings were measured at 492 nm using a microplate reader (SpectraMax M3; Molecular Devices, Sunnyvale, CA, USA) [21].

2.4.2. Biomass Measurement

Biomass quantification was assessed as described by Peeters et al. [20]. Firstly, biofilms (see Section 2.4 above) were fixed by adding 200 μL of 99% methanol for 15 min. The supernatant was then discarded. Microtiter plates were air-dried for 5 min and then 200 μL of 0.4% crystal violet solution (stock solution diluted in PBS; Sigma-Aldrich) were added to each well and the plates then incubated at room temperature for 20 min. After discarding the crystal violet solution, the wells were washed once with PBS to remove excess stain and the biomass in each well was then decolorized by adding 200 µL of 33% acetic acid for 5 min. One hundred microliters of the acetic acid solution were transferred to a new 96-well plate and the absorbance measured at 590 nm using a microplate reader (SpectraMax M3; Molecular Devices) [21].

2.5. Biofilm Architecture: Confocal Laser Scanning Microscopy (CLSM) Assay

Biofilms were formed on a polystyrene surface and treated as described above with different concentrations of micafungin (0.5–2.0 mg/L). Then, the biofilms were stained with Calcofluor white (Sigma-Aldrich) solution (5 µg/mL) for 1 h at room temperature and protected from the light [21–23]. Subsequently, the biofilms were washed twice with PBS and covered with *n*-propyl-gallate for observation using a confocal microscope (Leica TCS SP5 with OBS, Berlin, Germany). Fiji ImageJ2 software (UW-Madison LOCI, Madison, WI, USA), was used to obtain three-dimensional (3-D) reconstitutions of the biofilms [21,24]. In this way, image analysis was performed using *z*-series image stacks from five randomly chosen spots on each biofilm [21].

2.6. Literature Review

This exercise involved the compilation of available data regarding the susceptibility of the *C. haemulonii* species complex to echinocandins. The literature search was performed on 19 July 2020 using the following four databases: PubMed (https://pubmed.ncbi.nlm.nih.gov), Web of Science (https://webofknowledge.com), Google Scholar (https://scholar.google.com) and Scielo (https://scielo.org/). The term "Candida haemulonii" was added in the category "title/abstract" in the PubMed Advanced Search Builder and in the Web of Science databases, while in Google Scholar the search was conducted in the advanced search area, including the term "Candida haemulonii" and selecting the option "with the exact phrase in the title"; finally, for the Scielo database, we only used the search term "Candida haemulonii" in the general search. Papers available in English and published after the reclassification of the *C. haemulonii* complex by Cendejas-Bueno et al. [5] were selected. Subsequently, the list of results from each database was exported to the EndNote® software (version X1), using the "Output Records" tool in order to eliminate possibly duplicated references by means of the "Find Duplicates" tool. Finally, the papers were individually analyzed in order to select those that described either MIC or geometric-mean (GM)-MIC values of the *C. haemulonii* complex for echinocandins.

2.7. Statistics

All experiments were performed in triplicate, in three independent experimental sets. The results were analyzed statistically by the Analysis of Variance One-Way ANOVA (comparisons between three or more groups). All analyzes were performed using the GraphPad Prism5 program. For all analyses, *p* values of 0.05 or less were considered statistically significant.

3. Results and Discussion

3.1. Susceptibility of Planktonic Cells of the C. haemulonii Species Complex to Echinocandins

According to the breakpoints suggested in the M27S3 document published by CLSI, the planktonic cells of all clinical isolates of the *C. haemulonii* complex tested herein were considered susceptible to echinocandins, with MIC values ranging from 0.125 to 0.5 mg/L for caspofungin and 0.25–0.5 mg/L for micafungin (Table 1). For instance, a recent report described the successful use of caspofungin (MIC of ≤0.125 mg/L) in the treatment of a case of catheter-related candidemia caused by *C. haemulonii* in a pediatric patient in Mexico [25], whose fungal isolate exhibited in vitro high MICs for azoles (fluconazole MIC ≥ 256 mg/L, posaconazole ≥ 8 mg/L, itraconazole, ketoconazole and voriconazole ≥ 16 mg/L) and amphotericin B (MIC 1–2 mg/L). Some years before, a catheter-related candidemia in an adult patient hospitalized for a long period was only resolved when fluconazole treatment was replaced by caspofungin [4].

Table 1. MIC values of echinocandins against the *C. haemulonii* species complex studied herein.

Fungal Species	MIC (mg/L)	
Isolates	Caspofungin [b]	Micafungin
C. haemulonii		
LIP*Ch*2	0.5	0.25
LIP*Ch*3	0.5	0.5
LIP*Ch*4	0.5	0.5
LIP*Ch*7	0.25	0.25
LIP*Ch*12	0.125	0.25
GM-MIC [a]	**0.33**	**0.33**
Arithmetic mean	0.37	0.35
C. duobushaemulonii		
LIP*Ch*1	0.125	0.25
LIP*Ch*6	0.25	0.5
LIP*Ch*8	0.125	0.25
LIP*Ch*10	0.25	0.25
GM-MIC	**0.18**	**0.30**
Arithmetic mean	0.19	0.31
C. haemulonii var. *vulnera*		
LIP*Ch*5	0.25	0.25
LIP*Ch*9	0.25	0.25
LIP*Ch*11	0.5	0.25
GM-MIC	**0.32**	**0.25**
Arithmetic mean	0.33	0.25
Overall GM-MIC	**0.26**	**0.30**
Overall arithmetic mean	0.30	0.31

[a] GM-MIC, geometric mean-minimal inhibitory concentration. [b] Similar results were reported in our previously published paper [6]. Journal of Antimicrobial Chemotherapy (JAC) provided the permission to reproduce this set of results.

In general, echinocandins are highly active in vitro against species comprising the *C. haemulonii* complex [7,26–29], but the existence of isolates resistant to this class of antifungals has already been reported [4,5,30]. Herein, we conducted a careful review of the literature regarding the susceptibility of the *C. haemulonii* species complex to the three clinically available echinocandins, including only papers published after the species reclassification and the creation of the *C. haemulonii* complex [5]. Using the keyword "Candida haemulonii" in the search section, 148, 63, 46 and 5 publications were located from the Web of Science, PubMed, Google Scholar and Scielo databases, respectively (Table 2). However, only a small fraction of these published papers (varying from 12.2%–28.3%) cited the in vitro susceptibility profile of the *C. haemulonii* species complex against echinocandins. In this sense, we recovered a total of 21 distinct papers that fitted our established criteria and, for these reasons, they were selected for data extraction as follows: 5 (23.8%) papers studied the three members forming the *C. haemulonii* complex, 6 (28.6%) studied only two species (*C. haemulonii* and *C. duobushaemulonii*) and 10 (47.6%) studied only one species (*C. haemulonii*, $n = 6$, *C. duobushaemulonii*, $n = 3$, *C. haemulonii* var. *vulnera*, $n = 1$). Furthermore, 13 (61.9%) papers detailed the MIC value for each isolate investigated, while the remaining studies ($n = 8$; 38.1%) only presented the geometric mean (GM)-MIC and/or the range of MIC values for the fungal isolates against the test echinocandins. Finally, 12 (57.1%) papers tested the three echinocandins, 5 (23.8%) used two and 4 (19.1%) tested only one echinocandin, with caspofungin being the most frequently evaluated.

Table 2. Number of publications retrieved from database searches using the term "Candida haemulonii".

Database	Total Number of Papers	Number of Selected Papers *	References of the Selected Papers *
Web of Science	148	18	[5,7,25,29,31–44]
PubMed	63	16	[5,7,25,29,31–35,39–41,43–46]
Google Scholar	46	13	[5,7,25,29,31–33,35,36,40,44,46,47]
Scielo	5	1	[31]

The searches were conducted in PubMed (https://pubmed.ncbi.nlm.nih.gov), Web of Science (https://webofknowledge.com), Google Scholar (https://scholar.google.com/) and Scielo (https://scielo.org) on 19 July 2020. The term "Candida haemulonii" was added in the category "title/abstract" in the PubMed Advanced Search Builder and Web of Science; in Google Scholar the search was conducted in the advanced search area, including the term "Candida haemulonii" and selecting the option "with the exact phrase in the title"; in Scielo, we only searched for the term "Candida haemulonii" in the general search. Papers published after the reclassification of the C. haemulonii complex were included [5]. * Papers that evaluated the susceptibility of isolates of the C. haemulonii species complex to echinocandins.

The results emanating from this literature review revealed that micafungin and anidulafungin appeared to be more effective than caspofungin against the three species forming the C. haemulonii complex (Table 3) [5,7,25,29,31–47]. In this respect, 89.8% of the isolates of C. haemulonii exhibited susceptibility to caspofungin, while 96.3% and 98.4% were susceptible to micafungin and anidulafungin, respectively. Regarding C. duboushaemulonii, 95.5% of the isolates were susceptible to caspofungin, 99.1% to anidulafungin and 100.0% to micafungin. Finally, considering the clinical isolates of C. haemulonii var. vulnera, 85.0% were susceptible to caspofungin, 91.7% to micafungin and 97.1% to anidulafungin. Indeed, the MIC frequency distribution demonstrated that the modal MIC of echinocandins against the C. haemulonii complex was ≤0.12 mg/L in almost all cases (Table 4).

Table 3. Literature compilation regarding the distribution (%) of the susceptible (S) and non-susceptible (NS) isolates belonging to the C. haemulonii complex against echinocandins described in published papers available until 19 July 2020.

Fungal Species	Susceptibility Profile (%) *					
	Caspofungin		Micafungin		Anidulafungin	
	S	NS	S	NS	S	NS
C. haemulonii	89.8	10.2	96.3	3.7	98.4	1.6
	$n = 157$		$n = 136$		$n = 185$	
C. duobushaemulonii	95.5	4.5	100	0	99.1	0.9
	$n = 111$		$n = 105$		$n = 110$	
C. haemulonii var. vulnera	85.0	15.0	91.7	8.3	97.1	2.9
	$n = 20$		$n = 12$		$n = 35$	

* Antifungal susceptibility testing was interpreted according to the document M27-S3 published by CLSI; n, number of fungal isolates; the references used to construct this table were [5,7,25,29,31–47].

Comparing the GM-MIC values of our clinical isolates (Table 1) with those compiled from the literature reports (for these comparisons, we used the arithmetic mean of the GM-MIC values of the selected works, as summarized in Table 5), we observed that the GM-MIC values of caspofungin for our isolates of C. haemulonii, C. duobushaemulonii and C. haemulonii var. vulnera were higher than those reported in the literature (0.33 mg/L versus 0.18 mg/L for C. haemulonii, 0.18 mg/L versus 0.11 mg/L, for C. duobushaemulonii and 0.32 mg/L versus 0.21 mg/L for C. haemulonii var. vulnera). Similarly, GM-MIC values for micafungin calculated from the literature reports were lower than ours (0.18 mg/L versus 0.33 mg/L for C. haemulonii, 0.17 mg/L versus 0.30 mg/L for C. duobushaemulonii, and 0.13 mg/L versus 0.25 mg/L for C. haemulonii var. vulnera). Finally, based on the analysis of the literature data, anidulafungin also produced low GM-MIC values for the three fungal species of the

C. haemulonii complex (GM-MICs of 0.16, 0.32 and 0.06 mg/L for C. haemulonii, C. duobuhaemulonii and C. haemulonii var. vulnera, respectively).

Table 4. MIC distribution of C. haemulonii complex isolates obtained from the literature review against the three echinocandins.

Drug [a] Species	MIC (mg/L)												MIC_{50} [b]	MIC_{90} [c]
	≤0.015	0.03	0.06	0.12	0.25	0.5	1	2	4	8	16	>16	Range		
CAS															
Ch		<u>19</u>	17	14	12	6	1			1	1	14	0.03–>16	0.12	>16
Cd	3	14	18	<u>20</u>	9	4	1			1	1	3	≤0.015–>16	0.12	0.5
Chv				<u>2</u>	5	<u>4</u>						3	0.12–>16	0.25	>16
MCF															
Ch	8	12	<u>28</u>	8	4	1						4	≤0.015–>16	0.06	0.25
Cd	2	12	<u>36</u>	12	3	1							0.06–0.5	0.06	0.12
Chv			1	<u>4</u>								1	0.06–>16	0.12	0.12
ANF															
Ch	<u>27</u>	14	19	10	3	1		1				2	≤0.015–>16	0.03	0.12
Cd	11	8	<u>17</u>	16	15	4	3	1	1				≤0.015–4	0.12	0.5
Chv	<u>8</u>	1	4									1	≤0.015–>16	≤0.015	0.06

[a] CAS, caspofungin; MCF, micafungin; ANF, anidulafungin; [b] MIC_{50}, MIC at which 50% of isolates were inhibited; [c] MIC_{90}, MIC at which 90% of isolates were inhibited; Modal MICs are indicated with underlined numbers; MIC values of <0.03 were allocated as ≤0.015; Clinical and Laboratory Standards Institute (CLSI) document M27S3 suggests the following breakpoints for echinocandins against Candida spp.: susceptible ≤ 2 mg/L and non-susceptible > 2 mg/L; the references used to construct this table were [5,29,31,34,35,38–42,44,46,47].

Table 5. Literature review on the antifungal susceptibility of different isolates of the C. haemulonii complex to echinocandins.

Reference Number	Fungal Species (Number of Isolates)	GM-MIC (Range) *		
		Caspofungin	Micafungin	Anidulafungin
[5] •	Ch (n = 19)	11.10 [(#)] (0.25–>16)	0.17 [(#)] (<0.03–>16)	0.06 [(#)] (<0.03–>16)
	Cd (n = 7)	5.38 [(#)] (0.5–>16)	0.06 (0.06–0.12)	0.08 [(#)] (<0.03–4)
	Chv (n = 4)	11.31 [(#)] (0.5–16)	0.40 [(#)] (0.06–>16)	0.20 [(#)] (<0.03–>16)
[29] •	Ch (n = 14)	0.12 (0.125–0.5)	-	0.015 (0.015–0.015)
	Cd (n = 9)	0.22 [(#)] (0.06–16)	-	0.06 (0.015–0.5)
	Chv (n = 8)	0.26 (0.125–0.5)	-	0.016 (0.015–0.03)
[33] •	Ch (n = 6)/Chv (n = 1)	0.18 (0.06–1)	0.27 (0.125–1)	0.45 (0.25–1)
	Cd (n = 8)	0.13 (0.06–0.25)	0.38 (0.125–1)	0.54 (0.5–1)
[7] •	Ch (n = 26)	ND (0.03–0.5)	ND (0.06–0.5)	ND (0.015–0.5)
	Cd (n = 5)	ND (0.06–0.12)	ND (0.06–0.12)	ND (0.06–0.25)
[35] ○	Ch (n = 3)	0.5 (0.5–0.5)	0.19 (0.12–0.5)	0.03 (0.03–0.03)
[39] ○	Cd (n = 2)	-	0.12 (0.06–0.25)	0.04 (0.03–0.06)
[40] ○	Ch (n = 3)	0.10 (0.06–0.125)	0.20 (0.125–0.25)	-
[44] ○	Ch (n = 38)	0.06 [(#)] (0.03–16)	0.04 (<0.08–0.12)	0.05 (0.03–0.25)
	Cd (n = 55)	0.07 (0.016–0.5)	0.06 (0.016–0.25)	0.13 (0.016–2)
[32] •	Ch (n = 7)	0.19 (0.06–1)	0.28 (0.125–1)	0.44 (0.25–1)
	Cd (n = 5)	0.14 (0.06–0.25)	0.35 (0.125–1)	0.56 (0.5–1)
[45] •	Ch (n = 21)	-	-	0.10 (0.06–0.25)
	Cd (n = 13)	-	-	0.10 (0.03–0.5)
	Chv (n = 15)	-	-	0.13 (0.03–0.25)
[43] •	Ch (n = 32)	0.104 (ND)	0.106 (ND)	0.103 (ND)
[36] •	Ch (n = 16)	0.13[(#)] (0.015–8)	0.11[(#)] (0.03–8)	0.09 (0.015–0.5)
	Cd (n = 3)	5.03[(#)] (1–16)	0.06 (0.015–0.06)	0.79 (0.5–2)
	Chv (n = 5)	0.12 (0.06–0.25)	0.14 (0.12–0.25)	0.05 (0.015–0.12)
[42] ○	Ch (n = 4)	0.06 (0.03–0.12)	-	-
[47] ○	Chv (n = 2)	0.25 (0.25–0.25)	0.12 (0.12–0.12)	0.06 (0.06–0.06)

Table 5. Cont.

Reference Number	Fungal Species (Number of Isolates)	GM-MIC (Range) *		
		Caspofungin	Micafungin	Anidulafungin
Arithmetic mean of overall GM-MIC, except for the resistant strains[#]				
	Ch	0.18 ± 0.15	0.18 ± 0.09	0.16 ± 0.18
	Cd	0.11 ± 0.04	0.17 ± 0.15	0.32 ± 0.30
	Chv	0.21 ± 0.08	0.13 ± 0.01	0.06 ± 0.05

* GM-MIC, geometric mean of the minimal inhibitory concentrations expressed in mg/L; • Values of GM-MIC obtained directly from the papers; ○ Values of GM-MIC calculated by us from the MIC values for each isolate mentioned in the articles; Ch, C. haemulonii; Cd, C. duobushaemulonii; Chv, C. haemulonii var. vulnera; n, number of isolates studied; arithmetic mean of overall GM-MIC calculated from the GM-MIC of the different papers; ND, not determined; -, no isolates were tested.

In summary, the majority of literature reported GM-MIC concentration values of <0.5 mg/L for the three echinocandins against the *C. haemulonii* species complex. Nevertheless, two works warranted specific attention: Cendejas-Bueno et al. [5], in which the GM-MIC values for caspofungin for the three members of the *C. haemulonii* complex were disproportionately high in comparison to our present results and those given in the other literature publications; and Isla et al. [36], in which the GM-MIC value obtained for caspofungin against the *C. duobushaemulonii* isolates was considerably higher (Table 5). A possible explanation for the high MIC values found in the aforementioned papers is the possible occurrence of paradoxical growth effect (also known as the Eagle effect), that is characterized by reduced activity of the antifungal agents at high concentrations. In fact, Cendejas-Bueno et al. [5] stressed this discussion in their study, but in a superficial way. A recent study conducted with 106 clinical isolates of *C. auris* demonstrated that the vast majority of isolates were susceptible to the echinocandins; however, they exhibited different intensities of paradoxical growth effect in the presence of caspofungin, whilst four isolates were resistant to echinocandins and had a mutation in hot spot region 1 of the *FKS* gene [48]. Interestingly, those isolates presenting paradoxical growth effect were susceptible to caspofungin at doses used in human treatment, while those with *FKS1* mutation were still resistant in a murine model of invasive candidiasis, demonstrating that only the isolates with the mutations display in vivo echinocandin resistance [48].

3.2. Effects of Echinocandins on the Biofilm Formed by C. haemulonii Species Complex

In order to evaluate the effects of echinocandins (caspofungin and micafungin) on the viability and biomass of the biofilms formed by the clinical isolates of the *C. haemulonii* complex, the mature biofilms were firstly incubated with different concentrations of the antifungals and then analyzed. The metabolic activity of viable fungal cells was assessed by their ability to reduce XTT to formazan, whilst the decrease in biofilm biomass was measured spectroscopically by looking at the incorporation of crystal violet into methanol-fixed, non-viable cells (Figures 1 and 2). In general, the test echinocandins were found to be more efficient at reducing cell viability than decreasing the biomass of the *C. haemulonii* complex biofilms.

The decrease of both viability and biomass parameters by caspofungin was isolate-dependent. At the lowest concentration used (0.25 mg/L) this echinocandin caused a statistically significant reduction in the viability of all of the fungal cells tested ($p < 0.05$; One-way ANOVA analysis of variance, Dunnett's multiple comparison test), varying from 30–80% among the different isolates (Figure 1). However, caspofungin was unable to reduce the biomass of some of the *C. haemulonii* isolates (LIPCh2, LIPCh3 and LIPCh4) even at the highest concentration used. Nevertheless, for the remaining fungal isolates the drug caused a biomass reduction of up to 60% (mainly against the *C. duobushaemulonii* isolates) (Figure 2). The isolates LIP*Ch*2 (*C. haemulonii*), LIP*Ch*1 (*C. duobushaemulonii*) and LIP*Ch*5 (*C. haemulonii* var. *vulnera*) were less susceptible to caspofungin at the higher concentrations (Figure 1).

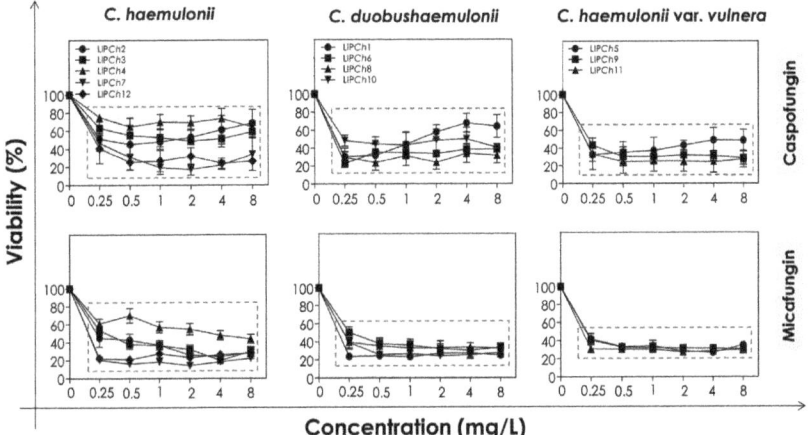

Figure 1. Cell viability of biofilms formed by clinical isolates comprising the *C. haemulonii* complex exposed to different concentrations of echinocandins (caspofungin and micafungin). The results were assessed spectroscopically (492 nm) by XTT reduction and expressed as the mean of metabolic activity percentages compared to untreated biofilms (control), which correspond to 100%. The graphs exhibit the mean ± standard deviation of three independent experiments. The dashed boxes represent the concentrations of echinocandins that caused statistically significant reduction of cell viability in relation to the respective control ($p < 0.05$; One-way ANOVA analysis of variance, Dunnett's multiple comparison test).

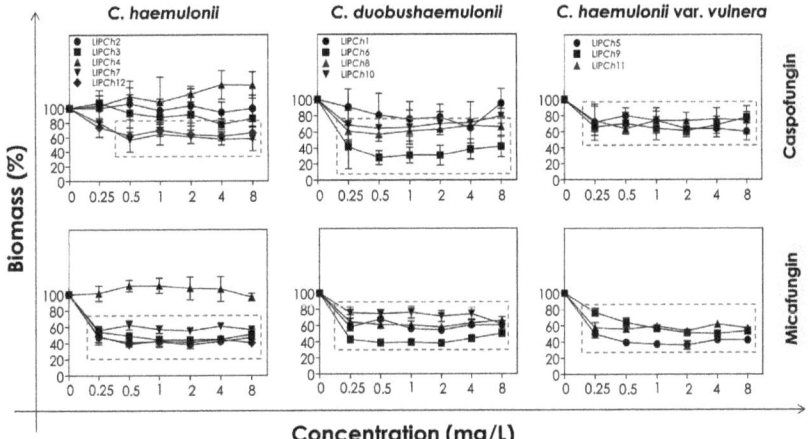

Figure 2. Biomass of biofilms formed by clinical isolates comprising the *C. haemulonii* species complex exposed to different concentrations of echinocandins (caspofungin and micafungin). The amount of crystal violet incorporated by the cells was assessed spectroscopically (absorbance at 590 nm) and the results expressed as the mean of biomass percentages compared to untreated biofilms (control), which correspond to 100%. The graphs show the mean ± standard deviation of three independent experiments. The dashed boxes represent the concentrations of echinocandins that caused a statistically significant reduction in biomass in relation to the respective control ($p < 0.05$; One-way ANOVA analysis of variance, Dunnett's multiple comparison test).

Micafungin proved to be more effective than caspofungin at disturbing both biofilm viability and biomass. A decrease in biofilm viability of up to 60% was seen among most of the clinical isolates, especially against *C. duobushaemulonii* and *C. haemulonii* var. *vulnera* (Figure 1). Unlike caspofungin, micafungin showed a decrease of up to 60% on the biofilm biomass of *C. haemulonii* isolates, with the exception of isolate LIP*Ch*4, which forms a very dense and robust biofilm (Figure 2). For the *C. duobushaemulonii* and *C. haemulonii* var. *vulnera* isolates, micafungin reduced biomass in the range 20–60% (Figure 2). In summary, the lowest concentration of micafungin used was able to significantly reduce the cell viability and the biomasses of biofilms formed by all of the test isolates, expect for the biomass of one isolate.

The determination of MBEC, which was defined as the lowest antifungal concentration able to reduce the biofilm viability in 50% [19], revealed that the biofilms of all isolates remained susceptible to echinocandins, with the exception of the isolate LIP*Ch*4 of *C. haemulonii* (Table 6). This fact could be explained by the ability of the isolate LIP*Ch*4 to form very robust biofilm on polystyrene in comparison with the other isolates [18,21], hampering the action of echinocandins due to the high amount of fungal cells-forming the biofilm architecture as well as due to the high production of extracellular matrix that can block the antifungal penetration into the biofilm structure.

Table 6. Minimal biofilm eradication concentration (MBEC) to echinocandins against *C. haemulonii* complex.

Echinocandins	MBEC (mg/L)											
	C. haemulonii Isolates					*C. duobushaemulonii* Isolates				*C. haemulonii* var. *vulnera* Isolates		
	Ch2	Ch3	Ch4	Ch7	Ch12	Ch1	Ch6	Ch8	Ch10	Ch5	Ch9	Ch11
Caspofungin	0.5	2	>8	0.25	0.25	<0.25	<0.25	<0.25	0.25	0.25	0.25	0.25
Micafungin	0.25	0.5	8	<0.25	<0.25	<0.25	0.5	0.25	0.25	0.25	<0.25	<0.25

As micafungin was more active than caspofungin against the mature biofilms formed by the *C. haemulonii* species complex it was chosen for further studies. In order to verify the 3-D organization of the biofilms following exposure to micafungin two isolates of *C. haemulonii* were selected: LIP*Ch*3, to represent the isolates having susceptible biofilms, and LIP*Ch*4, to represent isolates forming resistant biofilms. CLSM analysis was conducted using Calcofluor white, which binds to the chitin in the fungal cell wall, to evidence the biofilm biomass. The CLSM analysis corroborated the results observed by crystal violet approach, with the lowest antifungal concentration used causing a drastic reduction in the biofilm biomass of LIP*Ch*3, whilst even the highest concentration of micafungin failed to affect the biofilm formed by LIP*Ch*4 (Figure 3).

Until now, no information has been available in the literature regarding the activity of conventional antifungal agents against the biofilm formed by the *C. haemulonii* species complex. A recent study conducted with *C. auris*, which belongs to the *C. haemulonii* clade, showed that, despite the susceptibility of planktonic cells to echinocandins and amphotericin B, the biofilms were not vulnerable, exhibiting MBECs which were 512-fold higher than their planktonic MIC counterparts [19]. Actually, the biofilm formed by *C. auris* is not as robust as those arising from *C. albicans* and *C. glabrata*, but its tolerance to the major classes of antifungal agents is notable, especially for amphotericin B and micafungin, which are the recommended antifungal therapeutics for infections caused by *C. albicans* biofilms [49]. The antifungal tolerance of the *C. auris* biofilm has been shown to be phase-dependent, with the mature biofilms resistant to the three available antifungal drug classes [50]. On the other hand, micafungin has been shown to be effective against both planktonic and biofilm-forming *C. albicans* cells, while its effectiveness against *C. parapsilosis* was considered to be moderate [51]. Additionally, micafungin concentrations >2 mg/L prevented the regrowth of *Candida* biofilm cells [51]. Regarding the *C. parapsilosis* complex, caspofungin was more active against biofilms of *C. orthopsilosis* than *C. parapsilosis* sensu strictu, with 20% and 86% of isolates resistant to this antifungal, respectively, suggesting that a treatment of catheter-related candidemia caused by *C. orthopsilosis* with caspofungin would be more effective than against *C. parapsilosis* sensu strictu [52]. A study, conducted with five different *Candida* species recovered from cases of bloodstream infections demonstrated both species-specific and drug-specific differences in *Candida* biofilms regarding their susceptibility to echinocandins [53]. In this sense, while *C. albicans* and *C. krusei* biofilms were susceptible to the three clinically available echinocandins, *C. lusitaniae*, *C. guilliermondii* and *C. parapsilosis* were quite resistant to them [53]. In addition, micafungin seemed to be the most effective echinocandin against *C. parapsilosis* biofilms, presenting lower MBECs against this *Candida* species in comparison to caspofungin and anidulafungin [53]. These observations reinforce the need to determine the correct identification of the actual fungal species causing the candidiasis infection and, further, to assess its antifungal susceptibility profile against both planktonic and biofilm-forming cells in order to choose the best therapeutic option for each case.

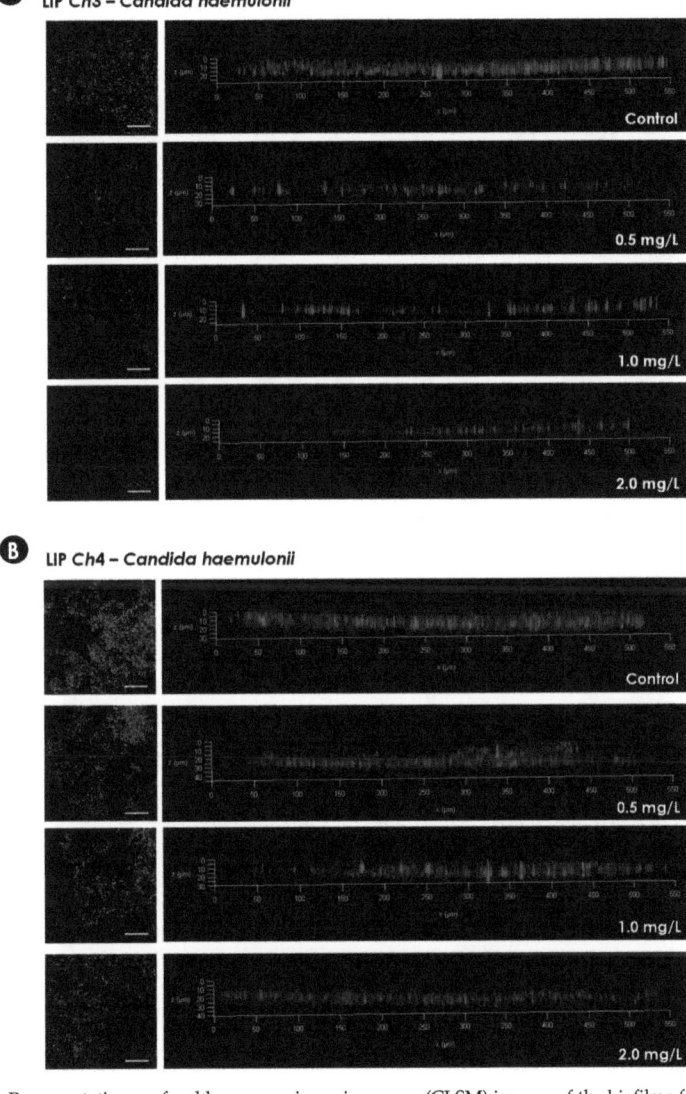

Figure 3. Representative confocal laser scanning microscopy (CLSM) images of the biofilms formed by *C. haemulonii* on a polystyrene surface. Yeasts (200 μL containing 10^6 cells) were placed to interact with the

polystyrene for 48 h at 37 °C. Subsequently, the supernatant fluids were removed and washed with PBS, and 200 µL of RPMI 1640 medium containing different concentrations of micafungin were added. The biofilms were incubated at 37 °C for an additional 48 h. Afterwards, the supernatant fluids were carefully removed again, and the wells were washed twice with PBS to remove non-adherent cells. Finally, the biofilms were stained with Calcofluor white in order to evidence the fungal biomass. The panels on the left represent the top view images of the fungal biofilms visualized by Confocal Laser Scanning Microscopy (CLSM) (bars represent 5 µm). The graphs on the right represent the three-dimensional reconstruction of the biofilms formed. The isolate LIPCh3 of *C. haemulonii* (**A**) was chosen to represent susceptible biofilms, while the isolate LIPCh4 of *C. haemulonii* (**B**) represents resistant biofilms.

Furthermore, we observed that one isolate of each species forming the *C. haemulonii* complex showed a smaller reduction in cell viability when incubated in the presence of higher concentrations of the echinocandins. This phenomenon is called paradoxical growth, and it corresponds to the decreased sensitivity to echinocandins in the presence of concentrations higher than the MIC values. To date, the evidence strongly suggests that this paradoxical effect is more commonly associated with caspofungin than either micafungin or anidulafungin [54]. This effect has already been documented for biofilms formed by other *Candida* species, such as *C. albicans* [53,55], *C. parapsilosis* [53], *C. tropicalis* [55] and *C. dubliniensis* [56].

To finalize, we recognize some of the limitations associated with the present study, such as the limited number of isolates used and the exclusion of anidulafungin. The experiments were conducted with only 12 clinical isolates of the *C. haemulonii* complex due to the difficulties in obtaining more isolates, since it is quite a rare fungal complex. Additionally, we tested only two of the three echinocandins currently in clinical use, and this was because at the time the experiments were conducted anidulafungin was not available for scientific research purposes.

4. Conclusions

In addition to their own clinical conditions, hospitalized patients are at constant risk of acquiring contagions associated with the hospital environment. Biofilm-related *Candida* infections represent an important and worrisome threat to these patients, and there is a limited number of available antifungal agents of sufficient potency to break down these highly resistant structures. In this sense, echinocandins are considered highly active against various *Candida* species and the results presented herein reinforce the potential of echinocandins to treat biofilm-related infections caused by the emergent and multidrug-resistant species comprising the *C. haemulonii* complex.

Author Contributions: All authors conceived and designed the experiments. L.S.R. performed the experiments. All authors analyzed the data. M.H.B. and A.L.S.S. contributed reagents/materials/analysis tools. All authors wrote and revised the paper. All authors contributed to the research and approved the final version of the manuscript. All authors agree to be accountable for all aspects of the work. All authors have read and agreed to the published version of the manuscript.

Funding: This work was supported by grants from Fundação Carlos Chagas Filho de Amparo à Pesquisa do Estado do Rio de Janeiro (FAPERJ) and Conselho Nacional de Desenvolvimento Científico e Tecnológico (CNPq) and Coordenação de Aperfeiçoamento de Pessoal de Nível Superior (CAPES—Financial code 001).

Acknowledgments: The authors would like to thank Denise Rocha de Souza (UFRJ) for technical assistance in the experiments and Grasiella Matioszek (UFRJ) for confocal analyses. The authors would like to thank Malachy McCann (Department of Chemistry at the National University of Ireland Maynooth—NUIM, Ireland) for his valuable contribution to the critical review and editing of English.

Conflicts of Interest: The authors declare no conflict of interest.

References

1. Khan, Z.U.; Al-Sweih, N.A.; Ahmad, S.; Al-Kazemi, N.; Khan, S.; Joseph, L.; Chandy, R. Outbreak of fungemia among neonates caused by *Candida haemulonii* resistant to amphotericin B, itraconazole, and fluconazole. *J. Clin. Microbiol.* **2007**, *45*, 2025–2027. [CrossRef] [PubMed]
2. Pfaller, M.A.; Diekema, D.J.; Gibbs, D.L.; Newell, V.A.; Ellis, D.; Tullio, V.; Rodloff, A.; Fu, W.; Ling, T.A. Results from the ARTEMIS DISK Global Antifungal Surveillance Study, 1997 to 2007: A 10.5-year analysis of susceptibilities of *Candida* Species to fluconazole and voriconazole as determined by CLSI standardized disk diffusion. *J. Clin. Microbiol.* **2010**, *48*, 1366–1377. [CrossRef] [PubMed]
3. Gomez-Lopez, A.; Buitrago, M.J.; Rodriguez-Tudela, J.L.; Cuenca-Estrella, M. in vitro antifungal susceptibility pattern and ergosterol content in clinical yeast strains. *Rev. Iberoam. Micol.* **2011**, *28*, 100–103. [CrossRef]
4. Kim, S.; Ko, K.S.; Moon, S.Y.; Lee, M.S.; Lee, M.Y.; Son, J.S. Catheter-related candidemia caused by *Candida haemulonii* in a patient in long-term hospital care. *J. Korean Med. Sci.* **2011**, *26*, 297–300. [CrossRef]
5. Cendejas-Bueno, E.; Kolecka, A.; Alastruey-Izquierdo, A.; Theelen, B.; Groenewald, M.; Kostrzewa, M.; Cuenca-Estrella, M.; Gomez-Lopez, A.; Boekhout, T. Reclassification of the *Candida haemulonii* complex as *Candida haemulonii* (*C. haemulonii* group I), *C. duobushaemulonii* sp. nov. (*C. haemulonii* group II), and *C. haemulonii* var. *vulnera* var. nov.: Three multiresistant human pathogenic yeasts. *J. Clin. Microbiol.* **2012**, *50*, 3641–3651. [CrossRef] [PubMed]
6. Ramos, L.S.; Figueiredo-Carvalho, M.H.; Barbedo, L.S.; Ziccardi, M.; Chaves, A.L.; Zancope-Oliveira, R.M.; Pinto, M.R.; Sgarbi, D.B.; Dornelas-Ribeiro, M.; Branquinha, M.H.; et al. *Candida haemulonii* complex: Species identification and antifungal susceptibility profiles of clinical isolates from Brazil. *J. Antimicrob. Chemother.* **2015**, *70*, 111–115. [CrossRef] [PubMed]
7. Hou, X.; Xiao, M.; Chen, S.C.; Wang, H.; Cheng, J.W.; Chen, X.X.; Xu, Z.P.; Fan, X.; Kong, F.; Xu, Y.C. Identification and antifungal susceptibility profiles of *Candida haemulonii* species complex clinical isolates from a Multicenter Study in China. *J. Clin. Microbiol.* **2016**, *54*, 2676–2680. [CrossRef] [PubMed]
8. Shapiro, R.S.; Robbins, N.; Cowen, L.E. Regulatory circuitry governing fungal development, drug resistance, and disease. *Microbiol. Mol. Biol. Rev.* **2011**, *75*, 213–267. [CrossRef] [PubMed]
9. Pappas, P.G.; Kauffman, C.A.; Andes, D.R.; Clancy, C.J.; Marr, K.A.; Ostrosky-Zeichner, L.; Reboli, A.C.; Schuster, M.G.; Vazquez, J.A.; Walsh, T.J.; et al. Clinical Practice Guideline for the management of candidiasis: 2016 update by the Infectious Diseases Society of America. *Clin. Infect. Dis.* **2015**, *62*, e1–e50. [CrossRef] [PubMed]
10. Chen, S.C.; Slavin, M.A.; Sorrell, T.C. Echinocandin antifungal drugs in fungal infections: A comparison. *Drugs* **2011**, *71*, 11–41. [CrossRef]
11. Kuhn, D.M.; George, T.; Chandra, J.; Mukherjee, P.K.; Ghannoum, M.A. Antifungal susceptibility of *Candida* biofilms: Unique efficacy of amphotericin B lipid formulations and echinocandins. *Antimicrob. Agents Chemother.* **2002**, *46*, 1773–1780. [CrossRef] [PubMed]
12. Choi, H.W.; Shin, J.H.; Jung, S.I.; Park, K.H.; Cho, D.; Kee, S.J.; Shin, M.G.; Suh, S.P.; Ryang, D.W. Species-specific differences in the susceptibilities of biofilms formed by *Candida* bloodstream isolates to echinocandin antifungals. *Antimicrob. Agents Chemother.* **2007**, *51*, 1520–1523. [CrossRef] [PubMed]
13. Lazzell, A.L.; Chaturvedi, A.K.; Pierce, C.G.; Prasad, D.; Uppuluri, P.; Lopez-Ribot, J.L. Treatment and prevention of *Candida albicans* biofilms with caspofungin in a novel central venous catheter murine model of candidiasis. *J. Antimicrob. Chemother.* **2009**, *64*, 567–570. [CrossRef] [PubMed]
14. CLSI. *Reference Method for Broth Dilution Antifungal Susceptibility Testing of Yeasts, CLSI Standard M27*, 4th ed.; CLSI: Wayne, PA, USA, 2017.
15. CLSI. *Reference Method for Broth Dilution Antifungal Susceptibility Testing of Yeasts. Third Informational Supplement, CLSI Document M27-S3*; CLSI: Wayne, PA, USA, 2018; Volume 28.
16. CLSI. *Reference Method for Broth Dilution Antifungal Susceptibility Testing of Yeasts. Fourth Informational Supplement, CLSI Document M27S4*; CLSI: Wayne, PA, USA, 2012.
17. CLSI. CLSI Document M60. In *Performance Standards for Antifungal Susceptibility Testing of Yeasts*, 2nd ed.; CLSI: Wayne, PA, USA, 2020; Volume 40.
18. Ramos, L.S.; Oliveira, S.S.C.; Souto, X.M.; Branquinha, M.H.; Santos, A.L.S. Planktonic growth and biofilm formation profiles in *Candida haemulonii* species complex. *Med. Mycol.* **2017**, *55*, 785–789. [CrossRef] [PubMed]

19. Romera, D.; Aguilera-Correa, J.J.; Gadea, I.; Vinuela-Sandoval, L.; Garcia-Rodriguez, J.; Esteban, J. *Candida auris*: A comparison between planktonic and biofilm susceptibility to antifungal drugs. *J. Med. Microbiol.* **2019**, *68*, 1353–1358. [CrossRef] [PubMed]
20. Peeters, E.; Nelis, H.J.; Coenye, T. Comparison of multiple methods for quantification of microbial biofilms grown in microtiter plates. *J. Microbiol. Methods* **2008**, *72*, 157–165. [CrossRef]
21. Ramos, L.S.; Mello, T.P.; Branquinha, M.H.; Santos, A.L.S. Biofilm formed by *Candida haemulonii* species complex: Structural analysis and extracellular matrix composition. *J. Fungi* **2020**, *6*, 46. [CrossRef]
22. Chandra, J.; Mukherjee, P.K.; Ghannoum, M.A. In vitro growth and analysis of *Candida* biofilms. *Nat. Protoc.* **2008**, *3*, 1909–1924. [CrossRef]
23. Ramage, G.; Rajendran, R.; Sherry, L.; Williams, C. Fungal biofilm resistance. *Int. J. Microbiol.* **2012**, *2012*, 528521. [CrossRef]
24. Beauvais, A.; Schmidt, C.; Guadagnini, S.; Roux, P.; Perret, E.; Henry, C.; Paris, S.; Mallet, A.; Prevost, M.C.; Latge, J.P. An extracellular matrix glues together the aerial-grown hyphae of *Aspergillus fumigatus*. *Cell. Microbiol.* **2007**, *9*, 1588–1600. [CrossRef]
25. Reséndiz-Sánchez, J.; Ortiz-Alvarez, J.; Casimiro-Ramos, A.; Hernandez-Rodriguez, C.; Villa-Tanaca, L. First report of a catheter-related bloodstream infection by *Candida haemulonii* in a children's hospital in Mexico City. *Int. J. Infect. Dis.* **2020**, *92*, 123–126. [CrossRef] [PubMed]
26. Kim, M.N.; Shin, J.H.; Sung, H.; Lee, K.; Kim, E.C.; Ryoo, N.; Lee, J.S.; Jung, S.I.; Park, K.H.; Kee, S.J.; et al. *Candida haemulonii* and closely related species at 5 university hospitals in Korea: Identification, antifungal susceptibility, and clinical features. *Clin. Infect. Dis.* **2009**, *48*, e57–e61. [CrossRef] [PubMed]
27. Ruan, S.Y.; Kuo, Y.W.; Huang, C.T.; Hsiue, H.C.; Hsueh, P.R. Infections due to *Candida haemulonii*: Species identification, antifungal susceptibility and outcomes. *Int. J. Antimicrob. Agents* **2010**, *35*, 85–88. [CrossRef] [PubMed]
28. Crouzet, J.; Sotto, A.; Picard, E.; Lachaud, L.; Bourgeois, N. A case of *Candida haemulonii* osteitis: Clinical features, biochemical characteristics, and antifungal resistance profile. *Clin. Microbiol. Infect.* **2011**, *17*, 1068–1070. [CrossRef]
29. De Almeida, J.N., Jr.; Assy, J.G.; Levin, A.S.; Del Negro, G.M.; Giudice, M.C.; Tringoni, M.P.; Thomaz, D.Y.; Motta, A.L.; Abdala, E.; Pierroti, L.C.; et al. *Candida haemulonii* complex species, Brazil, January 2010–March 2015. *Emerg. Infect. Dis.* **2016**, *22*, 561–563. [CrossRef] [PubMed]
30. Muro, M.D.; Motta Fde, A.; Burger, M.; Melo, A.S.; Dalla-Costa, L.M. Echinocandin resistance in two *Candida haemulonii* isolates from pediatric patients. *J. Clin. Microbiol.* **2012**, *50*, 3783–3785. [CrossRef]
31. Almeida, J.N., Jr.; Motta, A.L.; Rossi, F.; Abdala, E.; Pierrotti, L.C.; Kono, A.S.; Diz Mdel, P.; Benard, G.; Del Negro, G.M. First report of a clinical isolate of *Candida haemulonii* in Brazil. *Clinics* **2012**, *67*, 1229–1231. [CrossRef]
32. Kathuria, S.; Singh, P.K.; Sharma, C.; Prakash, A.; Masih, A.; Kumar, A.; Meis, J.F.; Chowdhary, A. Multidrug-resistant *Candida auris* misidentified as *Candida haemulonii*: Characterization by matrix assisted laser desorption ionization-time of flight mass spectrometry and DNA sequencing and its antifungal susceptibility profile variability by Vitek 2, CLSI broth microdilution, and Etest method. *J. Clin. Microbiol.* **2015**, *53*, 1823–1830. [CrossRef]
33. Kumar, A.; Prakash, A.; Singh, A.; Kumar, H.; Hagen, F.; Meis, J.F.; Chowdhary, A. *Candida haemulonii* species complex: An emerging species in India and its genetic diversity assessed with multilocus sequence and amplified fragment-length polymorphism analyses. *Emerg Microbes Infect.* **2016**, *5*, e49. [CrossRef]
34. Fang, S.Y.; Wei, K.C.; Chen, W.C.; Lee, S.J.; Yang, K.C.; Wu, C.S.; Sun, P.L. Primary deep cutaneous candidiasis caused by *Candida duobushaemulonii* in a 68-year-old man: The first case report and literature review. *Mycoses* **2016**, *59*, 818–821. [CrossRef]
35. Ben-Ami, R.; Berman, J.; Novikov, A.; Bash, E.; Shachor-Meyouhas, Y.; Zakin, S.; Maor, Y.; Tarabia, J.; Schechner, V.; Adler, A.; et al. Multidrug-resistant *Candida haemulonii* and *C. auris*, Tel Aviv, Israel. *Emerg. Infect. Dis.* **2017**, *23*. [CrossRef] [PubMed]
36. Isla, G.; Taverna, C.G.; Szusz, W.; Vivot, W.; García-Effron, G.; Davel, G. *Candida haemulonii* sensu lato: Update of the determination of susceptibility profile in Argentina and literature review. *Curr. Fungal Infect. Rep.* **2017**, *11*, 203–208. [CrossRef]

37. Ramos, R.; Caceres, D.H.; Perez, M.; Garcia, N.; Castillo, W.; Santiago, E.; Borace, J.; Lockhart, S.R.; Berkow, E.L.; Hayer, L.; et al. Emerging multidrug-resistant *Candida duobushaemulonii* infections in Panama hospitals: Importance of laboratory surveillance and accurate identification. *J. Clin. Microbiol.* **2018**, *56*, e00371-18. [CrossRef] [PubMed]
38. Muñoz, J.F.; Gade, L.; Chow, N.A.; Loparev, V.N.; Juieng, P.; Berkow, E.L.; Farrer, R.A.; Litvintseva, A.P.; Cuomo, C.A. Genomic insights into multidrug-resistance, mating and virulence in *Candida auris* and related emerging species. *Nat. Commun.* **2018**, *9*, 5346. [CrossRef]
39. Frías-De-León, M.G.; Martinez-Herrera, E.; Acosta-Altamirano, G.; Arenas, R.; Rodriguez-Cerdeira, C. Superficial candidosis by *Candida duobushaemulonii*: An emerging microorganism. *Infect. Genet. Evol.* **2019**, *75*, 103960. [CrossRef]
40. Zhang, H.; Niu, Y.; Tan, J.; Liu, W.; Sun, M.A.; Yang, E.; Wang, Q.; Li, R.; Wang, Y.; Liu, W. Global screening of genomic and transcriptomic factors associated with phenotype differences between multidrug-resistant and -susceptible *Candida haemulonii* strains. *mSystems* **2019**, *4*. [CrossRef]
41. Di Luca, M.; Koliszak, A.; Karbysheva, S.; Chowdhary, A.; Meis, J.F.; Trampuz, A. Thermogenic characterization and antifungal susceptibility of *Candida auris* by microcalorimetry. *J. Fungi* **2019**, *5*, 103. [CrossRef]
42. Bastos, R.W.; Rossato, L.; Valero, C.; Lagrou, K.; Colombo, A.L.; Goldman, G.H. Potential of Gallium as an antifungal agent. *Front. Cell Infect. Microbiol.* **2019**, *9*, 414. [CrossRef]
43. Xiao, M.; Chen, S.C.; Kong, F.; Xu, X.L.; Yan, L.; Kong, H.S.; Fan, X.; Hou, X.; Cheng, J.W.; Zhou, M.L.; et al. Distribution and antifungal susceptibility of *Candida* species causing candidemia in China: An update from the CHIF-NET Study. *J. Infect. Dis.* **2020**, *221*, S139–S147. [CrossRef]
44. Gade, L.; Muñoz, J.F.; Sheth, M.; Wagner, D.; Berkow, E.L.; Forsberg, K.; Jackson, B.R.; Ramos-Castro, R.; Escandón, P.; Dolande, M.; et al. Understanding the emergence of multidrug-resistant *Candida*: Using Whole-Genome Sequencing to describe the population structure of *Candida haemulonii* species complex. *Front. Genet.* **2020**, *11*, 554. [CrossRef]
45. Lima, S.L.; Francisco, E.C.; De Almeida Júnior, J.N.; Santos, D.W.C.L.; Carlesse, F.; Queiroz-Telles, F.; Melo, A.S.A.; Colombo, A.L. Increasing prevalence of multidrug-resistant *Candida haemulonii* species complex among all yeast cultures collected by a reference laboratory over the past 11 years. *J. Fungi* **2020**, *6*, 110. [CrossRef] [PubMed]
46. Coles, M.; Cox, K.; Chao, A. *Candida haemulonii*: An emerging opportunistic pathogen in the United States? *IDCases* **2020**, *21*, e00900. [CrossRef] [PubMed]
47. Rodrigues, L.S.; Gazara, R.K.; Passarelli-Araujo, H.; Valengo, A.E.; Pontes, P.V.M.; Nunes-da-Fonseca, R.; De Souza, R.F.; Venancio, T.M.; Dalla-Costa, L.M. First genome sequences of two multidrug-resistant *Candida haemulonii* var. *vulnera* isolates from pediatric patients with candidemia. *Front. Microbiol.* **2020**, *11*. [CrossRef] [PubMed]
48. Kordalewska, M.; Lee, A.; Park, S.; Berrio, I.; Chowdhary, A.; Zhao, Y.; Perlin, D.S. Understanding echinocandin resistance in the emerging pathogen *Candida auris*. *Antimicrob. Agents Chemother.* **2018**, *62*, e00238-18. [CrossRef] [PubMed]
49. Sherry, L.; Ramage, G.; Kean, R.; Borman, A.; Johnson, E.M.; Richardson, M.D.; Rautemaa-Richardson, R. Biofilm-forming capability of highly virulent, multidrug-resistant *Candida auris*. *Emerg. Infect. Dis.* **2017**, *23*, 328–331. [CrossRef]
50. Kean, R.; Delaney, C.; Sherry, L.; Borman, A.; Johnson, E.M.; Richardson, M.D.; Rautemaa-Richardson, R.; Williams, C.; Ramage, G. Transcriptome assembly and profiling of *Candida auris* reveals novel insights into biofilm-mediated resistance. *mSphere* **2018**, *3*, e00334-18. [CrossRef]
51. Guembe, M.; Guinea, J.; Marcos-Zambrano, L.J.; Fernandez-Cruz, A.; Pelaez, T.; Munoz, P.; Bouza, E. Micafungin at physiological serum concentrations shows antifungal activity against *Candida albicans* and *Candida parapsilosis* biofilms. *Antimicrob. Agents Chemother.* **2014**, *58*, 5581–5584. [CrossRef]
52. Ziccardi, M.; Souza, L.O.; Gandra, R.M.; Galdino, A.C.; Baptista, A.R.; Nunes, A.P.; Ribeiro, M.A.; Branquinha, M.H.; Santos, A.L.S. *Candida parapsilosis* (sensu lato) isolated from hospitals located in the Southeast of Brazil: Species distribution, antifungal susceptibility and virulence attributes. *Int. J. Med. Microbiol.* **2015**, *305*, 848–859. [CrossRef]

53. Simitsopoulou, M.; Peshkova, P.; Tasina, E.; Katragkou, A.; Kyrpitzi, D.; Velegraki, A.; Walsh, T.J.; Roilides, E. Species-specific and drug-specific differences in susceptibility of *Candida* biofilms to echinocandins: Characterization of less common bloodstream isolates. *Antimicrob. Agents Chemother.* **2013**, *57*, 2562–2570. [CrossRef]
54. Melo, A.S.; Colombo, A.L.; Arthington-Skaggs, B.A. Paradoxical growth effect of caspofungin observed on biofilms and planktonic cells of five different *Candida* species. *Antimicrob. Agents Chemother.* **2007**, *51*, 3081–3088. [CrossRef]
55. Ferreira, J.A.; Carr, J.H.; Starling, C.E.; De Resende, M.A.; Donlan, R.M. Biofilm formation and effect of caspofungin on biofilm structure of *Candida* species bloodstream isolates. *Antimicrob. Agents Chemother.* **2009**, *53*, 4377–4384. [CrossRef] [PubMed]
56. Jacobsen, M.D.; Whyte, J.A.; Odds, F.C. *Candida albicans* and *Candida dubliniensis* respond differently to echinocandin antifungal agents in vitro. *Antimicrob. Agents Chemother.* **2007**, *51*, 1882–1884. [CrossRef] [PubMed]

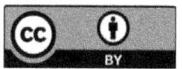

© 2020 by the authors. Licensee MDPI, Basel, Switzerland. This article is an open access article distributed under the terms and conditions of the Creative Commons Attribution (CC BY) license (http://creativecommons.org/licenses/by/4.0/).

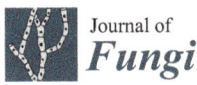

Review

Fungal Quorum-Sensing Molecules: A Review of Their Antifungal Effect against *Candida* Biofilms

Renátó Kovács [1,2,*] and László Majoros [1]

1. Department of Medical Microbiology, Faculty of Medicine, University of Debrecen, 4032 Debrecen, Hungary; major@med.unideb.hu
2. Faculty of Pharmacy, University of Debrecen, 4032 Debrecen, Hungary
* Correspondence: kovacs.renato@med.unideb.hu; Tel.: +0036-52-255-425; Fax: +0036-52-255-424

Received: 4 June 2020; Accepted: 30 June 2020; Published: 2 July 2020

Abstract: The number of effective therapeutic strategies against biofilms is limited; development of novel therapies is urgently needed to treat a variety of biofilm-associated infections. Quorum sensing is a special form of microbial cell-to-cell communication that is responsible for the release of numerous extracellular molecules, whose concentration is proportional with cell density. *Candida*-secreted quorum-sensing molecules (i.e., farnesol and tyrosol) have a pivotal role in morphogenesis, biofilm formation, and virulence. Farnesol can mediate the hyphae-to-yeast transition, while tyrosol has the opposite effect of inducing transition from the yeast to hyphal form. A number of questions regarding *Candida* quorum sensing remain to be addressed; nevertheless, the literature shows that farnesol and tyrosol possess remarkable antifungal and anti-biofilm effect at supraphysiological concentration. Furthermore, previous in vitro and in vivo data suggest that they may have a potent adjuvant effect in combination with certain traditional antifungal agents. This review discusses the most promising farnesol- and tyrosol-based in vitro and in vivo results, which may be a foundation for future development of novel therapeutic strategies to combat *Candida* biofilms.

Keywords: *Candida*; farnesol; tyrosol; biofilm; therapy; combination

1. Introduction

It has been estimated that there are 2.2 to 3.8 million fungal species worldwide; however, approximately 300 species have been described to cause human disease [1]. *Candida* species are among the most common human fungal pathogens. The annual incidence rate of *Candida*-associated bloodstream infections ranged from 9.5 to 14.4 per 100,000 in the United States of America [2]. This value ranged from 1.4 to 5.7 per 100,000 in Europe, depending on the country [3]. In the last two decades, the prevalence of resistant fungal infections has been steadily increasing due to the widespread use of antifungals in agriculture and veterinary and human medicine [4,5]. Global warming and anthropogenic effects have resulted in the emergence of previously little-known, potentially multi-resistant fungal pathogens in clinical practice, such as *Candida auris*, azole-resistant *Aspergillus* spp., or *Lomentospora prolificans*. These emerging pathogens have caused further challenges for therapy [6,7].

Several fungal species can switch their morphology from yeast to hyphal or pseudohyphal forms, which is coupled with biofilm formation and plays a pivotal role both in fungal virulence and in resistance to antifungals [8–10]. The increased number of biofilm-associated infections is exacerbated by a paucity of antifungal agents or therapeutic strategies in development that have unique mechanisms of action or possess alternative approaches, respectively [11]. Currently, the most promising antifungal agents are already in Phase 3 including ibrexafungerp [12], rezafungin [13], super bioavailable itraconazole [14], and VT-1161 [15]. Recently investigated alternative therapeutic approaches involve high-dose therapy with available antifungal agents [16–18], antifungal lock therapy [19], and combination-based therapies [20,21].

Based on in vitro and in vivo data, echinocandins and amphotericin B solutions are the most promising combination-based and/or antifungal lock strategies [19]. Further innovative therapeutic approaches may be the natural products-based treatments [22,23]. One of the more well-studied compounds is carbohydrate-derived fulvic acid as a heat stable colloidal material, which has an inhibitory effect on *Candida* and bacterial biofilm formation [24]. Moreover, a further alternative approach is the treatments disrupting quorum sensing. The usage of quorum sensing molecules at supraphysiological concentration may adversely influence the cell-to-cell communication in biofilms [25–27]. In addition, the quorum-sensing system can be inactivated, which is generally known as quorum quenching. Quorum quenching can be triggered by inhibiting the production of quorum sensing molecules, their detection by receptors or their degradation [28].

In this review, a detailed overview is provided of the recent status of quorum-sensing molecule-based therapeutic approaches and their potential future perspectives against *Candida* biofilms.

2. The Medical Importance of *Candida* Biofilms

Despite their importance, *Candida* biofilms remain a relatively underappreciated and understudied area. Therefore, effective therapeutic strategies against these sessile communities remain scarce. Biofilms are usually found in medical devices such as joint prostheses, pacemakers, urinary and central venous catheters, dentures, and mechanical heart valves, hindering the eradication of *Candida* infections [10]. In addition, several chronic *Candida*-related diseases are also associated with biofilm development [29]. Biofilm formation on the vaginal mucosa has been observed in in vivo models of vulvovaginal candidiasis [30]. Oral- and oesophageal mucosae-associated biofilms are a very important contributor to oral diseases caused by *Candida* species; gastrointestinal and urogenital tracts are also common sites of *Candida*-associated opportunistic infections [31]. *Candida* is one of the most commonly identified fungal genera in wounds whose environment can also promote the formation of biofilms [32]. A series of recent studies has indicated that strains defective in hyphal formation display significantly milder symptoms, highlighting the role of biofilm formation in pathogenesis of these chronic or recurrent infections [30,33].

These sessile communities exhibit five- to eightfold higher resistance to all licenced antifungal drugs when compared to their planktonic counterparts [10]. This high rate of resistance can be explained by the increased metabolic activity of cells in the early development phase of biofilm formation [10]. On the other hand, dormant, non-proliferating persister cells have also been observed, especially in mature biofilms, that have demonstrated high tolerance to antifungals [34]. Furthermore, the various *Candida* species can produce dense extracellular polymeric substances which serve as a solid barrier to prevent the diffusion of antifungal drugs and account for almost 90% of the biofilm dry mass [10]. As has been previously reported in the literature, sessile *Candida* communities exhibit an altered gene expression profile, including the upregulation of *CDR* and *MDR* genes which encode azole resistance transporter proteins, and pose further challenges for treatment [35].

To date, there is no definitive therapy against *Candida* biofilms; nevertheless, there are several promising in vitro, in vivo and clinical results. The increasing number of resistant *Candida* species and isolates highlight the need for new molecules with new targets. Alternative therapeutic approaches against multidrug-resistant fungal biofilms may be the result of a combination of traditional antifungal agents with quorum-sensing molecules [36].

3. Fungal Quorum Sensing

A major mechanism of microbial communication is a population density-dependent stimulus-response system called quorum sensing. This process occurs by the continuous release and monitoring of low molecular weight hormone-like secreted molecules (quorum-sensing molecules), which are not elementary in the central metabolism but have a variety of biological activities. The concentration of these quorum-sensing molecules is proportional with the size of population;

after reaching a critical threshold, a response is triggered leading to the coordinated expression or repression of quorum sensing-related target genes [37].

In the fungal kingdom, quorum sensing was a relatively unknown phenomenon until Hornby et al. (2001) described the effect of the isoprenoid farnesol on *Candida albicans* morphogenesis; this opened a new branch of science focusing on fungal quorum sensing [38]. At the same time, quorum sensing has been already reported in *Aspergillus* spp. [39] and *Penicillium* spp. [40]. To date, four main quorum-sensing molecules were described including farnesol, tyrosol, phenylethanol, and tryptophol, which have a remarkable effect on the regulation of morphogenesis (yeast to hyphae transition and vice versa), initiation of fungal apoptosis, and virulence [41].

Recently, several authors reported that certain quorum-sensing molecules may generate oxidative stress, especially at supraphysiological concentrations, which may have an antifungal effect [42–45]. The majority of data concerning fungal quorum sensing molecule-related therapeutic potential derived from *C. albicans* experiments, and these results cannot be always directly extrapolated to non-*albicans* species. Recently, the number of studies dealing with the effect of quorum-sensing molecules on non-*albicans* species has steadily increased, supporting the comprehensive understanding of the in vitro and in vivo antifungal effects exerted by these molecules.

4. Farnesol

4.1. Physiological Effect of Farnesol in Candida Species

Farnesol (3,7,11-trimethyl-2,6,10-dodecatriene-1-ol) was the first described *Candida*-derived quorum sensing molecule; it is released in *C. albicans* as a side product of the sterol synthetic pathway by dephosphorylation of farnesol pyrophosphate [38,46]. It is an acyclic sesquiterpene heat-stable molecule, which is produced primarily under aerobic conditions and it is unaffected by extreme pH and the type of carbon or nitrogen source [38,47]. Generally, the farnesol concentration is proportional to the colony-forming unit number [38]. Under physiological conditions, *C. albicans* isolates secrete a farnesol concentration with a mean of 35.6 µM (range: 13.7 to 58.5 µM) [48]. This concentration was 35 times higher than that secreted by non-*albicans* species, with the exception of *Candida dubliniensis*, which has demonstrated a concentration of 8.3 µM (range: 6.0 to 17.5 µM). All other non-albicans species excreted significantly lower farnesol concentrations, ranging from 0.4 to 1 µM [48]. These differences in excretion may be explained by the species-specific characteristics in sterol synthesis [49].

Based on a cDNA microarray analysis, a total of 274 genes were identified as responsive in *C. albicans*, with 104 genes up-regulated and 170 genes down-regulated [50]. Farnesol has an ability to influence *Candida* morphology, biofilm formation, drug efflux pump expression, apoptosis regulation, phagocytic response, surface hydrophobicity, iron metabolism, and heat-shock-related pathways [50–54]. One of the most prominent farnesol-associated effects is the induction of hypha-to-yeast transition and the inhibition of biofilm formation in various *Candida* species. It should be emphasized that 150-fold more farnesol is needed to block germ-tube formation in the presence of 10% serum, showing that it can bind to serum proteins at a high rate [55,56].

In view of this diverse role, it is not surprising that this compound influences several central signalling pathways in different *Candida* species. One of the best-studied farnesol-related pathways is the Ras1-cAMP-PKA cascade, where farnesol binds to the cyclase domain of the adenylyl cyclase *Cyr1*, influencing the level of intracellular cAMP [57]. Moreover, farnesol induces the cleavage of the small GTPase Ras1, resulting in a soluble Ras1; soluble Ras1 is a weak activator of *Cyr1* and supports the formation of yeast cells [58]. Furthermore, farnesol can directly inhibit the cAMP signalling pathway, supporting the hypha-to-yeast transition [59]. It is noteworthy that farnesol exposure stabilizes the *Nrg1* protein, which is the negative regulator of filamentation [60]. While farnesol was described first in *C. albicans*, it can inhibit filamentation and growth in other fungal species [27,61], including *Saccharomyces cerevisiae* [62], *Aspergillus niger* [63],

Aspergillus flavus [64], *Aspergillus nidulans* [65], *Penicillium expansum* [66], *Fusarium graminearum* [67], and *Paracoccidioides brasiliensis* [68].

Regarding reactive oxygen species production, the supraphysiological farnesol concentrations (200–300 µM) are stressful for most fungi, while the physiological concentrations (30–40 µM) protect them from stress [57]. In addition to the farnesol-related effect on growth in the case of different microbes, the molecule also has a relevant immunomodulator effect [57,69]. Farnesol can stimulate both macrophage chemokine synthesis or macrophage recruitment, and trigger activation of neutrophil granulocytes and monocytes. Farnesol exposure also influences the differentiation of monocytes into dendritic cells [57,69].

Farnesol has been reported to induce cell growth inhibition and/or apoptosis in tumor cells where the observed IC_{50} values varied widely for different tumor types and different cell lines [70]. Farnesol caused 100% cell death at >120 µM in A549 and H460 lung cancer cells [71]. Scheper et al. (2008) observed an IC_{50} value of 30 to 60 µM for farnesol on the primary human tongue squamous cell carcinoma cell lines (OSCC9, OSCC 25) [70]. Nagy et al. (2020) evaluated 10 µM, 50 µM, 150 µM, and 300 µM farnesol concentrations in terms of toxicity to the Caco-2 cell line, where no toxicity was observed with any concentration tested [45].

4.2. Antimicrobial Activity of Farnesol

At physiological concentrations, farnesol has no significant effect on *Candida* cells that have already begun hyphae development or biofilm formation [25,38]. However, prior results suggest that farnesol can cause biofilm degradation at supraphysiological concentrations, suggesting the potential use of this compound in biofilm-associated infections [36]. In addition, several authors have published studies demonstrating contribution of farnesol to reduced azole resistance of *Candida* cells, including in biofilms [72]. This phenomenon can be explained by the modulation of *Cdr1* efflux pumps, reactive oxygen species production, or changes in glutathione homeostasis [38,61,72]. Furthermore, farnesol has an effect on genes connected to ergosterol synthesis [46]. Dižová et al. (2018) observed that the presence of 200 µM farnesol down-regulated the *ERG20*, *ERG11* and *ERG9* genes. However, this farnesol concentration supplemented with 0.5 mg/L fluconazole restored the original expression level of *ERG20* and *ERG11*. Interestingly, the physiological farnesol concentration (~30 µM) only slightly influences the expression of these genes in 48 h-old biofilms [73]. Chen et al. (2018) reported that *CYR1* and *PDE2* regulate resistance mechanisms against various antifungals in *C. albicans* biofilms. However, farnesol can diminish the resistance of *C. albicans* biofilms by regulating the expression of the gene *CYR1* and *PDE2* [74]. Yu et al. (2012) observed that the sterol biosynthetic pathway may contribute to the inhibitory effects of farnesol, as the transcription levels of the *ERG11*, *ERG25*, *ERG6*, *ERG3*, and *ERG1* genes decreased following farnesol exposure [75]. Jabra-Rizk et al. (2006) showed that farnesol concentrations of 30–50 mM decrease the fluconazole MICs for *C. albicans* and *C. dubliniensis* from resistant values to a susceptible dose-dependent range, while concentrations of 100–300 mM resulted in fluconazole susceptibility [76].

One of the first major breakthroughs in combination-based experiments with farnesol and antifungals was published by Katragkou et al. (2015), who found a significant synergy against *C. albicans* 48 h-old biofilms between fluconazole, amphotericin B, and micafungin in the presence of farnesol [26]. The highest synergistic effect was observed in the case of micafungin combined with farnesol using fractional inhibitory concentration index determination and Bliss independence analysis. Based on the Bliss model, the observed effects were 39–52% higher compared to the expected efficacy if the drugs had been acting independently [26]. It should be noted that synergism was observed only in the case of farnesol/micafungin and farnesol/fluconazole based on calculated fractional inhibitory concentration indices, suggesting the usage of multiple analytical approaches for investigation of drug-drug interaction [26].

Regarding non-albicans species, Kovács et al. (2016) showed that farnesol consistently enhanced the activity of caspofungin and micafungin, as concordantly shown in two independent experimental settings (chequerboard dilution and time–kill experiments) [27]. Fernández-Rivero et al. (2017) reported that a supraphysiological farnesol concentration (300 µM) improved the activity of amphotericin B against *Candida tropicalis* biofilms but did not affect anidulafungin [77]. Two recent studies by Nagy et al. concluded that farnesol significantly enhanced the activity of echinocandins and triazoles against one-day-old *C. auris* biofilms in vitro, suggesting an alternative approach to overcome the previously well-documented azole and echinocandin resistance of *C. auris* biofilms [45,78].

Animal experiments with farnesol raised several questions in terms of in vivo applicability of this compound. In one of the first in vivo studies, Navarathna et al. (2007) concluded that the physiological farnesol production may play a pivotal role as a virulence factor in fungal pathogenesis; furthermore, exogenous oral and intraperitoneal farnesol administration (20 mM) enhances the mortality of mice in their systemic mouse model [79]. Contrary to these results, Hisajima et al. (2008) observed a protective effect against *C. albicans* in their oral candidiasis mouse model [80]. It should be noted that there was a 1000-fold difference between the administered farnesol dosages (9 µM/mouse) in the experiments of Hisajima et al. (2008) [80] compared to experiments performed by Navarathna et al. (2007) (20 mM/mouse) [79]. In addition, they reported a potential gastrointestinal tract-related farnesol effect including moderate bodyweight reduction and reduced *Candida* faeces burden [80]. A cocktail of *Candida*-derived regulatory alcohols combined with nanomolar amounts of farnesol was reported to have a similar protective effect by Martins et al. (2012) in their murine model of disseminated candidiasis [81]. Bozó et al. (2016) did not find a farnesol-related protective effect against vaginal *C. albicans* infection [82], in contrast to the findings of Hisajima et al. (2008) [80]. However, both administered farnesol regimens enhanced the activity of 5 mg/kg daily fluconazole treatment against fluconazole-resistant *C. albicans* strain [82]. Similar fluconazole resistance reversion was observed in the case of planktonic cells by Jabra-Rizk et al. (2006) [76] and Cordeiro et al. (2013) [83]. Fernandes Costa et al. (2019) used nanoparticles containing farnesol alone or in combination with miconazole; nanoparticles containing farnesol inhibited yeast-to-hyphae transition at concentrations greater than or equal to 240 µM [84]. In addition, chitosan nanoparticles containing miconazole (33 mg/L) and farnesol (2.1 mM) inhibited fungal proliferation and decreased the pathogenicity of mouse vulvovaginitis infection [84]. Nagy et al. (2020) demonstrated that a daily treatment with 75 µM farnesol decreased the *C. auris* kidney burden in their immunocompromised systemic mouse model, especially when inocula was pre-exposed to farnesol [45].

The farnesol-exerted antifungal activity can be explained by the higher level of reactive oxygen species, especially in the case of non-*albicans* species [43,45]. Furthermore, farnesol has an amphiphilic property which allows for its integration into cell membranes, influencing membrane fluidity and integrity. In the case of *Candida parapsilosis* and *C. dubliniensis*, farnesol affected the cellular polarization and membrane permeability [61,76,85]. These observations can help further elucidate the antifungal effect.

Farnesol has a remarkable antibacterial effect alone or in combination with traditional antibacterial agents as demonstrated by in vitro investigations. Jabra-Rizk et al. (2006) observed that farnesol treatment (100 µM) increases the activity of gentamicin against *Staphylococcus aureus* biofilms [86]. Gomes et al. (2009) showed that farnesol exposure (300 µM) produced a relatively long post-antimicrobial effect (>8 h) against *Staphylococcus epidermidis* [87], while Pammi et al. (2011) observed that farnesol exposure at a concentration of 500 µM significantly inhibited the *S. epidermidis* biofilm formation in vitro [88]. A clear synergistic interaction was observed between farnesol and nafcillin or vancomycin against *S. epidermidis* sessile cells [88]. Additionally, it potentiates the activity of beta-lactam antibiotics against antibiotic-resistant bacterium species [89]. Castelo-Branco et al. (2012) showed a potent antimicrobial effect exerted by exogenous farnesol exposure against mature *Burkholderia pseudomallei* biofilms [90]. Additionally, it increased the activity of amoxicillin, ceftazidime, doxycycline, and sulfamethoxazole-trimethoprim, which are routinely administered for the treatment of melioidoses [91]. Farnesol also had a synergizing effect against ciprofloxacin-resistant *Pseudomonas aeruginosa* biofilms when used in combination with ciprofloxacin [92]. In vivo data also supports the antibacterial efficacy of farnesol. It has been observed that 6.7 mM farnesol treatment significantly decreased the *S. epidermidis* associated catheter infection and systemic dissemination [88].

Based on several studies, farnesol has a remarkable effect in *Candida*-bacterium mixed biofilms. *C. albicans*-derived farnesol has also been shown to have an effect on the response of *S. aureus* to antibiotics in mixed species biofilms. Farnesol exposure results in a significant decrease in staphyloxantin, which is an important virulence factor of this bacterium [42]. Černáková et al. (2018) showed that 200 µM farnesol has an inhibitory effect on *C. albicans* growth in mixed-species biofilms with *Streptococcus mutans* [93]. Cugini et al. (2010) examined the *C. albicans*-*P. aeruginosa* mixed species biofilms, where the *C. albicans*-derived farnesol enhanced *P. aeruginosa* quinolone signal production in a LasR-defective strain [94].

5. Tyrosol

5.1. Physiological Effect of Tyrosol in Candida Species

Tyrosol (2-(4-hydoxyphenyl)-ethanol) is a tyrosine-derived molecule which is synthetized via either tyramine or 4-hydroxyphenylacetaldehyde [95,96]. In the case of *C. albicans*, it is released into the growth medium continuously during the exponential growth phase and is capable of decreasing the duration of the lag phase before cells begin germination. The accumulation of tyrosol in the culture medium is proportional to the rise of fungal cell number. While the molecule stimulates filamentation, it exclusively promotes germ tube formation in conditions that normally induce these physiological processes [95,96]. Tyrosol exposure influences cell cycle regulation, DNA replication, and chromosome segregation in *C. albicans* [95]. Additionally, it was shown to have an inhibitory effect on neutrophil granulocytes by interfering with the oxidative stress response of these phagocytes [97,98]. Significantly more tyrosol was secreted by *C. albicans* (range: 21.01 ± 0.76 to 53.40 ± 1.73 µM/1.6×10^7–5.3×10^7 cells/mL) and *C. tropicalis* (range: 41.21 ± 1.21 to 48.63 ± 3.83 µM/2.6×10^7–2.7×10^7 cells/mL) than by *Candida glabrata* (range: 1.3 ± 0.17 to 3.26 ± 0.33 µM/2.7×10^7–5.5×10^7 cells/mL) or *C. parapsilosis* (range: 1.59 ± 0.29 to 3.04 ± 0.43 µM/1.7×10^7–2.3×10^7 cells/mL), suggesting a possible link with virulence [99]. Tyrosol plays a pivotal role in biofilm production, where it can stimulate hypha production of *C. albicans*, especially between two and six hours of biofilm development. *C. albicans* biofilms released at least 50% more tyrosol when compared to planktonic cells [96].

Regarding non-*albicans* species, tyrosol has been recognized as inducing the biofilm-forming ability of *C. auris* to grow as yeast or pseudohyphae [96]. Based on RNA-Seq analysis, tyrosol treatment resulted in 261 and 181 differentially expressed genes with at least a 1.5-fold increase or decrease in expression in *C. parapsilosis*, respectively; however, the initial adherence was not affected by the presence of tyrosol [43]. Interestingly, the ortholog of the *C. albicans CZF1* gene, which is a key transcription factor of biofilm development in *C. parapsilosis*, was upregulated following tyrosol exposure [43,100]. Nevertheless, Jakab et al. (2019) did not observe higher rates of biofilm formation in the presence of tyrosol [43]. In *C. parapsilosis*, tyrosol exposure overexpressed the active efflux pumps and caused an enhanced oxidative stress response, while inhibiting growth, ribosome biogenesis, and virulence. Surprisingly, its metabolism was modulated toward glycolysis and ethanol fermentation [43]. Monteiro et al. (2015) reported that tyrosol exposure did not induce increased adhesion in *C. glabrata* [101].

Regarding tyrosol related toxic effect, initial cytotoxicity was observed at concentrations of >10 mM, 3 mM, 5 mM and >15 mM for human gingival fibroblasts (GN61), human gingival epithelial cells (S-G), human salivary gland carcinoma cells (HSG$_1$) and colon adenocarcinomas cell line (Caco-2), respectively [43,102].

5.2. Antimicrobial Activity of Tyrosol

Tyrosol is a relatively understudied molecule compared to farnesol in terms of potential antifungal or anti-biofilm activity; despite this, a few studies have examined the potential use of tyrosol in monotherapy or in combination with traditional antifungal agents against *Candida* species [36,72].

Arias et al. (2016) showed that tyrosol treatment at concentrations ranging from 100 to 200 mM exerted a significant reduction in metabolic activity against *C. albicans* and *C. glabrata* two-day-old oral biofilms, which was proportional to a reduction in cell number [103]. Do Vale et al. (2017) showed that tyrosol alone at concentrations of 50 and 90 mM demonstrated inhibition of the planktonic growth of *C. albicans* and *C. glabrata* cells, respectively [104]. However, tyrosol does not significantly reduce metabolic activity or the number of cells for one-day-old oral biofilms; in addition, the nature of interaction of tyrosol with chlorohexidine gluconate was indifferent. Nevertheless, 1.25 mM tyrosol with 0.00725 mM chlorhexidine gluconate showed a synergistic interaction in reducing the number of hyphae formed [104]. A combination of tyrosol and farnesol has been explored for oral *Candida* isolates for both planktonic and sessile growth. This combination showed synergy against *C. glabrata*, indicating that this combination may contribute to the development of oral care products against *Candida* species [105].

In another study, tyrosol showed anti-biofilm activity against denture-derived *C. albicans* isolates. However, it has been shown that the single use of tyrosol cannot decrease hydrolytic enzymes on oral *C. albicans* [106]. Shanmughapriya et al. (2014) observed that tyrosol treatment caused a 25% and a 50% reduction in intrauterine device-derived *Candida krusei* and *C. tropicalis* biofilm production at concentrations of 40 μM and 80 μM, respectively [107]. In addition, amphotericin B combined with tyrosol showed a remarkable inhibitory effect against these non-*albicans* biofilms. A concentration of 4 mg/L amphotericin B in the presence of 80 μM tyrosol exerted approximately 90% inhibition in biofilm formation [107]. Cordeiro et al. (2015) showed that the addition of tyrosol significantly reduced the MICs for amphotericin B, fluconazole, and itraconazole against planktonic *C. albicans* and *C. tropicalis* [108]. Furthermore, exogenous tyrosol alone was able to significantly reduce the biofilm formation of these species at concentrations ranging from 125 to 250 mM. At these concentrations, tyrosol decreased the metabolic activity of growing biofilms by approximately 24 and 30% for *C. albicans* and *C. tropicalis*, respectively. Reduction of metabolic activity was more pronounced when tyrosol was combined with traditional antifungal drugs including amphotericin B, fluconazole, and itraconazole. It should be noted that application of amphotericin B with tyrosol markedly decreased the metabolic activity of mature biofilms (35%) [108]. Kovács et al. (2017) reported that tyrosol may be used as an adjuvant agent with caspofungin or micafungin in alternative treatment strategies [109]. Regarding the in vivo antifungal effect of tyrosol, Jakab et al. (2019) reported that daily treatment with 15 mM tyrosol decreased the fungal tissue burden in their immunocompromised mouse model [43]. In this study, the expression of *ALS6*, which has a pivotal role in adhesion, was significantly reduced by tyrosol treatment. Furthermore, downregulation of the expression of *FAD2* and *FAD3* may also contribute to decreased virulence and kidney fungal burden. The well-documented antifungal effects exerted by tyrosol may be explained by the enhanced oxidative stress and the inhibition of virulence-related genes, growth, and ribosome biogenesis. In addition, tyrosol can alter the metabolism of *Candida* cells toward fermentation [43].

Data on the potential antibacterial effects of tyrosol remain scarce. Arias et al. (2016) found a potential anti-biofilm activity of tyrosol against *S. mutans* in single and mixed species biofilms with *C. albicans* or *C. glabrata* developed on acrylic resin and hydroxyapatite surfaces [103]. Their results may contribute to the development of innovative topical therapies focusing on biofilm-associated oral diseases. Abdel-Rhman et al. (2016) reported substantial antibacterial activity of tyrosol against *S. aureus*; moreover, tyrosol increased susceptibility to gentamicin, amikacin, and ciprofloxacin at subinhibitory concentrations ranging from 3.5 to 14.3 mM [110]. Tyrosol treatment can also influence *S. aureus* virulence, decreasing the production of protease and lipase enzymes and limiting the ability to form biofilms [110]. In the case of *P. aeruginosa*, tyrosol strongly inhibited haemolysin and protease production [111].

6. Future Remarks

Paradoxically, medical advancement has resulted in an increasing number of immunocompromised individuals susceptible to *Candida* infections. The incidence and mortality rate related to systemic

Candida infections has remained unchanged, despite the advances in the field of antifungal therapy. Based on recent comprehensive epidemiological studies, the high incidence and mortality may be attributed to sessile *Candida* populations, namely biofilms, which show high resistance against environmental factors, immune responses, and traditional antifungal therapy. Although there is no definitive solution or highly effective therapeutic recommendation against *Candida* biofilms, there are many promising therapeutic strategies including antifungal "lock" therapy, photodynamic inactivation, and the use of natural products or synthetic peptides with antifungal activity. A further solution may be the utilization of quorum-sensing molecules alone or in combination with traditional antifungal agents; however, there are numerous open questions as to their exact action or the interaction between quorum-sensing molecules and the host. In addition, the full understanding of quorum sensing in non-*albicans* species has remained unelucidated. In this review, we provided an overview on the current status of studies focusing on anti-biofilm activity of farnesol and tyrosol. Hopefully, these in vitro and in vivo results can be implemented in therapeutic practice as soon as possible to overcome *Candida* biofilm-related infections.

Author Contributions: Conceptualization, methodology and writing were performed by R.K. and L.M. All authors have read and agreed to the published version of the manuscript.

Funding: R.K. was supported by the EFOP-3.6.3-VEKOP-16-2017-00009 program and by a FEMS Research and Training Grant (FEMS-GO-2019-502).

Conflicts of Interest: L.M. received conference travel grants from Cidara, MSD, Astellas and Pfizer. All other authors report no conflicts of interest.

References

1. Hawksworth, D.L.; Lücking, R. Fungal Diversity Revisited: 2.2 to 3.8 Million Species. *Microbiol. Spectr.* **2017**, *5*. [CrossRef]
2. Magill, S.S.; O'Leary, E.; Janelle, S.J.; Thompson, D.L.; Dumyati, G.; Nadle, J.; Wilson, L.E.; Kainer, M.A.; Lynfield, R.; Greissman, S.; et al. Changes in Prevalence of Health Care-Associated Infections in U.S. Hospitals. *N. Engl. J. Med.* **2018**, *379*, 1732–1744. [CrossRef] [PubMed]
3. Quindós, G. Epidemiology of candidaemia and invasive candidiasis. A changing face. *Rev. Iberoam. Micol.* **2014**, *31*, 42–48. [CrossRef] [PubMed]
4. Wiederhold, N.P. Antifungal resistance: Current trends and future strategies to combat. *Infect. Drug Resist.* **2017**, *10*, 249–259. [CrossRef]
5. Kontoyiannis, D.P. Antifungal Resistance: An Emerging Reality and A Global Challenge. *J. Infect. Dis.* **2017**, *216* (Suppl. 3), S431–S435. [CrossRef]
6. Casadevall, A.; Kontoyiannis, D.P.; Robert, V. On the Emergence of *Candida auris*: Climate Change, Azoles, Swamps, and Birds. *MBio* **2019**, *10*, e01397-19. [CrossRef]
7. Friedman, D.Z.P.; Schwartz, I.S. Emerging Fungal Infections: New Patients, New Patterns, and New Pathogens. *J. Fungi* **2019**, *5*, 67. [CrossRef]
8. Silva, S.; Rodrigues, C.F.; Araújo, D.; Rodrigues, M.E.; Henriques, M. *Candida* Species Biofilms' Antifungal Resistance. *J. Fungi* **2017**, *3*, 8. [CrossRef]
9. De Barros, P.P.; Rossoni, R.D.; De Souza, C.M.; Scorzoni, L.; Fenley, J.C.; Junqueira, J.C. *Candida* Biofilms: An Update on Developmental Mechanisms and Therapeutic Challenges [published online ahead of print, 2020 Apr 10]. *Mycopathologia* **2020**. [CrossRef]
10. Cavalheiro, M.; Teixeira, M.C. Candida Biofilms: Threats, Challenges, and Promising Strategies. *Front. Med.* **2018**, *5*, 28. [CrossRef]
11. Nett, J.E. Future directions for anti-biofilm therapeutics targeting *Candida*. *Expert Rev. Anti Infect. Ther.* **2014**, *12*, 375–382. [CrossRef] [PubMed]
12. Davis, M.R.; Donnelley, M.A.; Thompson, G.R. Ibrexafungerp: A novel oral glucan synthase inhibitor [published online ahead of print, 2019 Jul 25]. *Med. Mycol.* **2019**, myz083. [CrossRef]
13. Pfaller, M.A.; Carvalhaes, C.; Messer, S.A.; Rhomberg, P.R.; Castanheira, M. Activity of a Long-Acting Echinocandin, Rezafungin, and Comparator Antifungal Agents Tested against Contemporary Invasive Fungal Isolates (SENTRY Program, 2016 to 2018). *Antimicrob. Agents Chemother.* **2020**, *64*, e00099-20. [CrossRef] [PubMed]

14. Nield, B.; Larsen, S.R.; Van Hal, S.J. Clinical experience with new formulation SUBA®-itraconazole for prophylaxis in patients undergoing stem cell transplantation or treatment for haematological malignancies. *J. Antimicrob. Chemother.* **2019**, *74*, 3049–3055. [CrossRef]
15. Warrilow, A.G.; Hull, C.M.; Parker, J.E.; Garvey, E.P.; Hoekstra, W.J.; Moore, W.R.; Schotzinger, R.J.; Kelly, D.E.; Kelly, S.L. The clinical candidate VT-1161 is a highly potent inhibitor of *Candida albicans* CYP51 but fails to bind the human enzyme. *Antimicrob. Agents Chemother.* **2014**, *58*, 7121–7127. [CrossRef]
16. Samaranayake, Y.H.; Ye, J.; Yau, J.Y.; Cheung, B.P.; Samaranayake, L.P. In vitro method to study antifungal perfusion in *Candida* biofilms. *J. Clin. Microbiol.* **2005**, *43*, 818–825. [CrossRef]
17. Kuhn, D.M.; George, T.; Chandra, J.; Mukherjee, P.K.; Ghannoum, M.A. Antifungal susceptibility of *Candida* biofilms: Unique efficacy of amphotericin B lipid formulations and echinocandins. *Antimicrob. Agents Chemother.* **2002**, *46*, 1773–1780. [CrossRef]
18. Pappas, P.G.; Kauffman, C.A.; Andes, D.R.; Clancy, C.J.; Marr, K.A.; Ostrosky-Zeichner, L.; Reboli, A.C.; Schuster, M.G.; Vazquez, J.A.; Walsh, T.J.; et al. Executive Summary: Clinical Practice Guideline for the Management of Candidiasis: 2016 Update by the Infectious Diseases Society of America. *Clin. Infect. Dis.* **2016**, *62*, 409–417. [CrossRef]
19. Walraven, C.J.; Lee, S.A. Antifungal lock therapy. *Antimicrob. Agents Chemother.* **2013**, *57*, 1–8. [CrossRef]
20. Kovács, R.; Nagy, F.; Tóth, Z.; Bozó, A.; Balázs, B.; Majoros, L. Synergistic effect of nikkomycin Z with caspofungin and micafungin against *Candida albicans* and *Candida parapsilosis* biofilms. *Lett. Appl. Microbiol.* **2019**, *69*, 271–278. [CrossRef]
21. Wall, G.; Chaturvedi, A.K.; Wormley, F.L., Jr.; Wiederhold, N.P.; Patterson, H.P.; Patterson, T.F.; Lopez-Ribot, J.L. Screening a Repurposing Library for Inhibitors of Multidrug-Resistant *Candida auris* Identifies Ebselen as a Repositionable Candidate for Antifungal Drug Development. *Antimicrob. Agents Chemother.* **2018**, *62*, e01084-18. [CrossRef] [PubMed]
22. Pedroso, R.; Balbino, B.L.; Andrade, G.; Dias, M.; Alvarenga, T.A.; Pedroso, R.; Pimenta, L.P.; Lucarini, R.; Pauletti, P.M.; Januário, A.H.; et al. In Vitro and In Vivo Anti-*Candida* spp. Activity of Plant-Derived Products. *Plants* **2019**, *8*, 494. [CrossRef] [PubMed]
23. Souza, C.M.; Pereira Junior, S.A.; Moraes, T.; Damasceno, J.L.; Amorim Mendes, S.; Dias, H.J.; Stefani, R.; Tavares, D.C.; Martins, C.H.; Crotti, A.E.; et al. Antifungal activity of plant-derived essential oils on *Candida tropicalis* planktonic and biofilms cells. *Med. Mycol.* **2016**, *54*, 515–523. [CrossRef] [PubMed]
24. Sherry, L.; Jose, A.; Murray, C.; Williams, C.; Jones, B.; Millington, O.; Bagg, J.; Ramage, G. Carbohydrate Derived Fulvic Acid: An in vitro Investigation of a Novel Membrane Active Antiseptic Agent against Candida albicans Biofilms. *Front. Microbiol.* **2012**, *3*, 116. [CrossRef]
25. Ramage, G.; Saville, S.P.; Wickes, B.L.; López-Ribot, J.L. Inhibition of *Candida albicans* biofilm formation by farnesol, a quorum-sensing molecule. *Appl. Environ. Microbiol.* **2002**, *68*, 5459–5463. [CrossRef]
26. Katragkou, A.; McCarthy, M.; Alexander, E.L.; Antachopoulos, C.; Meletiadis, J.; Jabra-Rizk, M.A.; Petraitis, V.; Roilides, E.; Walsh, T.J. In vitro interactions between farnesol and fluconazole, amphotericin B or micafungin against *Candida albicans* biofilms. *J. Antimicrob. Chemother.* **2015**, *70*, 470–478. [CrossRef]
27. Kovács, R.; Bozó, A.; Gesztelyi, R.; Domán, M.; Kardos, G.; Nagy, F.; Tóth, Z.; Majoros, L. Effect of caspofungin and micafungin in combination with farnesol against *Candida parapsilosis* biofilms. *Int. J. Antimicrob. Agents.* **2016**, *47*, 304–310. [CrossRef]
28. Weiland-Bräuer, N.; Malek, I.; Schmitz, R.A. Metagenomic quorum quenching enzymes affect biofilm formation of Candida albicans and Staphylococcus epidermidis. *PLoS ONE* **2019**, *14*, e0211366. [CrossRef]
29. Nobile, C.J.; Johnson, A.D. *Candida albicans* Biofilms and Human Disease. *Annu. Rev. Microbiol.* **2015**, *69*, 71–92. [CrossRef]
30. Harriott, M.M.; Lilly, E.A.; Rodriguez, T.E.; Fidel, P.L.; Noverr, M.C. *Candida albicans* forms biofilms on the vaginal mucosa. *Microbiology* **2010**, *156 Pt 12*, 3635–3644. [CrossRef]
31. Ganguly, S.; Mitchell, A.P. Mucosal biofilms of *Candida albicans*. *Curr. Opin. Microbiol.* **2011**, *14*, 380–385. [CrossRef] [PubMed]
32. Kalan, L.; Loesche, M.; Hodkinson, B.P.; Heilmann, K.; Ruthel, G.; Gardner, S.E.; Grice, E.A. Redefining the Chronic-Wound Microbiome: Fungal Communities Are Prevalent, Dynamic, and Associated with Delayed Healing. *MBio* **2016**, *7*, e01058-16. [CrossRef] [PubMed]

33. Ramage, G.; VandeWalle, K.; López-Ribot, J.L.; Wickes, B.L. The filamentation pathway controlled by the Efg1 regulator protein is required for normal biofilm formation and development in *Candida albicans*. *FEMS Microbiol. Lett.* **2002**, *214*, 95–100. [CrossRef]
34. Lewis, K. Persister cells, dormancy and infectious disease. *Nat. Rev. Microbiol.* **2007**, *5*, 48–56. [CrossRef] [PubMed]
35. Ramage, G.; Bachmann, S.; Patterson, T.F.; Wickes, B.L.; López-Ribot, J.L. Investigation of multidrug efflux pumps in relation to fluconazole resistance in *Candida albicans* biofilms. *J. Antimicrob. Chemother.* **2002**, *49*, 973–980. [CrossRef] [PubMed]
36. Mehmood, A.; Liu, G.; Wang, X.; Meng, G.; Wang, C.; Liu, Y. Fungal Quorum-Sensing Molecules and Inhibitors with Potential Antifungal Activity: A Review. *Molecules* **2019**, *24*, 1950. [CrossRef]
37. Albuquerque, P.; Casadevall, A. Quorum sensing in fungi—A review. *Med. Mycol.* **2012**, *50*, 337–345. [CrossRef] [PubMed]
38. Hornby, J.M.; Jensen, E.C.; Lisec, A.D.; Tasto, J.J.; Jahnke, B.; Shoemaker, R.; Dussault, P.; Nickerson, K.W. Quorum sensing in the dimorphic fungus *Candida albicans* is mediated by farnesol. *Appl. Environ. Microbiol.* **2001**, *67*, 2982–2992. [CrossRef]
39. Sorrentino, F.; Roy, I.; Keshavarz, T. Impact of linoleic acid supplementation on lovastatin production in *Aspergillus terreus* cultures. *Appl. Microbiol. Biotechnol.* **2010**, *88*, 65–73. [CrossRef]
40. Raina, S.; Odell, M.; Keshavarz, T. Quorum sensing as a method for improving sclerotiorin production in *Penicillium sclerotiorum*. *J. Biotechnol.* **2010**, *148*, 91–98. [CrossRef]
41. Wongsuk, T.; Pumeesat, P.; Luplertlop, N. Fungal quorum sensing molecules: Role in fungal morphogenesis and pathogenicity. *J. Basic Microbiol.* **2016**, *56*, 440–447. [CrossRef] [PubMed]
42. Vila, T.; Kong, E.F.; Ibrahim, A.; Piepenbrink, K.; Shetty, A.C.; McCracken, C.; Bruno, V.; Jabra-Rizk, M.A. *Candida albicans* quorum-sensing molecule farnesol modulates staphyloxanthin production and activates the thiol-based oxidative-stress response in *Staphylococcus aureus*. *Virulence* **2019**, *10*, 625–642. [CrossRef] [PubMed]
43. Jakab, Á.; Tóth, Z.; Nagy, F.; Nemes, D.; Bácskay, I.; Kardos, G.; Emri, T.; Pócsi, I.; Majoros, L.; Kovács, R. Physiological and Transcriptional Responses of *Candida parapsilosis* to Exogenous Tyrosol. *Appl. Environ. Microbiol.* **2019**, *85*, e01388-19. [CrossRef]
44. Shirtliff, M.E.; Krom, B.P.; Meijering, R.A.; Peters, B.M.; Zhu, J.; Scheper, M.A.; Harris, M.L.; Jabra-Rizk, M.A. Farnesol-induced apoptosis in *Candida albicans*. *Antimicrob. Agents Chemother.* **2009**, *53*, 2392–2401. [CrossRef]
45. Nagy, F.; Vitális, E.; Jakab, Á.; Borman, A.M.; Forgács, L.; Tóth, Z.; Majoros, L.; Kovács, R. In vitro and in vivo Effect of Exogenous Farnesol Exposure against *Candida auris*. *Front. Microbiol.* **2020**, *11*, 957. [CrossRef] [PubMed]
46. Hornby, J.M.; Kebaara, B.W.; Nickerson, K.W. Farnesol biosynthesis in *Candida albicans*: Cellular response to sterol inhibition by zaragozic acid B. *Antimicrob. Agents Chemother.* **2003**, *47*, 2366–2369. [CrossRef] [PubMed]
47. Westwater, C.; Balish, E.; Schofield, D.A. *Candida albicans*-conditioned medium protects yeast cells from oxidative stress: A possible link between quorum sensing and oxidative stress resistance. *Eukaryot Cell* **2005**, *4*, 1654–1661. [CrossRef]
48. Weber, K.; Sohr, R.; Schulz, B.; Fleischhacker, M.; Ruhnke, M. Secretion of E,E-farnesol and biofilm formation in eight different *Candida* species [published correction appears in Antimicrob Agents Chemother. 2009 Feb;53(2):848]. *Antimicrob. Agents Chemother.* **2008**, *52*, 1859–1861. [CrossRef]
49. Nickerson, K.W.; Atkin, A.L.; Hornby, J.M. Quorum sensing in dimorphic fungi: Farnesol and beyond. *Appl. Environ. Microbiol.* **2006**, *72*, 3805–3813. [CrossRef]
50. Cao, Y.Y.; Cao, Y.B.; Xu, Z.; Ying, K.; Li, Y.; Xie, Y.; Zhu, Z.Y.; Chen, W.S.; Jiang, Y.Y. cDNA microarray analysis of differential gene expression in *Candida albicans* biofilm exposed to farnesol. *Antimicrob. Agents Chemother.* **2005**, *49*, 584–589. [CrossRef]
51. Sharma, M.; Prasad, R. The quorum-sensing molecule farnesol is a modulator of drug efflux mediated by ABC multidrug transporters and synergizes with drugs in *Candida albicans*. *Antimicrob. Agents Chemother.* **2011**, *55*, 4834–4843. [CrossRef] [PubMed]
52. Léger, T.; Garcia, C.; Ounissi, M.; Lelandais, G.; Camadro, J.M. The metacaspase (Mca1p) has a dual role in farnesol-induced apoptosis in *Candida albicans*. *Mol. Cell Proteom.* **2015**, *14*, 93–108. [CrossRef]
53. Enjalbert, B.; Whiteway, M. Release from quorum-sensing molecules triggers hyphal formation during *Candida albicans* resumption of growth. *Eukaryot Cell* **2005**, *4*, 1203–1210. [CrossRef] [PubMed]
54. Uppuluri, P.; Mekala, S.; Chaffin, W.L. Farnesol-mediated inhibition of *Candida albicans* yeast growth and rescue by a diacylglycerol analogue. *Yeast* **2007**, *24*, 681–693. [CrossRef] [PubMed]

55. Weber, K.; Schulz, B.; Ruhnke, M. The quorum-sensing molecule E,E-farnesol—Its variable secretion and its impact on the growth and metabolism of *Candida* species. *Yeast* **2010**, *27*, 727–739. [CrossRef]
56. Langford, M.L.; Hasim, S.; Nickerson, K.W.; Atkin, A.L. Activity and toxicity of farnesol towards *Candida albicans* are dependent on growth conditions. *Antimicrob. Agents Chemother.* **2010**, *54*, 940–942. [CrossRef]
57. Polke, M.; Leonhardt, I.; Kurzai, O.; Jacobsen, I.D. Farnesol signalling in *Candida albicans*-more than just communication. *Crit. Rev. Microbiol.* **2018**, *44*, 230–243. [CrossRef]
58. Piispanen, A.E.; Grahl, N.; Hollomon, J.M.; Hogan, D.A. Regulated proteolysis of *Candida albicans* Ras1 is involved in morphogenesis and quorum sensing regulation. *Mol. Microbiol.* **2013**, *89*, 166–178. [CrossRef]
59. Lindsay, A.K.; Deveau, A.; Piispanen, A.E.; Hogan, D.A. Farnesol and cyclic AMP signaling effects on the hypha-to-yeast transition in *Candida albicans*. *Eukaryot Cell* **2012**, *11*, 1219–1225. [CrossRef]
60. Lu, Y.; Su, C.; Unoje, O.; Liu, H. Quorum sensing controls hyphal initiation in *Candida albicans* through Ubr1-mediated protein degradation. *Proc. Natl. Acad. Sci. USA* **2014**, *111*, 1975–1980. [CrossRef]
61. Rossignol, T.; Logue, M.E.; Reynolds, K.; Grenon, M.; Lowndes, N.F.; Butler, G. Transcriptional response of *Candida parapsilosis* following exposure to farnesol [published correction appears in Antimicrob Agents Chemother. 2008 Jun;52(6):2296]. *Antimicrob. Agents Chemother.* **2007**, *51*, 2304–2312. [CrossRef] [PubMed]
62. Fairn, G.D.; Macdonald, K.; McMaster, C.R. A chemogenomic screen in *Saccharomyces cerevisiae* uncovers a primary role for the mitochondria in farnesol toxicity and its regulation by the Pkc1 pathway. *J. Biol. Chem.* **2007**, *282*, 4868–4874. [CrossRef] [PubMed]
63. Lorek, J.; Pöggeler, S.; Weide, M.R.; Breves, R.; Bockmühl, D.P. Influence of farnesol on the morphogenesis of *Aspergillus niger*. *J. Basic Microbiol.* **2008**, *48*, 99–103. [CrossRef] [PubMed]
64. Wang, X.; Wang, Y.; Zhou, Y.; Wei, X. Farnesol induces apoptosis-like cell death in the pathogenic fungus *Aspergillus flavus*. *Mycologia* **2014**, *106*, 881–888. [CrossRef] [PubMed]
65. Semighini, C.P.; Hornby, J.M.; Dumitru, R.; Nickerson, K.W.; Harris, S.D. Farnesol-induced apoptosis in *Aspergillus nidulans* reveals a possible mechanism for antagonistic interactions between fungi. *Mol. Microbiol.* **2006**, *59*, 753–764. [CrossRef]
66. Liu, P.; Luo, L.; Guo, J.; Liu, H.; Wang, B.; Deng, B.; Long, C.A.; Cheng, Y. Farnesol induces apoptosis and oxidative stress in the fungal pathogen *Penicillium expansum*. *Mycologia* **2010**, *102*, 311–318. [CrossRef]
67. Semighini, C.P.; Murray, N.; Harris, S.D. Inhibition of *Fusarium graminearum* growth and development by farnesol. *FEMS Microbiol. Lett.* **2008**, *279*, 259–264. [CrossRef]
68. Derengowski, L.S.; De-Souza-Silva, C.; Braz, S.V.; Mello-De-Sousa, T.M.; Báo, S.N.; Kyaw, C.M.; Silva-Pereira, I. Antimicrobial effect of farnesol, a *Candida albicans* quorum sensing molecule, on *Paracoccidioides brasiliensis* growth and morphogenesis. *Ann. Clin. Microbiol. Antimicrob.* **2009**, *8*, 13. [CrossRef]
69. Hargarten, J.C.; Moore, T.C.; Petro, T.M.; Nickerson, K.W.; Atkin, A.L. Candida albicans Quorum Sensing Molecules Stimulate Mouse Macrophage Migration. *Infect. Immun.* **2015**, *83*, 3857–3864. [CrossRef]
70. Scheper, M.A.; Shirtliff, M.E.; Meiller, T.F.; Peters, B.M.; Jabra-Rizk, M.A. Farnesol, a fungal quorum-sensing molecule triggers apoptosis in human oral squamous carcinoma cells. *Neoplasia* **2008**, *10*, 954–963. [CrossRef]
71. Wang, Z.; Chen, H.T.; Roa, W.; Finlay, W. Farnesol for aerosol inhalation: Nebulization and activity against human lung cancer cells. *J. Pharm. Pharm. Sci.* **2003**, *6*, 95–100. [PubMed]
72. Rodrigues, C.F.; Černáková, L. Farnesol and Tyrosol: Secondary Metabolites with a Crucial quorum-sensing Role in *Candida* Biofilm Development. *Genes* **2020**, *11*, 444. [CrossRef] [PubMed]
73. Dižová, S.; Černáková, L.; Bujdáková, H. The impact of farnesol in combination with fluconazole on *Candida albicans* biofilm: Regulation of ERG20, ERG9, and ERG11 genes. *Folia Microbiol.* **2018**, *63*, 363–371. [CrossRef] [PubMed]
74. Chen, S.; Xia, J.; Li, C.; Zuo, L.; Wei, X. The possible molecular mechanisms of farnesol on the antifungal resistance of *C. albicans* biofilms: The regulation of CYR1 and PDE2. *BMC Microbiol.* **2018**, *18*, 203. [CrossRef]
75. Yu, L.H.; Wei, X.; Ma, M.; Chen, X.J.; Xu, S.B. Possible inhibitory molecular mechanism of farnesol on the development of fluconazole resistance in *Candida albicans* biofilm. *Antimicrob. Agents Chemother.* **2012**, *56*, 770–775. [CrossRef]
76. Jabra-Rizk, M.A.; Shirtliff, M.; James, C.; Meiller, T. Effect of farnesol on *Candida dubliniensis* biofilm formation and fluconazole resistance. *FEMS Yeast Res.* **2006**, *6*, 1063–1073. [CrossRef]
77. Fernández-Rivero, M.E.; Del Pozo, J.L.; Valentín, A.; De Diego, A.M.; Pemán, J.; Cantón, E. Activity of Amphotericin B and Anidulafungin Combined with Rifampicin, Clarithromycin, Ethylenediaminetetraacetic Acid, N-Acetylcysteine, and Farnesol against *Candida tropicalis* Biofilms. *J. Fungi* **2017**, *3*, 16. [CrossRef]

78. Nagy, F.; Tóth, Z.; Daróczi, L.; Székely, A.; Borman, A.M.; Majoros, L.; Kovács, R. Farnesol increases the activity of echinocandins against *Candida auris* biofilms. *Med. Mycol.* **2020**, *58*, 404–407. [CrossRef]
79. Navarathna, D.H.; Hornby, J.M.; Krishnan, N.; Parkhurst, A.; Duhamel, G.E.; Nickerson, K.W. Effect of farnesol on a mouse model of systemic candidiasis, determined by use of a DPP3 knockout mutant of *Candida albicans*. *Infect. Immun.* **2007**, *75*, 1609–1618. [CrossRef]
80. Hisajima, T.; Maruyama, N.; Tanabe, Y.; Ishibashi, H.; Yamada, T.; Makimura, K.; Nishiyama, Y.; Funakoshi, K.; Oshima, H.; Abe, S. Protective effects of farnesol against oral candidiasis in mice. *Microbiol. Immunol.* **2008**, *52*, 327–333. [CrossRef]
81. Martins, M.; Lazzell, A.L.; Lopez-Ribot, J.L.; Henriques, M.; Oliveira, R. Effect of exogenous administration of *Candida albicans* autoregulatory alcohols in a murine model of hematogenously disseminated candidiasis. *J. Basic Microbiol.* **2012**, *52*, 487–491. [CrossRef]
82. Bozó, A.; Domán, M.; Majoros, L.; Kardos, G.; Varga, I.; Kovács, R. The in vitro and in vivo efficacy of fluconazole in combination with farnesol against *Candida albicans* isolates using a murine vulvovaginitis model. *J. Microbiol.* **2016**, *54*, 753–760. [CrossRef] [PubMed]
83. Cordeiro, R.A.; Teixeira, C.E.; Brilhante, R.S.; Castelo-Branco, D.S.; Paiva, M.A.; Giffoni Leite, J.J.; Lima, D.T.; Monteiro, A.J.; Sidrim, J.J.; Rocha, M.F.; et al. Minimum inhibitory concentrations of amphotericin B, azoles and caspofungin against *Candida* species are reduced by farnesol. *Med. Mycol.* **2013**, *51*, 53–59. [CrossRef] [PubMed]
84. Fernandes Costa, A.; Evangelista Araujo, D.; Santos Cabral, M.; Teles Brito, I.; Borges de Menezes Leite, L.; Pereira, M.; Correa Amaral, A. Development, characterization, and in vitro-in vivo evaluation of polymeric nanoparticles containing miconazole and farnesol for treatment of vulvovaginal candidiasis. *Med. Mycol.* **2019**, *57*, 52–62. [CrossRef]
85. Funari, S.S.; Prades, J.; Escribá, P.V.; Barceló, F. Farnesol and geranylgeraniol modulate the structural properties of phosphatidylethanolamine model membranes. *Mol. Membr. Biol.* **2005**, *22*, 303–311. [CrossRef] [PubMed]
86. Jabra-Rizk, M.A.; Meiller, T.F.; James, C.E.; Shirtliff, M.E. Effect of farnesol on *Staphylococcus aureus* biofilm formation and antimicrobial susceptibility. *Antimicrob. Agents Chemother.* **2006**, *50*, 1463–1469. [CrossRef] [PubMed]
87. Gomes, F.I.; Teixeira, P.; Azeredo, J.; Oliveira, R. Effect of farnesol on planktonic and biofilm cells of *Staphylococcus epidermidis*. *Curr. Microbiol.* **2009**, *59*, 118–122. [CrossRef]
88. Pammi, M.; Liang, R.; Hicks, J.M.; Barrish, J.; Versalovic, J. Farnesol decreases biofilms of *Staphylococcus epidermidis* and exhibits synergy with nafcillin and vancomycin. *Pediatr. Res.* **2011**, *70*, 578–583. [CrossRef]
89. Kim, C.; Hesek, D.; Lee, M.; Mobashery, S. Potentiation of the activity of β-lactam antibiotics by farnesol and its derivatives. *Bioorg. Med. Chem. Lett.* **2018**, *28*, 642–645. [CrossRef]
90. Brilhante, R.S.; Valente, L.G.; Rocha, M.F.; Bandeira, T.J.; Cordeiro, R.A.; Lima, R.A.; Leite, J.J.; Ribeiro, J.F.; Pereira, J.F.; Castelo-Branco, D.S.; et al. Sesquiterpene farnesol contributes to increased susceptibility to β-lactams in strains of *Burkholderia pseudomallei*. *Antimicrob. Agents Chemother.* **2012**, *56*, 2198–2200. [CrossRef]
91. Castelo-Branco, D.S.; Riello, G.B.; Vasconcelos, D.C.; Guedes, G.M.; Serpa, R.; Bandeira, T.J.; Monteiro, A.J.; Cordeiro, R.A.; Rocha, M.F.; Sidrim, J.J.; et al. Farnesol increases the susceptibility of *Burkholderia pseudomallei* biofilm to antimicrobials used to treat melioidosis. *J. Appl. Microbiol.* **2016**, *120*, 600–606. [CrossRef] [PubMed]
92. Bandara, H.M.; Herpin, M.J.; Kolacny, D., Jr.; Harb, A.; Romanovicz, D.; Smyth, H.D. Incorporation of Farnesol Significantly Increases the Efficacy of Liposomal Ciprofloxacin against *Pseudomonas aeruginosa* Biofilms in Vitro. *Mol. Pharm.* **2016**, *13*, 2760–2770. [CrossRef] [PubMed]
93. Černáková, L.; Jordao, L.; Bujdáková, H. Impact of farnesol and Corsodyl® on *Candida albicans* forming dual biofilm with *Streptococcus mutans*. *Oral Dis.* **2018**, *24*, 1126–1131. [CrossRef] [PubMed]
94. Cugini, C.; Morales, D.K.; Hogan, D.A. *Candida albicans*-produced farnesol stimulates *Pseudomonas* quinolone signal production in LasR-defective *Pseudomonas aeruginosa* strains. *Microbiology* **2010**, *156*, 3096–3107. [CrossRef]
95. Chen, H.; Fujita, M.; Feng, Q.; Clardy, J.; Fink, G.R. Tyrosol is a quorum-sensing molecule in *Candida albicans*. *Proc. Natl. Acad. Sci. USA* **2004**, *101*, 5048–5052. [CrossRef]
96. Alem, M.A.; Oteef, M.D.; Flowers, T.H.; Douglas, L.J. Production of tyrosol by *Candida albicans* biofilms and its role in quorum sensing and biofilm development. *Eukaryot. Cell* **2006**, *5*, 1770–1779. [CrossRef]
97. Bigagli, E.; Cinci, L.; Paccosi, S.; Parenti, A.; D'Ambrosio, M.; Luceri, C. Nutritionally relevant concentrations of resveratrol and hydroxytyrosol mitigate oxidative burst of human granulocytes and monocytes and the production of pro-inflammatory mediators in LPS-stimulated RAW 264.7 macrophages. *Int. Immunopharmacol.* **2017**, *43*, 147–155. [CrossRef]

98. Rigacci, S.; Stefani, M. Nutraceutical Properties of Olive Oil Polyphenols. An Itinerary from Cultured Cells through Animal Models to Humans. *Int. J. Mol. Sci.* **2016**, *17*, 843. [CrossRef]
99. Cremer, J.; Vatou, V.; Braveny, I. 2,4-(hydroxyphenyl)-ethanol, an antioxidative agent produced by *Candida* spp., impairs neutrophilic yeast killing in vitro. *FEMS Microbiol. Lett.* **1999**, *170*, 319–325. [CrossRef]
100. Holland, L.M.; Schröder, M.S.; Turner, S.A.; Taff, H.; Andes, D.; Grózer, Z.; Gácser, A.; Ames, L.; Haynes, K.; Higgins, D.G.; et al. Comparative phenotypic analysis of the major fungal pathogens *Candida parapsilosis* and *Candida albicans*. *PLoS Pathog.* **2014**, *10*, e1004365. [CrossRef]
101. Monteiro, D.R.; Feresin, L.P.; Arias, L.S.; Barão, V.A.; Barbosa, D.B.; Delbem, A.C. Effect of tyrosol on adhesion of *Candida albicans* and *Candida glabrata* to acrylic surfaces. *Med. Mycol.* **2015**, *53*, 656–665. [CrossRef] [PubMed]
102. Babich, H.; Visioli, F. In vitro cytotoxicity to human cells in culture of some phenolics from olive oil. *Farmaco* **2003**, *58*, 403–407. [CrossRef]
103. Arias, L.S.; Delbem, A.C.; Fernandes, R.A.; Barbosa, D.B.; Monteiro, D.R. Activity of tyrosol against single and mixed-species oral biofilms. *J. Appl. Microbiol.* **2016**, *120*, 1240–1249. [CrossRef]
104. Do Vale, L.R.; Delbem, A.; Arias, L.S.; Fernandes, R.A.; Vieira, A.; Barbosa, D.B.; Monteiro, D.R. Differential effects of the combination of tyrosol with chlorhexidine gluconate on oral biofilms. *Oral Dis.* **2017**, *23*, 537–541. [CrossRef] [PubMed]
105. Monteiro, D.R.; Arias, L.S.; Fernandes, R.A.; Deszo da Silva, L.F.; De Castilho, M.; Da Rosa, T.O.; Vieira, A.; Straioto, F.G.; Barbosa, D.B.; Delbem, A. Antifungal activity of tyrosol and farnesol used in combination against *Candida* species in the planktonic state or forming biofilms. *J. Appl. Microbiol.* **2017**, *123*, 392–400. [CrossRef] [PubMed]
106. Monteiro, D.R.; Arias, L.S.; Fernandes, R.A.; Straioto, F.G.; Barros Barbosa, D.; Pessan, J.P.; Delbem, A. Role of tyrosol on *Candida albicans*, *Candida glabrata* and *Streptococcus mutans* biofilms developed on different surfaces. *Am. J. Dent.* **2017**, *30*, 35–39.
107. Shanmughapriya, S.; Sornakumari, H.; Lency, A.; Kavitha, S.; Natarajaseenivasan, K. Synergistic effect of amphotericin B and tyrosol on biofilm formed by *Candida krusei* and *Candida tropicalis* from intrauterine device users. *Med. Mycol.* **2014**, *52*, 853–861. [CrossRef]
108. Cordeiro, R.; Teixeira, C.E.; Brilhante, R.S.; Castelo-Branco, D.S.; Alencar, L.P.; De Oliveira, J.S.; Monteiro, A.J.; Bandeira, T.J.; Sidrim, J.J.; Moreira, J.L.; et al. Exogenous tyrosol inhibits planktonic cells and biofilms of *Candida* species and enhances their susceptibility to antifungals. *FEMS Yeast Res.* **2015**, *15*, fov012. [CrossRef] [PubMed]
109. Kovács, R.; Tóth, Z.; Nagy, F.; Daróczi, L.; Bozó, A.; Majoros, L. Activity of exogenous tyrosol in combination with caspofungin and micafungin against *Candida parapsilosis* sessile cells. *J. Appl. Microbiol.* **2017**, *122*, 1529–1536. [CrossRef]
110. Abdel-Rhman, S.H.; Rizk, D.E. Effect of tyrosol on *Staphylococcus aureus* antimicrobial susceptibility, biofilm formation and virulence factors. *Afr. J. Microbiol. Res.* **2016**, *10*, 687–693. [CrossRef]
111. Abdel-Rhman, S.H.; El-Mahdy, A.M.; El-Mowafy, M. Effect of Tyrosol and Farnesol on Virulence and Antibiotic Resistance of Clinical Isolates of *Pseudomonas aeruginosa*. *Biomed. Res. Int.* **2015**, *2015*, 456463. [CrossRef] [PubMed]

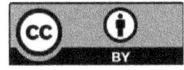

© 2020 by the authors. Licensee MDPI, Basel, Switzerland. This article is an open access article distributed under the terms and conditions of the Creative Commons Attribution (CC BY) license (http://creativecommons.org/licenses/by/4.0/).

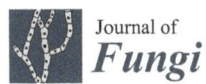

Article

Biofilm Formed by *Candida haemulonii* Species Complex: Structural Analysis and Extracellular Matrix Composition

Lívia S. Ramos [1], Thaís P. Mello [1], Marta H. Branquinha [1] and André L. S. Santos [1,2,*]

[1] Laboratório de Estudos Avançados de Microrganismos Emergentes e Resistentes (LEAMER), Departamento de Microbiologia Geral, Instituto de Microbiologia Paulo de Góes (IMPG), Universidade Federal do Rio de Janeiro (UFRJ), Rio de Janeiro 21941-901, Brazil; liviaramos2@yahoo.com.br (L.S.R.); thaispdmello@gmail.com (T.P.M.); mbranquinha@micro.ufrj.br (M.H.B.)
[2] Programa de Pós-Graduação em Bioquímica (PPGBq), Instituto de Química (IQ), UFRJ, Rio de Janeiro 21941-909, Brazil
* Correspondence: andre@micro.ufrj.br; Tel.: +55-21-3938-0366

Received: 6 March 2020; Accepted: 1 April 2020; Published: 3 April 2020

Abstract: *Candida haemulonii* species complex (*C. haemulonii*, *C. duobushaemulonii*, and *C. haemulonii* var. *vulnera*) has emerged as opportunistic, multidrug-resistant yeasts able to cause fungemia. Previously, we showed that *C. haemulonii* complex formed biofilm on polystyrene. Biofilm is a well-known virulence attribute of *Candida* spp. directly associated with drug resistance. In the present study, the architecture and the main extracellular matrix (ECM) components forming the biofilm over polystyrene were investigated in clinical isolates of the *C. haemulonii* complex. We also evaluated the ability of these fungi to form biofilm on catheters used in medical arena. The results revealed that all fungi formed biofilms on polystyrene after 48 h at 37 °C. Microscopic analyses demonstrated a dense network of yeasts forming the biofilm structure, with water channels and ECM. Regarding ECM, proteins and carbohydrates were the main components, followed by nucleic acids and sterols. Mature biofilms were also detected on late bladder (siliconized latex), nasoenteric (polyurethane), and nasogastric (polyvinyl chloride) catheters, with the biomasses being significantly greater than on polystyrene. Collectively, our results demonstrated the ability of the *C. haemulonii* species complex to form biofilm on different types of inert surfaces, which is an incontestable virulence attribute associated with devices-related candidemia in hospitalized individuals.

Keywords: *Candida haemulonii* complex; biofilm; extracellular matrix; catheter; polystyrene; virulence

1. Introduction

Candida haemulonii, *Candida duobushaemulonii*, and *Candida haemulonii* var. *vulnera* form a fungal complex (named *C. haemulonii* complex) that is represented by emergent, opportunistic yeasts able to cause human infections with a wide range of clinical manifestations, varying from superficial to deep-seated infections, especially in individuals with immunocompromising health conditions [1]. In this sense, the main isolation sites of the *C. haemulonii* species complex described in the literature are blood, foot ulcers, nails, bones, skin wounds, and vagina; however, there are reports of isolates obtained from other body fluids such as cerebrospinal fluid, bronchoalveolar lavage, vaginal discharge, pleural effusion, peritoneal and ascitic fluids, bile, and urine [1–15].

The multidrug-resistance profile of the *C. haemulonii* species complex has been highlighted by many research groups worldwide, making it a challenge to treat such infections, which is aggravated by the immunological status of the majority of target patients. Although the knowledge about this fungal complex has been growing in recent years, many aspects related to its virulence need to be better investigated. In this sense, biofilm formation is an unquestionable and well-known virulence attribute associated with both bacterial and fungal infections around the world. Biofilm formation by the *C. haemulonii* species complex has already been reported based on the use of classical methodologies [1,7,16], but there is lack of information about the characteristics of the biofilm formed by these fungi. Indeed, it is believed that biofilm lifestyle is the preferred organization mode of microorganisms in nature, which is characterized by a highly complex structured community of microorganisms that interact with each other and with a biotic/abiotic surface, covered by a self-produced extracellular matrix (ECM) composed mainly of proteins, polysaccharides, lipids, nucleic acids, minerals, and water [17,18]. Functionally, the ECM plays an important role in the biofilm maintenance, architecture, and dynamic, being responsible for conferring protection against external stressors, such as host immune responses (both humoral and cellular components) and drugs (either disinfectants or antimicrobial agents), which directly impact the treatment, especially that of seriously ill patients [18,19].

Biofilm-related infections are considered a huge problem in healthcare settings worldwide [20]. Many chronic infections caused by both bacteria and fungi have been associated to biofilm mode of growth, including lung infections (e.g., fungal ball) and chronic leg wounds [20]. *Candida* species, for example, can form biofilm on a variety of medical devices, and it is well-known that catheter-related fungemia is associated with high morbidity and mortality rates among patients in healthcare services, despite the consequent financial burden related to this situation [20]. *C. haemulonii* complex has already been associated to cases of catheter-related fungemia in both pediatric and elderly patients [6,21], and the catheter, in this scenario, acts as a gateway to the infection development as well as to its chronicity.

In the present study, we aimed to investigate the architecture of the biofilm formed by 12 clinical isolates comprising the *C. haemulonii* species complex (*C. haemulonii*, n = 5; *C. duobushaemulonii*, n = 4; and *C. haemulonii* var. *vulnera*, n = 3) on polystyrene, with a special focus on the study of the chemical composition of their ECM. Additionally, we evaluated and compared the ability of these fungal isolates to form biofilm on different medical devices commonly applied in clinical settings, such as nasogastric, late bladder, and nasoenteric catheters made of polyvinyl chloride, siliconized latex, and polyurethane, respectively.

2. Materials and Methods

2.1. Microorganisms and Growth Conditions

A total of 12 clinical isolates recovered from patients from Brazilian hospitals between 2005 and 2013 and identified by molecular approaches as belonging to the *C. haemulonii* species complex were used in the present work [10]. Some relevant data about the fungal isolates are summarized in Table 1. Fungal cells were cultured in Sabouraud dextrose medium (under the following conditions: 37 °C for 48 h at 200 rpm) and then used in all the experiments. The yeast cells were quantified using a Neubauer chamber.

2.2. Biofilm Formation on Polystyrene

Fungal cell suspensions in Sabouraud broth (200 μL containing 10^6 yeasts) were transferred into each well of a flat-bottom 96-well polystyrene microtiter plate, and then incubated without agitation at 37 °C for 48 h. Plate wells containing only culture medium were used to set up the reader as blanks. The supernatant fluids were removed by pipetting and, subsequently, the plate wells were washed three times with phosphate-buffered saline (PBS, pH 7.2) to remove nonadherent cells. The measurements of biofilm parameters (biomass, metabolic activity, and ECM) were then performed as described below.

Table 1. Clinical isolates used in the present work.

Species Code (GenBank Acession Number)	Isolation Site
Candida haemulonii	
LIP*Ch*2 (KJ476194)	Cutaneous (sole of the foot)
LIP*Ch*3 (KJ476195)	Cutaneous (toe nail)
LIP*Ch*4 (KJ476196)	Cutaneous (finger nail)
LIP*Ch*7 (KJ476199)	Cutaneous (toe nail)
LIP*Ch*12 (KJ476204)	Fluid (blood)
Candida duobushaemulonii	
LIP*Ch*1 (KJ476193)	Cutaneous (finger nail)
LIP*Ch*6 (KJ476198)	Cutaneous (toe nail)
LIP*Ch*8 (KJ476200)	Fluid (blood)
LIP*Ch*10 (KJ476202)	Fluid (bronchoalveolar lavage)
Candida haemulonii var. *vulnera*	
LIP*Ch*5 (KJ476197)	Cutaneous (toe nail)
LIP*Ch*9 (KJ476201)	Fluid (urine)
LIP*Ch*11 (KJ476203)	Fluid (blood)

2.3. Biofilm Parameters

2.3.1. Biomass

Biomass quantification was performed as described by Peeters et al. [22]. Firstly, methanol at 99% (200 µL) was used to fix the biofilms for 15 min at room temperature, then the supernatant was discarded, and the plates were air-dried during 5 min. Afterwards, the plates were incubated for 20 min at room temperature with 0.4% crystal violet solution (200 µL; stock solution diluted in PBS; Sigma-Aldrich, St Louis, MO, USA). The plate wells were finally washed once with PBS in order to remove the excess of staining and the bound dye was then eluted with 33% acetic acid (200 µL) for 5 min. The acetic acid solution (100 µL) was transferred to a new 96-well plate and the absorbance was measured using a microplate reader at 590 nm (SpectraMax M3; Molecular Devices, Sunnyvale, CA, USA).

2.3.2. Metabolic Activity

The metabolic activity of the biofilm was determined using a colorimetric assay able to measure the metabolic reduction of 2,3-bis (2-methoxy-4-nitro-5-sulfophenyl)-5-[(phenylamino) carbonyl]-2H-tetrazolium hydroxide (XTT; Sigma-Aldrich, St Louis, MO, USA) to a water-soluble brown formazan product [22]. The XTT/menadione solution was prepared by dissolving 2 mg XTT in 10 mL of pre-warmed PBS, which was supplemented with 100 µL of a stock solution of menadione (0.4 mM in acetone). The XTT/menadione solution (200 µL) was added to the plate wells and incubated at 37°C for 3 h in the dark. Afterwards, 100 µL of supernatant from each well was transferred to a new microplate and the colorimetric changes were quantified using a microplate reader at 492 nm (SpectraMax M3; Molecular Devices, San Jose, CA, USA).

2.3.3. ECM

The biofilm ECM was quantified according to the method described by Choi et al. [23]. Briefly, 0.1% safranin (200 µL; Sigma-Aldrich, St Louis, MO, USA) diluted in PBS was used to stain the nonfixed biofilms, at room temperature for 5 min. Afterwards, the plate wells were washed once with PBS and the bound dye was eluted with 30% acetic acid (200 µL). Supernatants (100 µL) were transferred to a new 96-well plate and absorbance was quantified using a microplate reader at 530 nm (SpectraMax M3; Molecular Devices, San Jose, CA, USA).

2.4. Biofilm Architecture

2.4.1. Confocal Laser Scanning Microscopy (CLSM)

Biofilms formed on polystyrene surface for 48 h at 37 °C were stained with 5 µg/mL of Calcofluor white (Sigma-Aldrich, San Luis, MO, USA) for 1 h at room temperature, protected from the light [24,25]. Subsequently, the biofilms were washed twice with PBS and covered with *n*-propylgallate for observation under a confocal microscope (Leica TCS SP5 with OBS, Berlin, Germany). Three-dimensional reconstitutions of biofilms were obtained by Fiji (ImageJ2, UW-Madison LOCI, Wisconsin, WI, USA) software [26]. The analysis of images was conducted using *z*-series image stacks from spots of each biofilm chosen randomly.

2.4.2. Scanning Electron Microscopy (SEM)

Biofilms formed on polystyrene coverslips (Nalgene, Thermo Fisher Scientific, Waltham, MA, USA), at 37 °C for 48 h, were fixed in a solution made of 2.5% glutaraldehyde in 0.1 M sodium cacodylate buffer, pH 7.2, at 4 °C overnight. Then, PBS was used to wash the systems, which were post-fixed with 2% osmium tetroxide for 2 h. Dehydration was done in graded concentrations of acetone (25%–100%). The critical point method was used to dry fungal biofilms, which were then mounted on stubs, coated with gold (20–30 nm), and analyzed using a JEOL JSM 6490LV scanning electron microscope [27,28].

2.5. Biofilm ECM Composition

2.5.1. Extraction of ECM

Biofilms formed on polystyrene for 48 h at 37 °C were washed three times with PBS to remove the medium and nonadherent cells. Then, 200 µL of 1.5 M NaCl was added to each well of the microtiter plate and incubated overnight at 4 °C [29]. Finally, the well contents were transferred to a clean tube and filtered through a 0.22-µm membrane (Millipore, São Paulo, SP, Brazil).

2.5.2. Chemical Quantification of the Main Biomolecules

The protein concentration was determined by the method described by Lowry et al. [30], using bovine serum albumin (BSA; Sigma-Aldrich, San Luis, MO, USA) as standard. The carbohydrate concentration was determined by the method described by Dubois et al. [31], with some modifications. Briefly, the experiment was carried out using a polystyrene 96-well microplate, in which 50 µL of the extracellular matrix, 150 µL of sulfuric acid, and 30 µL of 80% phenol were added. The standard curve was made with glucose (Sigma-Aldrich, San Luis, MO, USA). The plate was heated in a water bath for 10 min at 90 °C, and then incubated at room temperature for 5 min. Finally, the absorbance was measured at 530 nm using a microplate reader (SpectraMax M3; Molecular Devices, San Jose, CA, USA). The nucleic acids present in ECM were extracted with the Gentra® Puregene® Yeast and G+ Bacteria Kit (Qiagen®, Maryland, MD, USA), according to the manufacturer's protocol, and then quantified using a spectrophotometer (Nano-Vue PlusTM; GE Healthcare, Chicago, IL, USA). The sterol concentration was determined using the AmplexTM Red Cholesterol Assay kit (Thermo Fisher Scientific, Waltham, MA, USA), according to the manufacturer's instructions.

2.6. Biofilm Formation on Distinct Catheters Employed in Clinical Settings

In order to evaluate the ability of *C. haemulonii* species complex to form biofilm on common medical devices, a nasogastric catheter composed by polyvinyl chloride (Medsonda, Arapoti, PR, Brazil), a late bladder catheter composed by siliconized latex (Sisco, São Paulo, SP, Brazil), and a nasoenteric catheter composed by polyurethane (Solumed, Atuba-Pinhais, PR, Brazil) were selected. Autoclaved scissors were used to cut catheters into pieces of approximately 0.30, 0.70, and 0.36 cm^2, respectively, and placed on flat-bottom 96-well microplates. Fungal cell suspensions were placed on the catheters in flat-bottom 96-well plates (using polystyrene substratum as control) in Sabouraud medium (10^6 yeasts in 200 µL) at 37 °C for 48 h. Blank controls were prepared by adding only culture medium to the catheters. Then, the catheters were washed three times with PBS to remove nonadherent cells and carefully transferred to a new flat-bottom 96-well microplate, and then the biofilm biomass was measured as described earlier.

2.7. Statistics

All experiments were performed in triplicate, in three independent experimental sets. The results were analyzed statistically by Student's *t*-test (in the comparisons between two groups) and one-way analysis of variance (ANOVA) (in the comparisons between three or more groups). The correlation tests were determined by Pearson's correlation coefficient (r). All analyses were performed using the program GraphPad Prism5. In all analyses, *p*-values of 0.05 or less were considered statistically significant.

3. Results and Discussion

3.1. Biofilm on Polystyrene Surface: Classical Parameters

It is known that adhesion represents the first step for biofilm formation, which is an important virulence attribute described for several *Candida* species presenting medical implications [32,33]. The relevance of biofilm formation by *Candida* spp. lies the crucial characteristics such as greater resistance to antifungal drugs, host immune responses, and stress situations, resulting in difficulties in the treatment and possible persistence of the infectious process [17]. Taking this into consideration, initially, we confirmed the capacity of clinical isolates belonging to the *C. haemulonii* complex to form biofilm over a polystyrene surface [16]. In this set of experiments, three classical parameters related to biofilm formation were evaluated after 48 h of contact with polystyrene: (i) biomass by the incorporation of crystal violet in methanol-fixed cells, (ii) metabolic activity (cell viability) by reduction of XTT, and (iii) ECM by absorption of safranin, in the latter cases, using non-fixed fungal cells. All 12 clinical isolates comprising the *C. haemulonii* complex formed biofilm at different degrees, exhibiting a typical isolate-specific pattern (Figure 1A,C,E). Statistically significant differences were not observed, while the average measurements of the three biofilm parameters among the three fungal species forming the *C. haemulonii* complex were compared (Figure 1B,D,F). Biofilms revealed by the incorporation of crystal violet and safranin showed the presence of a network formed by yeasts and an exuberant ECM, respectively (data not shown).

Regarding the biofilm biomass, we observed that the average of biofilm formation on polystyrene by the clinical isolates studied herein was similar to that reported by Cendejas-Bueno et al. [1], who also studied clinical isolates of the *C. haemulonii* complex obtained from different isolation sites. The comparison of biofilm formation among the members of other *Candida* species complex has already been documented. In this sense, the three species of the *C. parapsilosis* complex (*C. parapsilosis* sensu strictu, *C. orthopsilosis*, and *C. metapsilosis*) exhibited similar abilities to produce mature biofilms on abiotic surfaces regarding biomass, viability, and three-dimensional architecture [34–36]. Regarding the *C. glabrata* complex, Figueiredo-Carvalho et al. [37] reported that biofilm biomass was significantly higher than *C. nivariensis*.

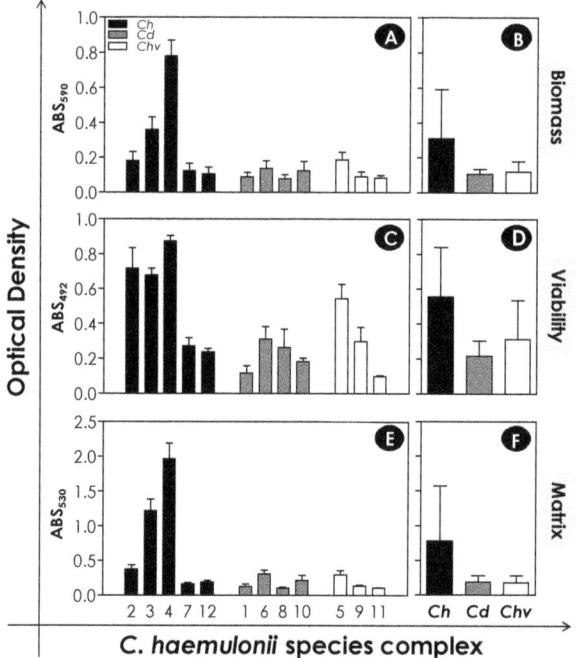

Figure 1. Biofilm formation by the *C. haemulonii* species complex on polystyrene surface. Yeasts (200 μL containing 10^6 cells) were placed to interact with polystyrene for 48 h at 37 °C. Afterwards, the systems were processed to detect fungal biomass by crystal violet incorporation in methanol-fixed biofilms at 590 nm, cell viability by the reduction of 2,3-bis (2-methoxy-4-nitro-5-sulfophenyl)-5-[(phenylamino) carbonyl]-2H-tetrazolium hydroxide (XTT) in formazan at 492 nm, and extracellular matrix by staining non-fixed biofilms with safranin at 530 nm. The results were expressed as absorbance (ABS) values per clinical isolate studied (**A,C,E**) and mean per fungal species (**B,D,F**). The results are shown as mean ± standard deviation of three independent experiments. The numbers on the X-axis of graphs represent each of the 12 clinical isolates of the *C. haemulonii* species complex studied, in which *Ch* means *C. haemulonii*, *Cd* means *C. duobushaemulonii*, and *Chv* means *C. haemulonii* var. *vulnera*.

3.2. CLSM Analysis

The three-dimensional organization as well as the biomass distribution in the biofilms formed by the clinical isolates comprising the *C. haemulonii* complex were analyzed by CLSM (Figure 2), which is a nondestructive technique that allows in situ visualization of the intact biofilm [38]. To do it, Calcofluor white was used to stain the yeasts owing to its affinity to chitin (which is a universal polysaccharide present in the fungal cell wall), evidencing the biofilm biomass as well as the ECM (Figure 2), which is evidenced by the diffuse marking between the yeasts, as previously proposed [39]. In addition, the three-dimensional representation of biofilms was used to determine their thickness, which ranged from 21.6 to 39.1 μm (overall mean = 28.3 ± 5.6 μm) for all clinical isolates studied. The biofilm thickness in each fungal species is as follows: *C. haemulonii*, 21.6 to 32.1 μm (overall mean = 26.1 ± 4.8 μm); *C. duobushaemulonii*, 25.9 to 39.1 μm (mean = 30.5 ± 5.8 μm); and *C. haemulonii* var. *vulnera*, 26.1 to 37.1 μm (mean = 29.1 ± 7.1 μm) (Figure 2). Some authors have documented different thicknesses of biofilms formed by *Candida* species, varying from 11 to 13 μm for *C. tropicalis* [40], 25 to 77 μm for *C. albicans* [39,41], 35.2 to 81.2 μm for *C. famata* [42], and 21 to 26 μm for *C. auris* [43]. In this sense, a variety of conditions can interfere with biofilm features, including isolate specificities, planktonic growth, initial inoculum concentration, and variability on biofilm-forming conditions (substratum, temperature, CO_2 tension, fluid flow, developmental timing, and medium used to support biofilm formation) [44].

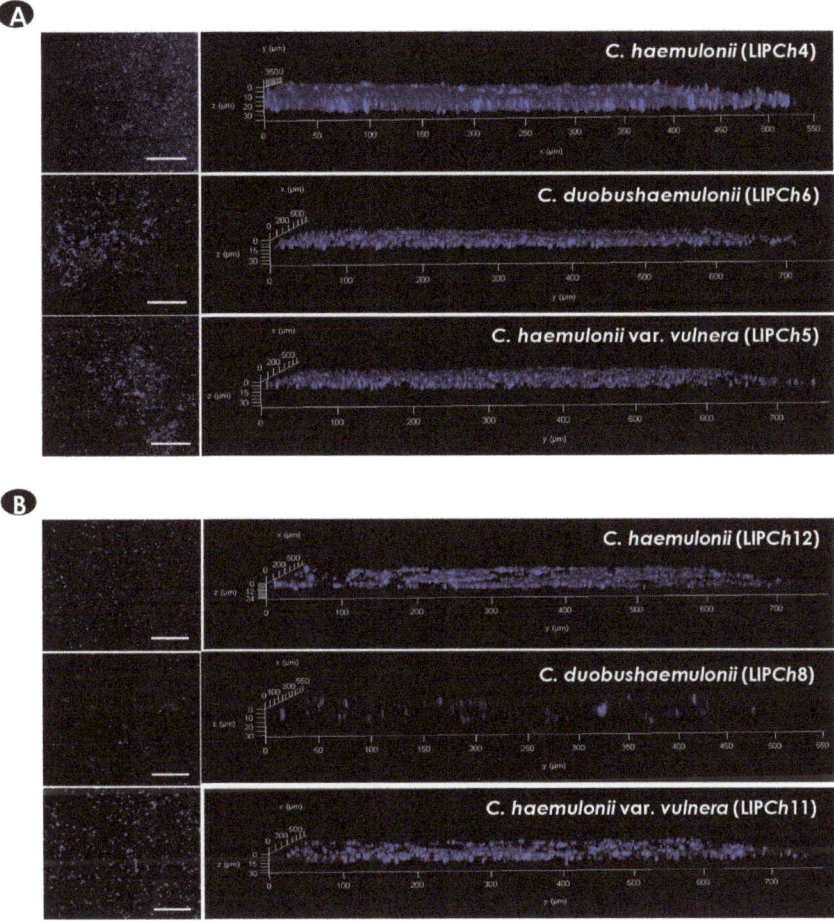

Figure 2. Representative confocal laser scanning microscopy (CLSM) images of the biofilms formed by the *C. haemulonii* species complex on polystyrene surface. Yeasts (200 µL containing 10^6 cells) were placed to interact with polystyrene for 48 h at 37 °C. Subsequently, the biofilms were stained with Calcofluor white, evidencing the fungal biomass. The panels on the left represent the top view images of the fungal biofilms visualized by CLSM; bars represent 5 µm. The graphs on the right represent the three-dimensional reconstruction of the biofilms formed by each species. The isolates *C. haemulonii* (LIPCh4), *C. duobushaemulonii* (LIPCh6), and *C. haemulonii* var. *vulnera* (LIPCh5), which formed the most robust biofilms (**A**), as well as the isolates *C. haemulonii* (LIPCh12), *C. duobushaemulonii* (LIPCh8), and *C. haemulonii* var. *vulnera* (LIPCh11), which formed the weakest biofilms (**B**), are shown.

3.3. SEM Analysis

SEM analysis was used to assess the biofilm ultrastructure and to evidence peculiar morphological characteristics. Mature biofilms of *C. haemulonii* species complex consisted of a dense network of yeast cells, while structures similar to pseudohyphae were scarcely observed in the majority of the isolates studied (Figure 3). As seen through other approaches, isolate-specific differences were also visualized in biofilm ultrastructure. In this sense, the biofilms formed by *C. haemulonii* isolates LIPC*h*3 and LIPC*h*4, for example, exhibited a continuous, intimately packed multilayer structure (Figure 3A–E), while in the remaining fungal isolates, the biofilms were formed by a predominantly discontinuous monolayer with cell aggregates (Figure 3G–I). Water channels could also be visualized (Figure 3J), as well as ECM, as exemplified by isolates of *C. haemulonii* (LIPC*h*4), *C. duobushaemulonii* (LIPC*h*6), and *C. haemulonii* var. *vulnera* (LIPC*h*5) (Figures 4A, 4B and 4C, respectively).

Similarly, Silva et al. [45] demonstrated that *C. glabrata* biofilms are also composed only by yeasts, while *C. parapsilosis* sensu strictu and *C. tropicalis* biofilms characteristics vary depending on the strain used. Those authors observed that some *C. parapsilosis* strains formed biofilms containing both yeast and pseudohypha morphologies, while others presented yeast cells only, and these findings showed no relation with the isolation site of each strain [45]. The majority of *C. tropicalis* isolates displayed only yeast cells, but a small number of isolates showed hyphal formation, especially appearing as long filaments [45]. The biofilm formed by *C. auris*, which is phylogenetically closer to the *C. haemulonii* species complex, is predominantly composed by budding yeast cells and occasionally pseudohyphae [46]. *C. albicans* biofilms, on the other hand, are classically composed by a basal yeast cell polylayer and an upper region formed by hyphal forms [44].

3.4. ECM Composition

The ECM of biofilms from different *Candida* species exhibits a heterogeneous nature, which has already been thought to be associated to the roles of these components in biofilm architecture and dynamics [47]. The main components of ECM biofilms from *Candida* spp. are proteins, carbohydrates, lipids, and nucleic acids. Several studies have documented the participation of ECM biofilm in adhesion to surfaces, structural maintenance, defense against external aggressors, signaling, and enzymatic issues; however, the enhanced antimicrobial resistance is the most clinically important phenotype of biofilm mode of growth, which is of special concern in hospital settings [25,38,48]. Herein, we investigated the main classic components of the ECM of *Candida* spp. biofilms: proteins, carbohydrates, nucleic acids, and sterols. Among the evaluated components, proteins (mean of 11.61 ± 8.09 µg/mL for *C. haemulonii*, 2.97 ± 1.16 µg/mL for *C. duobushaemulonii*, and 3.88 ± 2.04 µg/mL for *C. haemulonii* var. *vulnera*) were found in greater quantity in the chemically extracted ECM from mature biofilms of all the clinical isolates, followed by carbohydrates (mean of 4.39 ± 2.30 µg/mL for *C. haemulonii*, 3.20 ± 0.74 µg/mL for *C. duobushaemulonii*, and 2.79 ± 1.42 µg/mL for *C. haemulonii* var. *vulnera*); nucleic acids (mean of 0.093 ± 0.074 µg/mL for *C. haemulonii*, 0.026 ± 0.035 µg/mL for *C. duobushaemulonii*, and 0.048 ± 0.082 µg/mL for *C. haemulonii* var. *vulnera*); and, lastly, sterols (mean of 0.023 ± 0.006 µg/mL for *C. haemulonii*, 0.014 ± 0.005 µg/mL for *C. duobushaemulonii*, and 0.007 ± 0.005 µg/mL for *C. haemulonii* var. *vulnera*) (Figure 5). Sterol amounts in *C. haemulonii* isolates were significantly higher when compared with those in *C. haemulonii* var. *vulnera* ($p < 0.05$; one-way ANOVA, Tukey's multiple comparison test) (Figure 5).

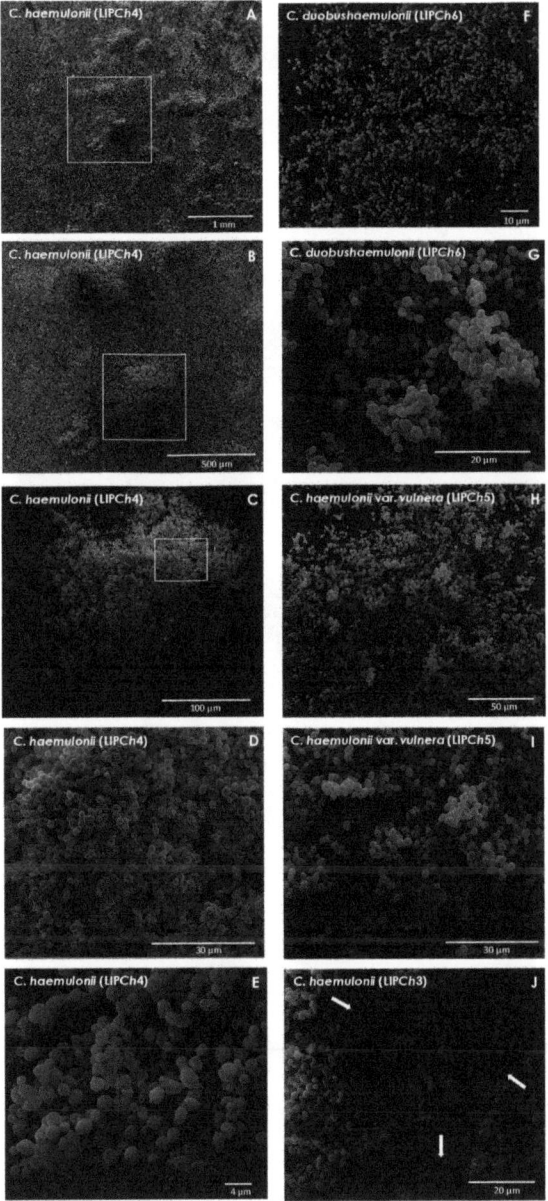

Figure 3. Representative low-magnification scanning electron microscopy (SEM) images of the biofilms formed by the *C. haemulonii* species complex on polystyrene surface. Yeasts (200 μL containing 10^6 cells) were placed to interact with polystyrene coverslips for 48 h at 37 °C, after which the coverslips were visualized using SEM. The images revealed a dense network of yeast cells. In the panel, the images on the left side exhibit different magnifications of the biofilm formed by the isolate LIP*Ch*4 of *C. haemulonii* (**A–E**) while on the right side, it is possible to see the biofilms of isolate LIP*Ch*6 of *C. duobushaemulonii* (**F,G**) and LIP*Ch*5 of *C. haemulonii* var. *vulnera* (**H,I**). Representative water channels are indicated by white arrows in the image of isolate LIP*Ch*3 of *C. haemulonii* (**J**). Note that the white square in (**A**) is the place that was chosen to be amplified and shown in (**B**), and this logic sequence was used in the left side images from (**A**) to (**D**).

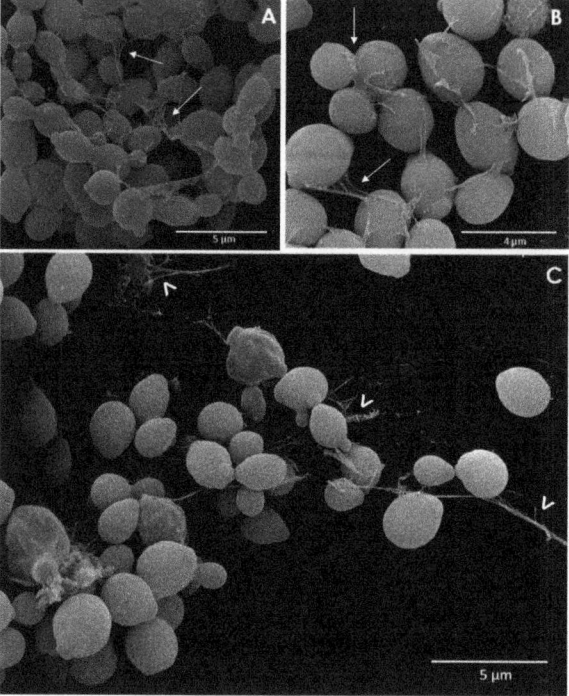

Figure 4. Representative high-magnification SEM images of the biofilms formed by the *C. haemulonii* species complex on polystyrene surface, focusing on the extracellular matrix (ECM). Yeasts (200 μL containing 10^6 cells) were placed to interact with polystyrene coverslips for 48 h at 37 °C, after which the coverslips were visualized using SEM. The ECM of biofilms of *C. haemulonii* LIPCh4 (**A**), *C. duobushaemulonii* LIPCh6 (**B**), and *C. haemulonii* var. *vulnera* LIPCh5 (**C**) are indicated by symbols. The images clearly reveal the presence of an ECM surrounding and holding the yeast cells together (white thin arrows) as well as connecting the yeasts with the polystyrene surface (white thick arrowheads).

Zarnowski et al. [47] described proteins and carbohydrates as the major components of *C. albicans* ECM biofilm, which included 458 distinct protein activities and three polysaccharides of functional importance (α-1,2 branched α-1,6-mannans associated with unbranched β-1,6-glucans forming a mannan-glucan complex, and β-1,3-glucans in a smaller part). Differences regarding non-*albicans Candida* species biofilms ECM composition were reported many years ago. In this sense, Silva et al. [45] documented that *C. parapsilosis* biofilm ECM exhibited high carbohydrate and low protein contents; on the other hand, *C. tropicalis* exhibited high contents of both carbohydrates and proteins, while *C. glabrata* showed low contents of both carbohydrates and proteins.

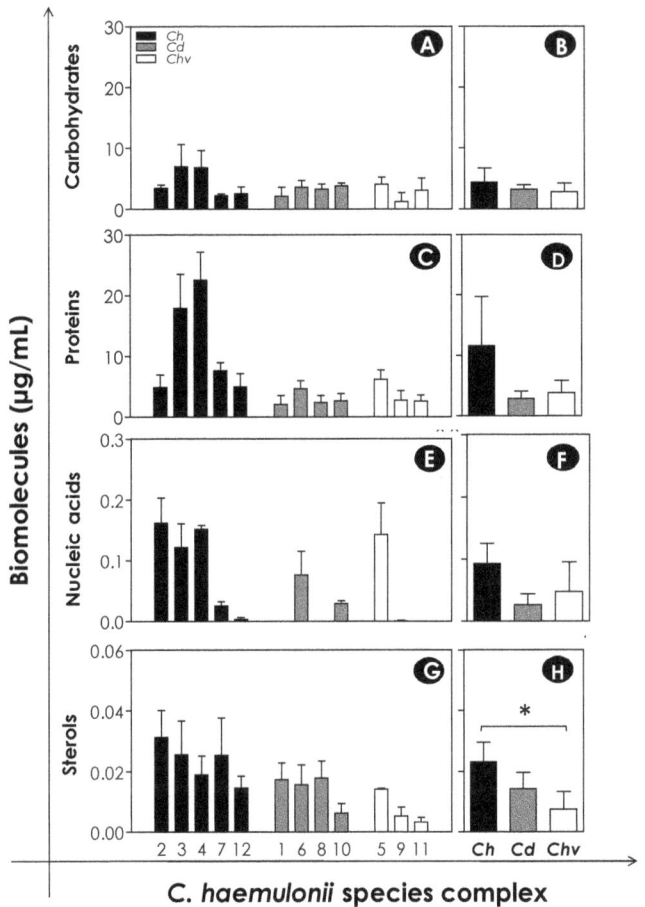

Figure 5. Main biomolecules forming the extracellular matrix (ECM) of the *C. haemulonii* species complex biofilms on polystyrene surface. Yeasts (200 μL containing 10^6 cells) were placed to interact with polystyrene for 48 h at 37 °C. After that, ECM was extracted and carbohydrates, proteins, nucleic acids, and sterols were quantified as detailed in methodology section. The results were expressed as concentration (μg/mL) of each biomolecule per clinical isolate studied (**A,C,E,G**) and mean concentration per fungal species (**B,D,F,H**). The results are shown as mean ± standard deviation of three independent experiments. The symbol (*) indicates *p*-values < 0.05 (one-way ANOVA, Tukey's multiple comparison test). The numbers on the X-axis of graphs represent each of the 12 clinical isolates of the *C. haemulonii* complex studied, in which *Ch* means *C. haemulonii*, *Cd* means *C. duobushaemulonii*, and *Chv* means *C. haemulonii* var. *vulnera*.

3.5. Biofilm Formation on Medical Devices

Catheter-related infections are considered a real problem in the medical arena around the world. Candidemia related to catheter use has already been reported in a variety of *Candida* species, including *C. haemulonii* species complex, resulting from the ability of this and other fungal pathogens to adhere to the catheter surface and, consequently, reach the bloodstream mainly of immunocompromised individuals [6]. For this reason, we decided to evaluate the *C. haemulonii* species complex biofilm formation capacity on the surface of different types of catheters currently used in the hospital environment—a latter bladder catheter made of siliconized latex, a nasoenteric catheter made of polyurethane, and a nasogastric catheter made of polyvinyl chloride. Biofilm formation on these materials was compared to that on polystyrene, a classical substratum used for biofilm analysis (Figure 1). The clinical isolates of the *C. haemulonii* complex were incubated for 48 h at 37 °C with the different materials and the biomass was measured by the incorporation of crystal violet. The results were expressed as absorbance (ABS_{590})/cm^2, as the catheters have different dimensions. Our results stressed that the biofilm formation was significantly bigger over the different catheter types when compared with polystyrene regarding all the clinical isolates tested, demonstrating the risk that these clinical isolates would represent in the hospital settings, especially in individuals using nasogastric, nasoenteric, and urinary catheters (Figure 6(aA,aC,aE)). Additionally, biofilm formation on polyurethane and polyvinyl chloride catheters was comparable, with no significant differences between them (Figure 6(aA,aC,aE)). When comparing the mean biofilm formation per species of the *C. haemulonii* complex between the different substrates, we observed that the biofilms formed on polyurethane and polyvinyl chloride catheters were significantly bigger than on polystyrene for both *C. haemulonii* and *C. duobushaemulonii*. Further, biofilms formed on polyvinyl chloride catheters were significantly bigger than on siliconized latex only for *C. haemulonii* (Figure 6(aB,aD)), while for *C. haemulonii* var. *vulnera*, no differences were observed (Figure 6(aF)). Additionally, in relation to the isolation site, cutaneous (fungal isolates LIPC*h*2, LIPC*h*3, LIPC*h*4, and LIPC*h*7 of *C. haemulonii*; LIPC*h*1 and LIPC*h*6 of *C. duobushaemulonii*; and LIPC*h*5 of *C. haemulonii* var. *vulnera*) versus fluids (fungal isolates LIPC*h*12 of *C. haemulonii*; LIPC*h*8 and LIPC*h*10 of *C. duobushaemulonii*; and LIPC*h*9 and LIPC*h*11 of *C. haemulonii* var. *vulnera*) (Table 1), we observed that biofilm formation on the polyurethane ($p = 0.0427$, unpaired Student's *t*-test) and polyvinyl chloride catheters ($p = 0.0472$, unpaired Student's *t*-test) by the isolates from cases of cutaneous candidiasis was significantly higher when compared with isolates obtained from body fluids (Figure 6b). However, for polystyrene and siliconized latex catheters, no statistically significant differences ($p > 0.05$) were observed in this regard (Figure 6b).

Estivill et al. [49], for example, demonstrated the ability of different *Candida* species (*C. albicans*, *C. parapsilosis*, *C. tropicalis*, *C. glabrata*, and *C. krusei*) to form biofilm on different catheter types, and as observed in our clinical isolates, the biofilms formed on the polyurethane and polyvinyl chloride catheters presented very close values for all species studied. Additionally, our group has previously demonstrated the ability of filamentous fungi from *Scedosporium* spp. and *Lomentospora prolificans* to form biofilm on these same catheters [50].

The biofilm formation capacity of *Candida* spp., with a special focus on *C. albicans*, on medical devices has been extensively studied over time. Indeed, the nature of substratum used really influences the biofilm formation. For example, *C. albicans* form better biofilms on soft materials of dentures than on acrylic surfaces [51]. Similarly, *C. albicans* form better biofilms in silicone elastomer and latex surfaces in comparison with polyvinyl chloride and, on the other hand, construct weaker biofilms on polyurethane and silicone [52]. Interestingly, chemical changes made on the surface of medical devices can also interfere in *C. albicans* biofilm formation. For instance, a significant reduction in biomass and metabolic activity of *C. albicans* biofilm was detected when fungal cells were putted to adhere on polyetherurethane covered with 6% of polyethylene oxide [53]. Such differences should be considered, when possible, in the choice of biomaterials to minimize the development of catheter-related *Candida* infections.

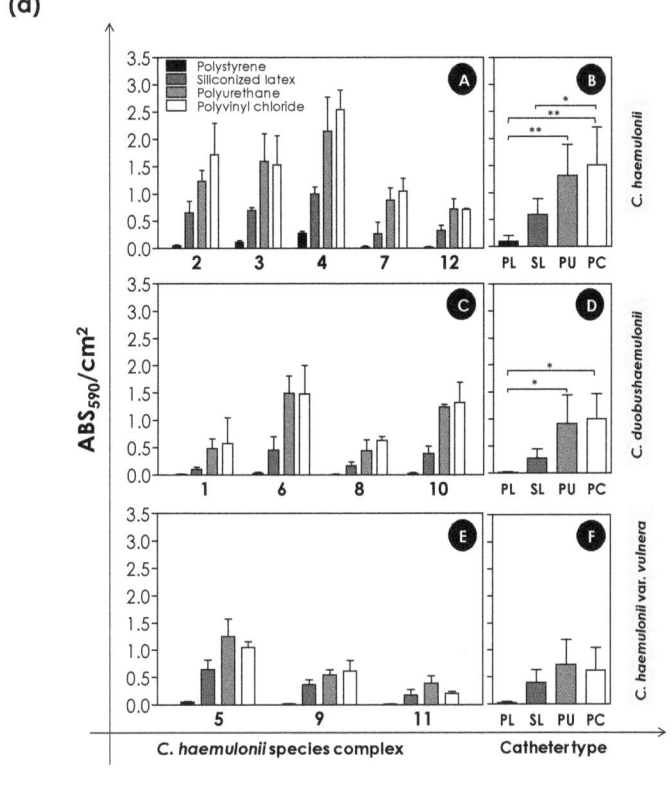

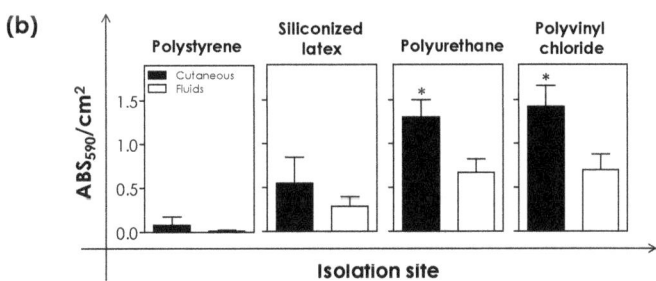

Figure 6. Biofilm formation on different catheter types by clinical isolates comprising the *C. haemulonii* complex. Fungal cells (200 µL containing 10^6 cells) were placed to interact with polystyrene (PL) and different types of catheters (siliconized latex, SL; polyurethane, PU; and polyvinyl chloride, PC) for 48 h at 37 °C. Subsequently, the biofilm biomass was measured by the crystal violet incorporation (590 nm). (a) The results were expressed as ABS_{590}/cm^2 for each clinical isolate studied (A,C,E) and mean per each catheter type (B,D,F). Values represent the mean ± standard deviation of three independent experiments. The (*) indicates *p*-values < 0.05 and (**) *p*-values < 0.01 (one-way ANOVA, Tukey's multiple comparison test). The numbers on the X-axis of the graphs represent each of the 12 clinical isolates of the *C. haemulonii* complex studied. (b) Comparison of biofilm biomass produced by the clinical isolates on polystyrene and each catheter type regarding the isolation sites (cutaneous and fluids). The 12 isolates were divided into two groups: cutaneous, including nail and skin (*n* = 7); and fluids, including blood, urine, and bronchoalveolar lavage (*n* = 5) (Table 1). (*) indicates *p*-values < 0.05 (unpaired Student's *t*-test).

4. Conclusions

Collectively, the present study demonstrated the ability of the *C. haemulonii* species complex to form biofilm on different types of inert substrates, which is an incontestable virulence attribute associated with catheter-related candidemia in hospitalized individuals, representing a serious problem especially when dealing with multidrug-resistant pathogens such as the *C. haemulonii* species complex. Additionally, our results provide new data about *C. haemulonii* species complex biofilm ECM composition.

Author Contributions: All authors conceived and designed the experiments. L.S.R. and T.P.M. performed the experiments. All authors analyzed the data. M.H.B. and A.L.S.S. contributed reagents/materials/analysis tools. All authors wrote and revised the paper. All authors contributed to the research and have read and agree to the published version of the manuscript.

Funding: This work was supported by grants from Fundação Carlos Chagas Filho de Amparo à Pesquisa do Estado do Rio de Janeiro (FAPERJ), Conselho Nacional de Desenvolvimento Científico e Tecnológico (CNPq), and Coordenação de Aperfeiçoamento de Pessoal de Nível Superior (CAPES - Financial code 001).

Acknowledgments: The authors would like to thank Denise Rocha de Souza (UFRJ) for technical assistance in the experiments and Grasiella Matioszek (UFRJ) for confocal analyses.

Conflicts of Interest: The authors declare no conflict of interest. The funders had no role in the design of the study; in the collection, analyses, or interpretation of data; in the writing of the manuscript, or in the decision to publish the results.

References

1. Cendejas-Bueno, E.; Kolecka, A.; Alastruey-Izquierdo, A.; Theelen, B.; Groenewald, M.; Kostrzewa, M.; Cuenca-Estrella, M.; Gomez-Lopez, A.; Boekhout, T. Reclassification of the *Candida haemulonii* complex as *Candida haemulonii* (*C. haemulonii* group I), *C. duobushaemulonii* sp. nov. (*C. haemulonii* group II), and *C. haemulonii* var. *vulnera* var. nov.: Three multiresistant human pathogenic yeasts. *J. Clin. Microbiol.* **2012**, *50*, 3641–3651. [CrossRef]
2. Khan, Z.U.; Al-Sweih, N.A.; Ahmad, S.; Al-Kazemi, N.; Khan, S.; Joseph, L.; Chandy, R. Outbreak of fungemia among neonates caused by *Candida haemulonii* resistant to amphotericin B, itraconazole, and fluconazole. *J. Clin. Microbiol.* **2007**, *45*, 2025–2027. [CrossRef]
3. Kim, M.N.; Shin, J.H.; Sung, H.; Lee, K.; Kim, E.C.; Ryoo, N.; Lee, J.S.; Jung, S.I.; Park, K.H.; Kee, S.J.; et al. *Candida haemulonii* and closely related species at 5 university hospitals in Korea: Identification, antifungal susceptibility, and clinical features. *Clin. Infect. Dis.* **2009**, *48*, e57–e61. [CrossRef] [PubMed]
4. Córdoba, S.; Vivot, W.; Bosco-Borgeat, M.E.; Taverna, C.; Szusz, W.; Murisengo, O.; Isla, G.; Davel, G. Species distribution and susceptibility profile of yeasts isolated from blood cultures: Results of a multicenter active laboratory-based surveillance study in Argentina. *Rev. Argent. Microbiol.* **2011**, *43*, 176–185. [CrossRef] [PubMed]
5. Crouzet, J.; Sotto, A.; Picard, E.; Lachaud, L.; Bourgeois, N. A case of *Candida haemulonii* osteitis: Clinical features, biochemical characteristics, and antifungal resistance profile. *Clin. Microbiol. Infect.* **2011**, *17*, 1068–1070. [CrossRef] [PubMed]
6. Kim, S.; Ko, K.S.; Moon, S.Y.; Lee, M.S.; Lee, M.Y.; Son, J.S. Catheter-related candidemia caused by *Candida haemulonii* in a patient in long-term hospital care. *J. Korean Med. Sci.* **2011**, *26*, 297–300. [CrossRef]
7. Oh, B.J.; Shin, J.H.; Kim, M.N.; Sung, H.; Lee, K.; Joo, M.Y.; Shin, M.G.; Suh, S.P.; Ryang, D.W. Biofilm formation and genotyping of *Candida haemulonii*, *Candida pseudohaemulonii*, and a proposed new species (*Candida auris*) isolates from Korea. *Med. Mycol.* **2011**, *49*, 98–102. [CrossRef]
8. Almeida, J.N., Jr.; Motta, A.L.; Rossi, F.; Abdala, E.; Pierrotti, L.C.; Kono, A.S.; Diz Mdel, P.; Benard, G.; Del Negro, G.M. First report of a clinical isolate of *Candida haemulonii* in Brazil. *Clinics (Sao Paulo)* **2012**, *67*, 1229–1231. [CrossRef]
9. Yuvaraj, A.; Rohit, A.; Koshy, P.J.; Nagarajan, P.; Nair, S.; Abraham, G. Rare occurrence of fatal *Candida haemulonii* peritonitis in a diabetic CAPD patient. *Ren. Fail.* **2014**, *36*, 1466–1467. [CrossRef]
10. Ramos, L.S.; Figueiredo-Carvalho, M.H.; Barbedo, L.S.; Ziccardi, M.; Chaves, A.L.; Zancope-Oliveira, R.M.; Pinto, M.R.; Sgarbi, D.B.; Dornelas-Ribeiro, M.; Branquinha, M.H.; et al. *Candida haemulonii* complex: Species identification and antifungal susceptibility profiles of clinical isolates from Brazil. *J. Antimicrob. Chemother.* **2015**, *70*, 111–115. [CrossRef]

11. Silva, C.M.; Carvalho-Parahym, A.M.; Macedo, D.P.; Lima-Neto, R.G.; Francisco, E.C.; Melo, A.S.; da Conceicao, M.S.M.; Juca, M.B.; Mello, L.R.; Amorim, R.M.; et al. Neonatal candidemia caused by *Candida haemulonii*: Case report and review of literature. *Mycopathologia* **2015**, *180*, 69–73. [CrossRef] [PubMed]
12. De Almeida, J.N., Jr.; Assy, J.G.; Levin, A.S.; Del Negro, G.M.; Giudice, M.C.; Tringoni, M.P.; Thomaz, D.Y.; Motta, A.L.; Abdala, E.; Pierroti, L.C.; et al. *Candida haemulonii* complex species, Brazil, January 2010-March 2015. *Emerg. Infect. Dis.* **2016**, *22*, 561–563. [CrossRef] [PubMed]
13. Boatto, H.F.; Cavalcanti, S.D.; Del Negro, G.M.; Girao, M.J.; Francisco, E.C.; Ishida, K.; Gompertz, O.F. *Candida duobushaemulonii*: An emerging rare pathogenic yeast isolated from recurrent vulvovaginal candidiasis in Brazil. *Mem. Inst. Oswaldo Cruz* **2016**, *111*, 407–410. [CrossRef] [PubMed]
14. Fang, S.Y.; Wei, K.C.; Chen, W.C.; Lee, S.J.; Yang, K.C.; Wu, C.S.; Sun, P.L. Primary deep cutaneous candidiasis caused by *Candida duobushaemulonii* in a 68-year-old man: The first case report and literature review. *Mycoses* **2016**, *59*, 818–821. [CrossRef] [PubMed]
15. Hou, X.; Xiao, M.; Chen, S.C.; Wang, H.; Cheng, J.W.; Chen, X.X.; Xu, Z.P.; Fan, X.; Kong, F.; Xu, Y.C. Identification and antifungal susceptibility profiles of *Candida haemulonii* species complex clinical isolates from a Multicenter Study in China. *J. Clin. Microbiol.* **2016**, *54*, 2676–2680. [CrossRef]
16. Ramos, L.S.; Oliveira, S.S.C.; Souto, X.M.; Branquinha, M.H.; Santos, A.L.S. Planktonic growth and biofilm formation profiles in *Candida haemulonii* species complex. *Med. Mycol.* **2017**, *55*, 785–789. [CrossRef]
17. Santos, A.L.S.; Mello, T.P.; Ramos, L.S.; Branquinha, M.H. Biofilm: A robust and efficient barrier to antifungal chemotherapy. *J. Antimicro* **2015**, *1*, e101. [CrossRef]
18. Borghi, E.; Borgo, F.; Morace, G. Fungal biofilms: Update on resistance. *Adv. Exp. Med. Biol.* **2016**, *931*, 37–47. [CrossRef]
19. Reichhardt, C.; Stevens, D.A.; Cegelski, L. Fungal biofilm composition and opportunities in drug discovery. *Future Med. Chem.* **2016**, *8*, 1455–1468. [CrossRef]
20. Percival, S.L.; Suleman, L.; Vuotto, C.; Donelli, G. Healthcare-associated infections, medical devices and biofilms: Risk, tolerance and control. *J. Med. Microbiol.* **2015**, *64*, 323–334. [CrossRef]
21. Giusiano, G.; Mangiaterra, M.; Garcia Saito, V.; Rojas, F.; Gomez, V.; Diaz, M.C. Fluconazole and itraconazole resistance of yeasts isolated from the bloodstream and catheters of hospitalized pediatric patients. *Chemotherapy* **2006**, *52*, 254–259. [CrossRef] [PubMed]
22. Peeters, E.; Nelis, H.J.; Coenye, T. Comparison of multiple methods for quantification of microbial biofilms grown in microtiter plates. *J. Microbiol. Methods* **2008**, *72*, 157–165. [CrossRef]
23. Choi, N.Y.; Kang, S.Y.; Kim, K.J. Artemisia princeps inhibits biofilm formation and virulence-factor expression of antibiotic-resistant bacteria. *BioMed Res. Int* **2015**, *2015*, 239519. [CrossRef] [PubMed]
24. Chandra, J.; Mukherjee, P.K.; Ghannoum, M.A. In vitro growth and analysis of *Candida* biofilms. *Nat. Protoc.* **2008**, *3*, 1909–1924. [CrossRef] [PubMed]
25. Ramage, G.; Rajendran, R.; Sherry, L.; Williams, C. Fungal biofilm resistance. *Int. J. Microbiol.* **2012**, *2012*, 528521. [CrossRef] [PubMed]
26. Beauvais, A.; Schmidt, C.; Guadagnini, S.; Roux, P.; Perret, E.; Henry, C.; Paris, S.; Mallet, A.; Prevost, M.C.; Latge, J.P. An extracellular matrix glues together the aerial-grown hyphae of *Aspergillus fumigatus*. *Cell. Microbiol.* **2007**, *9*, 1588–1600. [CrossRef] [PubMed]
27. Sangetha, S.; Zuraini, Z.; Suryani, S.; Sasidharan, S. In situ TEM and SEM studies on the antimicrobial activity and prevention of *Candida albicans* biofilm by *Cassia spectabilis* extract. *Micron* **2009**, *40*, 439–443. [CrossRef]
28. Mello, T.P.; Aor, A.C.; Goncalves, D.S.; Seabra, S.H.; Branquinha, M.H.; Santos, A.L. Assessment of biofilm formation by *Scedosporium apiospermum*, *S. aurantiacum*, *S. minutisporum* and *Lomentospora prolificans*. *Biofouling* **2016**, *32*, 737–749. [CrossRef]
29. Chiba, A.; Sugimoto, S.; Sato, F.; Hori, S.; Mizunoe, Y. A refined technique for extraction of extracellular matrices from bacterial biofilms and its applicability. *Microb. Biotechnol.* **2015**, *8*, 392–403. [CrossRef]
30. Lowry, O.H.; Rosebrough, N.J.; Farr, A.L.; Randall, R.J. Protein measurement with the Folin phenol reagent. *J. Biol. Chem.* **1951**, *193*, 265–275.
31. DuBois, M.; Gilles, K.A.; Hamilton, J.K.; Rebers, P.A.; Smith, F. Colorimetric method for determination of sugars and related substances. *Anal. Chem.* **1956**, *28*, 350–356. [CrossRef]

32. Sardi Jde, C.; Pitangui Nde, S.; Rodriguez-Arellanes, G.; Taylor, M.L.; Fusco-Almeida, A.M.; Mendes-Giannini, M.J. Highlights in pathogenic fungal biofilms. *Rev. Iberoam. Micol.* **2014**, *31*, 22–29. [CrossRef] [PubMed]
33. Tsui, C.; Kong, E.F.; Jabra-Rizk, M.A. Pathogenesis of *Candida albicans* biofilm. *Pathog Dis.* **2016**, *74*, ftw018. [CrossRef] [PubMed]
34. Lattif, A.A.; Mukherjee, P.K.; Chandra, J.; Swindell, K.; Lockhart, S.R.; Diekema, D.J.; Pfaller, M.A.; Ghannoum, M.A. Characterization of biofilms formed by *Candida parapsilosis*, *C. metapsilosis*, and *C. orthopsilosis*. *Int. J. Med. Microbiol.* **2010**, *300*, 265–270. [CrossRef] [PubMed]
35. Abi-Chacra, E.A.; Souza, L.O.; Cruz, L.P.; Braga-Silva, L.A.; Goncalves, D.S.; Sodre, C.L.; Ribeiro, M.D.; Seabra, S.H.; Figueiredo-Carvalho, M.H.; Barbedo, L.S.; et al. Phenotypical properties associated with virulence from clinical isolates belonging to the *Candida parapsilosis* complex. *FEMS Yeast Res.* **2013**, *13*, 831–848. [CrossRef]
36. Ziccardi, M.; Souza, L.O.; Gandra, R.M.; Galdino, A.C.; Baptista, A.R.; Nunes, A.P.; Ribeiro, M.A.; Branquinha, M.H.; Santos, A.L. *Candida parapsilosis* (sensu lato) isolated from hospitals located in the Southeast of Brazil: Species distribution, antifungal susceptibility and virulence attributes. *Int. J. Med. Microbiol.* **2015**, *305*, 848–859. [CrossRef]
37. Figueiredo-Carvalho, M.H.; Ramos Lde, S.; Barbedo, L.S.; Chaves, A.L.; Muramoto, I.A.; Santos, A.L.; Almeida-Paes, R.; Zancope-Oliveira, R.M. First description of *Candida nivariensis* in Brazil: Antifungal susceptibility profile and potential virulence attributes. *Mem. Inst. Oswaldo Cruz* **2016**, *111*, 51–58. [CrossRef]
38. Flemming, H.C.; Wingender, J. The biofilm matrix. *Nat. Rev. Microbiol.* **2010**, *8*, 623–633. [CrossRef]
39. Chandra, J.; Kuhn, D.M.; Mukherjee, P.K.; Hoyer, L.L.; McCormick, T.; Ghannoum, M.A. Biofilm formation by the fungal pathogen *Candida albicans*: Development, architecture, and drug resistance. *J. Bacteriol.* **2001**, *183*, 5385–5394. [CrossRef]
40. Ferreira, C.; Goncalves, B.; Vilas Boas, D.; Oliveira, H.; Henriques, M.; Azeredo, J.; Silva, S. *Candida tropicalis* biofilm and human epithelium invasion is highly influenced by environmental pH. *Pathog Dis.* **2016**, *74*. [CrossRef]
41. Mukherjee, P.K.; Chand, D.V.; Chandra, J.; Anderson, J.M.; Ghannoum, M.A. Shear stress modulates the thickness and architecture of *Candida albicans* biofilms in a phase-dependent manner. *Mycoses* **2009**, *52*, 440–446. [CrossRef] [PubMed]
42. Malm, A.; Chudzik, B.; Piersiak, T.; Gawron, A. Glass surface as potential in vitro substratum for *Candida famata* biofilm. *Ann. Agric. Environ. Med.* **2010**, *17*, 115–118. [PubMed]
43. Larkin, E.; Hager, C.; Chandra, J.; Mukherjee, P.K.; Retuerto, M.; Salem, I.; Long, L.; Isham, N.; Kovanda, L.; Borroto-Esoda, K.; et al. The emerging pathogen *Candida auris*: Growth phenotype, virulence factors, activity of antifungals, and effect of SCY-078, a novel glucan synthesis inhibitor, on growth morphology and biofilm formation. *Antimicrob. Agents Chemother.* **2017**, *61*. [CrossRef] [PubMed]
44. Soll, D.R.; Daniels, K.J. Plasticity of *Candida albicans* biofilms. *Microbiol. Mol. Biol. Rev.* **2016**, *80*, 565–595. [CrossRef] [PubMed]
45. Silva, S.; Henriques, M.; Martins, A.; Oliveira, R.; Williams, D.; Azeredo, J. Biofilms of non-*Candida albicans Candida* species: Quantification, structure and matrix composition. *Med. Mycol.* **2009**, *47*, 681–689. [CrossRef]
46. Sherry, L.; Ramage, G.; Kean, R.; Borman, A.; Johnson, E.M.; Richardson, M.D.; Rautemaa-Richardson, R. Biofilm-forming capability of highly virulent, multidrug-resistant *Candida auris*. *Emerg. Infect. Dis.* **2017**, *23*, 328–331. [CrossRef]
47. Zarnowski, R.; Westler, W.M.; Lacmbouh, G.A.; Marita, J.M.; Bothe, J.R.; Bernhardt, J.; Lounes-Hadj Sahraoui, A.; Fontaine, J.; Sanchez, H.; Hatfield, R.D.; et al. Novel entries in a fungal biofilm matrix encyclopedia. *mBio* **2014**, *5*, e01333-14. [CrossRef]
48. Branda, S.S.; Vik, S.; Friedman, L.; Kolter, R. Biofilms: The matrix revisited. *Trends Microbiol.* **2005**, *13*, 20–26. [CrossRef]
49. Estivill, D.; Arias, A.; Torres-Lana, A.; Carrillo-Munoz, A.J.; Arevalo, M.P. Biofilm formation by five species of *Candida* on three clinical materials. *J. Microbiol. Methods* **2011**, *86*, 238–242. [CrossRef]
50. Mello, T.P.; Oliveira, S.S.C.; Frases, S.; Branquinha, M.H.; Santos, A.L.S. Surface properties, adhesion and biofilm formation on different surfaces by *Scedosporium* spp. and *Lomentospora prolificans*. *Biofouling* **2018**, *34*, 800–814. [CrossRef]

51. Radford, D.R.; Sweet, S.P.; Challacombe, S.J.; Walter, J.D. Adherence of *Candida albicans* to denture-base materials with different surface finishes. *J. Dent.* **1998**, *26*, 577–583. [CrossRef]
52. Hawser, S.P.; Douglas, L.J. Biofilm formation by *Candida* species on the surface of catheter materials *in vitro*. *Infect. Immun.* **1994**, *62*, 915–921. [CrossRef] [PubMed]
53. Chandra, J.; Patel, J.D.; Li, J.; Zhou, G.; Mukherjee, P.K.; McCormick, T.S.; Anderson, J.M.; Ghannoum, M.A. Modification of surface properties of biomaterials influences the ability of *Candida albicans* to form biofilms. *Appl. Environ. Microbiol.* **2005**, *71*, 8795–8801. [CrossRef] [PubMed]

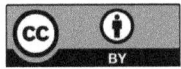

© 2020 by the authors. Licensee MDPI, Basel, Switzerland. This article is an open access article distributed under the terms and conditions of the Creative Commons Attribution (CC BY) license (http://creativecommons.org/licenses/by/4.0/).

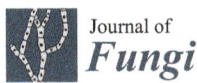

Review

Unraveling How *Candida albicans* Forms Sexual Biofilms

Austin M. Perry [1,2], Aaron D. Hernday [1] and Clarissa J. Nobile [1,*]

[1] Department of Molecular and Cell Biology, School of Natural Sciences, University of California, Merced, CA 95343, USA; aperry5@ucmerced.edu (A.M.P.); ahernday@ucmerced.edu (A.D.H.)
[2] Quantitative and Systems Biology Graduate Program, University of California, Merced, CA 95343, USA
* Correspondence: cnobile@ucmerced.edu; Tel.: +1-209-228-2427

Received: 21 December 2019; Accepted: 13 January 2020; Published: 15 January 2020

Abstract: Biofilms, structured and densely packed communities of microbial cells attached to surfaces, are considered to be the natural growth state for a vast majority of microorganisms. The ability to form biofilms is an important virulence factor for most pathogens, including the opportunistic human fungal pathogen *Candida albicans*. *C. albicans* is one of the most prevalent fungal species of the human microbiota that asymptomatically colonizes healthy individuals. However, *C. albicans* can also cause severe and life-threatening infections when host conditions permit (e.g., through alterations in the host immune system, pH, and resident microbiota). Like many other pathogens, this ability to cause infections depends, in part, on the ability to form biofilms. Once formed, *C. albicans* biofilms are often resistant to antifungal agents and the host immune response, and can act as reservoirs to maintain persistent infections as well as to seed new infections in a host. The majority of *C. albicans* clinical isolates are heterozygous (**a**/α) at the mating type-like (*MTL*) locus, which defines *Candida* mating types, and are capable of forming robust biofilms when cultured in vitro. These "conventional" biofilms, formed by *MTL*-heterozygous (**a**/α) cells, have been the primary focus of *C. albicans* biofilm research to date. Recent work in the field, however, has uncovered novel mechanisms through which biofilms are generated by *C. albicans* cells that are homozygous or hemizygous (**a**/**a**, **a**/Δ, α/α, or α/Δ) at the *MTL* locus. In these studies, the addition of pheromones of the opposite mating type can induce the formation of specialized "sexual" biofilms, either through the addition of synthetic peptide pheromones to the culture, or in response to co-culturing of cells of the opposite mating types. Although sexual biofilms are generally less robust than conventional biofilms, they could serve as a protective niche to support genetic exchange between mating-competent cells, and thus may represent an adaptive mechanism to increase population diversity in dynamic environments. Although conventional and sexual biofilms appear functionally distinct, both types of biofilms are structurally similar, containing yeast, pseudohyphal, and hyphal cells surrounded by an extracellular matrix. Despite their structural similarities, conventional and sexual biofilms appear to be governed by distinct transcriptional networks and signaling pathways, suggesting that they may be adapted for, and responsive to, distinct environmental conditions. Here we review sexual biofilms and compare and contrast them to conventional biofilms of *C. albicans*.

Keywords: biofilms; *Candida albicans*; sexual biofilms; pheromone-induced biofilms; mating type-like (*MTL*) locus; white cell; opaque cell; phenotypic states; pheromone signaling; biofilm formation; biofilm development

1. Introduction

Biofilms are communities of microbial cells that are attached to surfaces and encased in a protective substance called the extracellular matrix [1–5]. Biofilms readily form on surfaces that are biotic (e.g., organs, mucosal and epithelial layers, and teeth) and abiotic (e.g., dentures, catheters, and industrial materials) [1–5]. The biofilm growth state provides the microorganisms inside with a sheltered microenvironment that is buffered against fluctuations in the surrounding environment and is protected from predators, environmental stresses, and mechanical forces that microorganisms would normally encounter in the planktonic (or free-living/free-floating) growth state [1–5]. Due to these adaptive benefits, most microorganisms under natural settings have evolved to spend the majority of their existence in the biofilm growth state [1].

Biofilm formation is a key virulence factor for most pathogens, including *Candida albicans*, which is the most commonly encountered human fungal pathogen in clinical settings [3–7]. *C. albicans* causes a wide variety of infections, ranging from benign mucosal (e.g., yeast infections and thrush) to hematogenously disseminated (bloodstream) candidiasis [6,7]. *Candida* infections are notably serious in immunocompromised individuals, such as AIDS patients, patients undergoing chemotherapy, transplantation patients receiving immunosuppression therapy, and patients with implanted medical devices [8–10]. Although research on *C. albicans* has been ongoing for over 70 years, most work has historically focused on *C. albicans* in its planktonic growth state. Over the last 20 years, however, the biofilm growth state of *C. albicans* has become a major area of research focus. *C. albicans* can form biofilms on abiotic surfaces (e.g., dentures, intravenous catheters, and prosthetic devices), as well as biotic surfaces (e.g., mucosal layers in the oral cavity and genitourinary tract) [3–5]. Once established, the cells within a *C. albicans* biofilm are protected from the host immune response, mechanical perturbations, and chemical stresses, allowing *C. albicans* to persist in the host and potentially cause recalcitrant infections [3–5]. More recently, a specialized "sexual" form of *C. albicans* biofilm has been discovered; although structurally similar to "conventional" biofilms, these "sexual" biofilms have many distinct phenotypic characteristics and generate a unique microenvironment that supports *C. albicans* mating [11,12].

Best known as the most common cause of life-threatening fungal infections in hospital settings, *C. albicans* is also a normal commensal in the majority of healthy humans. Remarkably, *C. albicans* can asymptomatically colonize several diverse regions of the body, including the oral cavity, gastrointestinal tract, skin, and genitourinary tract of humans [13–16]. These niches vary dramatically in terms of pH, nutrient sources and availability, and oxygen content [17,18]. This adaptive plasticity is due, in part, to the ability of *C. albicans* to undergo distinct morphological transitions in response to environmental cues; the best characterized examples include the yeast to hyphal cell transition and the transition between two distinct phenotypic cell types, termed "white" and "opaque" [5,18,19]. We begin by reviewing the white-opaque transition as it is intimately intertwined with the formation of sexual biofilms and mating. Next, we review the pheromone signaling and responses that occur in both white and opaque cell types during sexual biofilm formation and mating. Lastly, we compare and contrast conventional and sexual biofilms and consider the mechanisms through which sexual biofilms may aid in the process of mating.

2. The White–Opaque Transition

White and opaque cell types are heritably maintained for many generations, and reversible switching between the two cell states occurs stochastically under standard laboratory growth conditions [19]. This balance between the white and opaque states is influenced by specific environmental cues that can bias the switch towards one cell type or the other, or even force all of the cells in a population to adopt the white cell phenotype [18–21]. Approximately 16% of the genome is differentially expressed between the white and opaque cell types, resulting in cells with dramatically different phenotypes and functional attributes [18,22–24]. The morphologies of each cell type are also distinct; white cells are spherical and smooth and give rise to white, dome shaped colonies, whereas opaque cells are oblong and pimpled and form flatter and darker colonies [18,19]. Each state displays distinct metabolic preferences, resulting in striking fitness differences under a variety of environmental conditions [25]. White and opaque cells also respond to environmental conditions in unique ways; for example, opaque cells, but not white cells, can be induced to form filaments in response to nitrogen or phosphate limitation, while white, but not opaque cells, are induced to form filaments in the presence of serum [26]. The two cell types also display distinct responses to alterations in temperature under standard laboratory growth conditions; white cells are stable at 37 °C, while opaque cells revert to the white state en masse at 37 °C [18]. Opaque cells, however, can be stabilized at 37 °C by specific environmental stimuli, such as anaerobic conditions, elevated carbon dioxide levels, N-acetylglucosamine, or nutrient limitations [20,21,27–31]. Interestingly, each cell type also interacts with the host immune system in different ways; for example, white cells secrete a macrophage chemoattractant while opaque cells do not, thus increasing the likelihood for opaque cells to escape macrophage engulfment, possibly allowing them to evade this aspect of the host innate immune response [32].

The ability to undergo the white to opaque transition is controlled by the configuration of a discrete region on chromosome 5 known as the Mating Type-Like (*MTL*) locus [33–35]. The *C. albicans MTL* locus can carry two distinct configurations, **a** and α, which consist of genes that specify the **a** and α mating types, respectively [35]. Most *C. albicans* clinical isolates (~97%) are diploid and exist in the *MTL*-heterozygous (**a**/α) configuration, however a few clinical isolates have been found to exist in the *MTL*-homozygous (**a**/**a** or α/α) configuration [33,34]. *MTL*-heterozygous strains express the sex genes *MTL***a**1 and *MTL*α2, the protein products of which form a heterodimer that directly represses the white to opaque transition by binding to the promoter region of *WOR1*, the master regulator of the opaque cell type, and repressing its transcription [33,36]. *MTL*-homozygous strains contain either *MTL***a**1 or *MTL*α2, but not both, and thus *WOR1* expression is derepressed and switching to the opaque state occurs stochastically at a rate of approximately once every 10^4 cell divisions [19,33,34,36]. The white state is considered to be the default cell type, and is often referred to as the "ground state" of the white-opaque switch, since it does not require activation of any known white to opaque transition regulators, while the opaque state is referred to as the "excited state" of the switch because it requires expression of Wor1, which results in activation of many additional regulatory and non-regulatory genes that are specific to the opaque state [22,37].

Although the vast majority (~97%) of *C. albicans* clinical isolates are heterozygous at the *MTL* locus, and were previously presumed to be "locked" in the white cell state [33,34], recent research has shown that the white to opaque switch may be a much more common occurrence in vivo than previously thought. For example, it is now appreciated that natural *MTL*-heterozygous isolates can undergo white to opaque switching in vitro under elevated levels of CO_2 and in the presence of N-acetylglucosamine, conditions that resemble that of the gastrointestinal tract; however, unlike *MTL*-homozygous opaque cells, these *MTL*-heterozygous opaque cells appear unable to mate [21]. In *MTL*-heterozygous cells, *HBR1*, which encodes a transcription factor that mediates the hemoglobin response, promotes expression of genes carried at the *MTL*α locus and thus indirectly reinforces the **a**1/α2-mediated repression of *WOR1* and ultimately the repression of white to opaque switching [38,39]. Deletion of one copy of *HBR1* in *MTL*-heterozygous cells results in a substantial reduction in *MTL***a**1 and *MTL*α2 mRNA expression levels and a slight upregulation of *MTL***a**1 gene expression; the resulting reduction in **a**1/α2 heterodimer levels allows these cells to behave like **a** cells in regards to switching and mating [38,39]. In another example, deletion of *OFR1*, which encodes a protein of unknown function, enables *MTL*-heterozygous white cells to switch to the opaque state and express both **a**- and α-specific pheromones and pheromone receptors, conferring *ofr1* mutants with the unique ability to mate with opaque cells of any *MTL* configuration [40]. In addition, an *MTL*-homozygous clinical isolate strain P94015, which was observed to drift between "white-like" and "opaque-like" cell states, was found to contain a homozygous nonsense mutation in *EFG1*, which encodes a known repressor of the white to opaque transition [41]. Taken together, physiologically relevant environmental cues, or spontaneously arising loss-of-function mutations, could enable naturally occurring strains to undergo white to opaque switching. Lastly, *MTL*-heterozygous cells can become *MTL*-homozygous through loss of heterozygosity on part or all of chromosome 5. This can occur through local gene conversion, homozygosis of an entire arm of the chromosome, or through spontaneous loss of one copy of chromosome 5 followed by duplication of the remaining homologous chromosome [42,43]. These loss of heterozygosity events have been shown to occur in response to a wide range of environmental conditions, including exposure to antifungal agents, growth in the presence of sorbose, oxidative stress, and temperature stress [42–46].

In addition to *MTL*-heterozygous cells becoming *MTL*-homozygous, *MTL*-homozygous cells can also become *MTL*-heterozygous through the *C. albicans* parasexual life cycle [47]. During parasex, *MTL*-homozygous opaque cells can become *MTL*-heterozygous by mating with *MTL*-homozygous cells of the opposite mating type; this is termed heterothallic mating [47–49]. Interestingly, opaque cells can also mate with opaque cells of the same mating type, termed homothallic mating, providing a means for genetic exchange within unisexual populations and even between clonal progeny of a single parent cell [50]. Generally, the parasexual life cycle requires that *MTL*-heterozygous white cells undergo loss of heterozygosity at the *MTL* locus followed by switching to the opaque cell state [33,51–53]. The resulting *MTL*-homozygous opaque cells secrete sex-specific pheromones that can cause opaque cells of the opposite mating type to extend mating projections towards the highest pheromone concentration gradient [53]. Once two mating projections fuse, the resulting conjugation bridge allows for nuclear fusion and the formation of a tetraploid nucleus [53]. This structure is stable for several cell divisions, thereby producing tetraploid progeny [49,53]. Specific environmental cues can cause the tetraploid cells to reduce their ploidy state via concerted chromosome loss, thereby completing the parasexual life cycle by producing diploid cells [48,49,54,55]. This concerted chromosome loss, however, can often result in aneuploidy, which is hypothesized to allow *C. albicans* to rapidly adapt to variable environments and harsh conditions [49,55]. While asexual reproduction (e.g., through budding) can benefit *C. albicans* populations by preserving well-adapted genotypes, parasex can generate novel allelic combinations to allow for rapid evolution in changing environments [48,54,55], which may contribute to the remarkable ability of *C. albicans* to colonize diverse niches in the body and to its overall success as a commensal and pathogen [49]. Despite these apparent benefits, parasex has thus far been reported to occur at low rates in vivo [27,47]. Given that ~97% of the *C. albicans* population in vivo is thought to be *MTL*-heterozygous [34], the probability that two *MTL*-homozygous white cells of opposite mating types undergo the multiple steps required for mating simultaneously, and within close enough proximity to detect mating pheromone, seems exceedingly low. Recent research, however, is beginning to uncover that homothallic mating occurs more frequent under specific in vitro environmental conditions, such as glucose starvation and oxidative stress, supporting the idea that homothallic mating may be more common than anticipated in vivo [56]. Intriguingly, parasexual mating is hypothesized to occur at high frequencies within sexual biofilms, which are formed by *MTL*-homozygous white cells in response to mating pheromone [11,12]. Like all *C. albicans* biofilms, the multilayer structure of the sexual biofilm is such that its innermost layers are likely to contain lower levels of oxygen and nutrients than the layers closer to its surface, and thus sexual biofilms could be a niche that supports homothallic mating.

Perhaps the most striking difference between the white and opaque cell types is that opaque cells can mate with other opaque cells, but form severely impaired biofilms, while white cells can form robust biofilms, but are unable to mate [11,12,33,47,52,57,58]. Generally, a *C. albicans* biofilm consists of a basal layer of yeast cells with hyphae and pseudohyphae extending away from the substrate to which they are adhered [5,59,60]. In recent years, it has been shown that *MTL*-heterozygous and *MTL*-homozygous white cells form different types of biofilms in response to different stimuli [11,12,57–59]. *MTL*-heterozygous (**a**/α) cells form robust biofilms in response to shear flow forces and various environmental conditions (e.g., temperature, shifts in pH, etc.), and are termed conventional biofilms [5]. Once formed, conventional biofilms are challenging to treat in clinical settings due to their recalcitrance to antifungal agents, mechanical forces, and the host immune response. Alternatively, sexual biofilms formed by *MTL*-homozygous (**a** or α) white cells in response to mating pheromone are less robust than conventional biofilms [11,12], but as discussed above, they may provide an adaptive niche for mating.

3. Pheromone Signaling and Response

3.1. Mating Pheromones

The **a** and α pheromones produced by *C. albicans*, encoded by *MF**a**1* and *MFα1* respectively, play essential roles in the processes of heterothallic and homothallic mating [50,61–63]. Opaque α cells constitutively express high levels of *MFα1*, producing a trimeric pheromone precursor peptide, whereas white α cells do not [62]. This α-pheromone precursor peptide is thought to be post-translationally modified by the Kex2 protease and Ste13 dipeptidyl aminopeptidase A, to result in two secreted and identical tridecapeptides with the sequence GFRLTNFGYFEPG and one tetradecapeptide with the sequence GFRLTNFGYFEPGK that represent the mature α pheromones; both the tridecapeptide and tetradecapeptide are capable of eliciting mating responses [62–68]. In contrast, **a** cells only weakly express *MF**a**1* under standard laboratory conditions [61]. However, when exposed to α-pheromone, white and opaque **a** cells highly express both *MF**a**1* and *MFα1* [50,58]. *MF**a**1* also encodes a precursor peptide which is predicted to be processed similarly to the **a**-pheromone of *Saccharomyces cerevisiae* [61,69,70]. Initial cleavage from the **a** pheromone precursor peptide is thought to occur via the Ste24 and Axl1 proteases [61,69]. The developing peptide is then further processed by the prenyl-group-adding enzymes Ram1 and Ram2, the prenyl-dependent protease Rce1, and the cysteine-carboxy methyltransferase Ste14 [61,69]. The mature **a**-pheromone is a prenylated tetradecapeptide with the sequence AVRSVSTGNCCSTC, and requires Hst6, an ABC transporter, to leave the cell [61,70,71]. Due to the structural simplicity of α-pheromone and the fact that α-pheromone can be more easily chemically synthesized relative to **a**-pheromone, most pheromone signaling experiments in the field are carried out using **a** cells and the addition of chemically synthesized α-pheromone.

Although both *MF**a**1* and *MFα1* are expressed in **a** cells in response to pheromone, α-pheromone is typically degraded by Bar1, an aspartyl protease, via a phenomenon known as "barrier activity" [72]. Barrier activity promotes heterothallic mating in ascomycetes by preventing pheromone hyperstimulation and by allowing for a recovery from cell cycle arrest [72]. It also inhibits the ability of *C. albicans* to undergo auto-pheromone stimulation and thus prevents homothallic mating. Deletion of *BAR1* in *C. albicans* allows for homothallic mating through an autocrine pathway where opaque **a** cells excrete α-pheromone, which then binds to Ste2, the α-pheromone receptor, on the same cell, leading to self-activation for mating [50]. In addition, glucose starvation and oxidative stress enable unisexual populations of opaque **a** cells to undergo homothallic mating despite high *BAR1* expression levels [56], resulting in auto-activated opaque cells that can mate with other opaque cells of the same mating type [50,56]. These findings suggest that certain strain backgrounds as well as specific niches in the human body can override the phenomenon of barrier activity, allowing for unisexual populations to become activated by pheromone [50,56]. This has important consequences for the parasexual lifecycle of *C. albicans* as homothallism allows for same-sex mating to occur within cell mixtures of the same mating types and between certain strains that are incompatible for heterothallic mating [50]. Given that this mechanism results in pheromone stimulation and mating for unisexual populations of opaque cells, a similar scenario could be envisioned within a sexual biofilm. The biofilm environment may even enhance the rate of homothallic mating by sequestering pheromone and possibly protecting pheromone from degradation within the biofilm structure [11,12]. In addition, within a biofilm, recently divided opaque cells would be held in close proximity to each other, increasing both the likelihood of finding a mate nearby and the frequency of mating between progeny of a single opaque cell. Given that *C. albicans* relies on generating aneuploid progeny for genetic diversity, rather than recombination during meiosis, homothallic mating between clones in this capacity could rapidly and efficiently introduce genetic diversity into a population [50,54,55].

3.2. Pheromone-Signaling Pathway Control

C. albicans employs a conserved Mitogen-Activated Protein Kinase (MAPK) signaling pathway to transduce pheromone signals and alter gene expression [73,74]. This pathway begins with the conserved mating type-specific G-protein coupled receptors (GPCRs), Ste2, expressed on **a** cells to recognize α-pheromone, and Ste3, expressed on α cells to recognize **a**-pheromone [73–75]. Activation of either GPCR results in the dissociation of the G_α subunit (Cag1) from the G_β subunit (Ste4), and the G_γ subunit (Ste18) of a heterotrimeric G-protein [73–76]. The G-protein subunits then activate Cst20, a kinase that activates the downstream MAPK cascade, consisting of Ste11, Hst7, and Cek1/Cek2 [73–75]. All kinases in this pathway, with the exception of Cst20, are held together in close proximity by the scaffolding protein Cst5 [73–75,77]. Cek1 and Cek2 then activate the transcription factor Cph1 in both white and opaque cells, resulting in the differential expression of white and opaque state-specific genes [58,73]. The activities of Cek1 and Cek2 are regulated by Cpp1, a MAP kinase phosphatase [78]. Interestingly, *STE4*, *CST5*, *CEK1*, and *CEK2* are expressed at lower levels in white cells than opaque cells [79], and their repression contributes to the sterility of white cells as white cells engineered to express *STE4*, *CST5*, and *CEK2* (*CEK1* was not tested) at levels similar to opaque cells have been shown to undergo mating at frequencies approaching that of opaque cells [79]. It is also interesting to note that Cek1 (rather than Cek2) appears to play a major role in opaque cell mating; opaque *cek1* mutants mate at much lower frequencies than opaque *cek2* mutants [78]. The precise contributions of Cek1 and Cek2 to the pheromone response in white and opaque cells is complex and an intriguing research area for future study. Nonetheless, we do know that G-protein signaling pathways, such as this one, are highly conserved among fungal pathogens and are involved in controlling several important developmental processes, including mating, filamentation, and virulence [80].

3.3. Differences Between the White and Opaque Cell Pheromone Responses

When opaque cells sense pheromone of the opposite mating type, they become activated for mating via the MAPK signaling pathway (described above). This pheromone stimulation can occur under a variety of different environmental conditions, including planktonic and biofilm conditions [58,61,62,68]. Interestingly, opaque cells have been observed to respond more efficiently to pheromone in media containing alternative carbon sources (e.g., Spider media) [68]. Additionally, the opaque cell pheromone response can be enhanced under a variety of environmental conditions by deletion of *GPA2*, which encodes a G-protein α-subunit that functions at the beginning of the cyclic AMP-protein kinase A (cAMP-PKA) pathway [68]. This finding suggests that mating may occur more frequently within certain (e.g., specific nutrient limiting) host niches and that there is likely crosstalk between the signaling pathways regulating pheromone (i.e., MAPK) and nutrient sensing (i.e., cAMP-PKA) responses.

The opaque cell pheromone response in C. albicans is mediated by the transcription factor Cph1, a homolog of the transcription factor Ste12 in S. cerevisiae that is activated by a MAPK signaling pathway and controls genes involved in mating [58,70,73,74,81–83]. In opaque cells responding to pheromone, Cph1 initiates a transcriptional response that results in an upregulation of genes involved in filamentation (e.g., *FGR23*), cell fusion (e.g., *FUS1*, *FIG1*), karyogamy (e.g., *KAR4*), MAPK signaling (e.g., *CEK1/2*), and adhesion and virulence (e.g., *HWP1/2*, *ECE1*, *SAP4/5/6*, *RBT1/4*) [52,53,58,62,68]. Interestingly, although opaque cells generally grow slower than white cells, genes involved in DNA replication and the cell cycle (e.g., *MCM6*, *MCM7*, *PRI2*, and *POL5a*) are specifically repressed in opaque cells responding to pheromone, suggesting that exposure to pheromone further slows progression out of the G1 phase of the cell cycle [52,53,58,62,68,84]. In opaque **a** cells, *STE2* is upregulated, and the α-pheromone receptor Ste2 becomes localized to the tip of growing cellular extensions known as mating projections or conjugation tubes [11,52,53,58,62]; mating projections are phenotypically similar to hyphae, but lack septa [52,53]. Not surprisingly, transcriptional profiling data revealed that opaque cells forming mating projections in response to pheromone upregulate a subset of the genes associated with filamentation and virulence that are upregulated by white cells forming hyphae in response to serum [62,85]. These findings indicate that there is overlap among genes expressed during hyphal formation and pheromone treatment, but that there are also several genes that are distinctly expressed in each process [62].

Although *C. albicans* white cells are unable to mate, **a** and α white cells still express pheromone receptors and are thought to respond to pheromone in a Cph1-dependent manner [11,58], albeit at a much slower rate than opaque cells [58]. For example, under standard sexual biofilm conditions, the transcriptional response of opaque cells four hours after pheromone exposure is comparable to that of white cells 24 h after pheromone exposure [58]. Interestingly, the pheromone response in white cells appears to occur primarily under sexual biofilm conditions; in fact, much of the response is lost when white cells are subjected to pheromone under planktonic conditions [52,68]. It is also interesting to note that similar to the pheromone response in opaque cells, sexual biofilm formation is highly dependent on nutrient levels [57,68,86], suggestive again of crosstalk between the pheromone response and nutrient sensing signaling pathways. Despite white cells being unable to mate, many genes involved in MAPK signaling and mating are upregulated in white cells responding to pheromone (e.g., *STE2*, *HST6*, *FIG1*, *FUS1*, *KAR4*), which may be an artefact derived from the co-option of Cph1 by white cells for biofilm formation [58]. In addition, many of the adhesion-, biofilm- and other virulence-associated genes upregulated in opaque cells responding to pheromone are similarly upregulated by white cells responding to pheromone in biofilms (e.g., *RBT1*, *HWP1/2*, *ECE1*, *PGA23/50*, *SAP5/6*) [58]. However, unlike opaque cells, white **a** cells do not experience a halt in their cell cycle upon exposure to α-pheromone [11,52]. Overall, in synthetic pheromone-stimulated biofilms, 116 genes are differentially expressed in both white and opaque cells, white cells uniquely differentially express 147 genes, and opaque cells uniquely differentially express 190 genes [58]. Given that Cph1 is believed to mediate both sexual biofilm formation in white cells and mating in opaque cells in response to pheromone, Cph1 may be involved in mediating a core pheromone response involving filamentation and adhesion that can be modified depending on the epigenetic state of the cell [58,73]. Over the course of evolutionary time, it appears that *C. albicans* has rewired aspects of cell–cell communication to be used for host–pathogen interactions, which may provide insight into the unique history of this opportunistic pathogen. Additional work on the regulatory controls of white and opaque cells may improve our understanding of how transcription factors drift to regulate novel functions.

4. Conventional and Sexual Biofilms

4.1. Properties of Conventional and Sexual Biofilms Compared

Conventional and sexual biofilms formed by *C. albicans* are both composed of yeast-form, pseudohyphal, and hyphal cells [5,12,60,86]. The *C. albicans* biofilm life cycle typically begins when planktonic yeast-form cells adhere to a substrate in response to specific environmental stimuli [4,5]. These yeast-form cells proliferate, resulting in a dense mat that is tightly anchored to its substrate. Hyphae and pseudohyphae then begin to grow and extend away from the substrate, providing architectural support for the biofilm. As the growing *C. albicans* biofilm matures, the cells within the biofilm produce extracellular matrix material, composed predominantly of proteins, polysaccharides, and DNA that surrounds all of the cells within the biofilm [4,5]. Once a mature biofilm is formed, daughter yeast-form cells disperse from the biofilm and revert to the planktonic growth state or form new biofilms elsewhere [4,5,87]. Although this generalized biofilm life cycle is common across all *C. albicans* biofilms, the configuration of the *MTL* locus and the phenotypic state of the cells play important roles in determining the environmental stimuli that induce biofilm formation as well as certain unique physical characteristics of the biofilms formed. *MTL*-heterozygous white cells form thick and resilient conventional biofilms in response to specific environmental stimuli, such as shear flow rate and host factors, whereas *MTL*-homozygous white cells form thinner and weaker sexual biofilms in response to mating pheromone [11,12,57,86].

Generally, microorganisms that exist in biofilms are protected from environmental stresses relative to microorganisms that exist planktonically [1]. The extracellular matrix surrounding both *C. albicans* conventional and sexual biofilms acts as a physical barrier inhibiting many compounds, such as antimicrobial agents, from penetrating into the deeper layers of the biofilm [3–5]. Mature conventional biofilms, in particular, are highly resilient to most forms of environmental stress, such as treatment with antifungal agents, exposure to mechanical forces, and attack by the host immune system [4,5]. In addition to the physical barrier provided by the matrix, the resilience of conventional biofilms to antifungal agents is also due to the fact that cells within conventional, but not sexual, biofilms upregulate drug efflux pumps (e.g., Cdr1/2, Mdr1), thereby prohibiting antifungal drugs from reaching lethal concentrations within the biofilm [58,60]. Consistent with this finding, sexual biofilms are much more easily permeated by a variety of compounds than conventional biofilms [12,59]. Interestingly, this phenotype can be partially rescued by the overexpression of *BCR1* [12,59], which encodes the biofilm master regulator of several downstream adhesins, suggesting that cell–cell and/or cell–substrate adherence may also contribute to the recalcitrance of conventional biofilms to antimicrobial compounds. Cells within conventional biofilms are also more tightly adhered to each other and their substrates compared to sexual biofilms [12,58,59]. These differences in adherence are likely due to the upregulation of genes involved in adhesion (e.g., *ALS3*) in conventional biofilms, which are less (if at all) upregulated in sexual biofilms [3–5,58,60]. Additional factors contributing to the drug resistance of conventional biofilms include variation in cell membrane sterol composition and the presence of metabolically dormant persister cells, which can display extreme tolerance to most classes of antifungal drugs [3,4,13,88,89]. We note that these two factors have only been studied in conventional biofilms, and thus whether or not they also are present in sexual biofilms is unknown, and an intriguing area of interest for future studies.

If sexual biofilms do not provide the same protective environment as conventional biofilms, why does *C. albicans* bother to form sexual biofilms in the first place? Given that ~97% of the *C. albicans* population in nature is thought to be *MTL*-heterozygous, the chance that two *MTL*-homozygous white cells of opposite mating types will exist in close enough proximity to undergo the complex steps involved to mate is seemingly unlikely [34]. Even if two opaque cells were in close enough proximity to one another, ambient forces would likely disrupt the pheromone concentration gradient before the cells could find one another and fuse. Since sexual biofilms are not nearly as thick or dense as conventional biofilms, these properties could enable opaque cells to extend mating projections through the biofilm towards other opaque cells, while still being sufficiently dense to maintain pheromone gradients and provide some stability against external forces [11,12]. Consistent with the idea that sexual biofilms provide an optimal environment for mating, white **a** cells produce their own pheromone when responding to α-pheromone, which promotes both homothallic and heterothallic mating [90]. In terms of the host response, white cells are preferentially phagocytosed by macrophages as compared to opaque cells and only white cells secrete a leukocyte chemoattractant [32,91]. Thus, white cells may protect mating opaque cells by acting as decoys to sequester infiltrating host cells [32]. Overall, by stabilizing pheromone gradients and providing an optimal environment for opaque cells to undergo mating, sexual biofilms may promote mating in specialized niches of the body that support white-opaque switching (e.g., the skin).

Cell heterogeneity resulting from the various microenvironments present throughout conventional biofilms is also likely to contribute to biofilm resilience [3]. These microenvironment differences lead to specific gene expression changes within cells in discreet environmental niches of the biofilm, resulting in widespread cellular heterogeneity throughout the biofilm architecture [92]. For example, the innermost regions of conventional biofilms are hypoxic and contain less nutrients and more waste products compared to the outermost regions of the biofilm [93]. These unique microenvironments also enable *C. albicans* to coexist and interact with specific microbial species. For example, the hypoxic inner regions of conventional *C. albicans* biofilms support the growth of obligate anaerobic bacteria, such as *Bacteroides fragilis* and *Clostridium perfringens* [3,93]. Although the microenvironments present in sexual biofilms have not been studied to date, because sexual biofilms are much thinner than conventional biofilms [12,59], there are likely to be fewer opportunities for microenvironments to form.

Nonetheless, given their phenotypic differences, the microenvironments of conventional and sexual biofilms are certainly distinct.

Interspecies interactions within polymicrobial biofilms between *C. albicans* and other species (mostly bacteria) have only been studied to date within the context of conventional *C. albicans* biofilms. These interactions can be beneficial or antagonistic in nature. A large proportion of research to date has focused on the beneficial interactions between *C. albicans* and *Staphylococcus* species, such as *Staphylococcus aureus*; these two species are often co-isolated from biofilm infections with high mortality rates in clinical settings [94]. Although these two species can form biofilms independently, initial attachment of *C. albicans* cells to surfaces is enhanced when *C. albicans* is co-inoculated with *S. aureus* [95]. In mature polymicrobial biofilms of *S. aureus* and *C. albicans*, *S. aureus* cells can be found adhered to *C. albicans* hyphae and are present throughout the biofilm structure [95–97]. *S. aureus* is, in fact, known to specifically recognize and bind to the adhesin Als3 on the cell surface of *C. albicans* hyphae, and consistent with this, cells of *C. albicans als3* mutants have been found to interact with significantly fewer *S. aureus* cells than wild-type *C. albicans* cells [96]. Interestingly, *ALS3* expression is reduced in sexual biofilms compared to conventional biofilms [58,60], and thus one may hypothesize that *S. aureus* and *C. albicans* are less likely to co-localize in the context of sexual biofilms. Other structural components of *C. albicans* biofilms are also known to play roles in mixed-species interactions. For example, β-glucans present in the extracellular matrix of *C. albicans* biofilms were found to aid methicillin-resistant *S. aureus* (MRSA) strains in surviving vancomycin, one of the few antibiotics effective against MRSA [3,98]. In terms of antagonistic interactions, *Enterococcus faecalis* can secrete EntV, a bacteriocin that inhibits conventional *C. albicans* biofilm formation [3,99]. In another example, *Pseudomonas aeruginosa* can secrete a 12-carbon acyl homoserine lactone that hinders *C. albicans* filamentation and conventional biofilm formation by mimicking farnesol, a quorum sensing molecule produced by *C. albicans* that modulates filamentation [100,101]. *P. aeruginosa* can also release phenazines that specifically inhibit *C. albicans* filamentation and conventional biofilm formation [102]. Overall, given that sexual and conventional biofilms have different physical and biochemical properties, the interactions of these two biofilm systems with other microorganisms are likely to differ considerably.

Conventional and sexual biofilms also differ in their interactions with the host immune response. Neutrophils and mononuclear leukocytes are important host players against fungal infections [103,104]. When neutrophils recognize *C. albicans* cells, they activate a number of antimicrobial defenses, including phagocytosis, degranulation, the release of reactive oxygen species (ROS), and the release of web-like neutrophil extracellular traps (NETs) [103]. In general, neutrophils are very effective at killing planktonic *C. albicans* yeast and hyphal cells [105], where these antimicrobial mechanisms work efficiently. When it comes to *C. albicans* conventional biofilms, however, neutrophils are generally unable to penetrate beyond the outermost regions of the biofilm, ROS are not produced, and NETs are not released [3,4,59,106,107]. This biofilm-specific recalcitrance to neutrophils is largely due to the presence of the extracellular matrix, as physical disruption of the matrix in conventional biofilms restores the ability of neutrophils to release NETs [106]. Consistently, neutrophils are able to release NETs and kill *C. albicans* cells within a biofilm formed by the *C. albicans pmr1* mutant, which is unable to produce matrix mannan [106]. Interestingly, in the presence of a sexual biofilm, neutrophils can penetrate into the innermost layers of the biofilm [59], although whether NETs are released, and fungal cells are killed is unknown. Based on this information, one would hypothesize that sexual biofilms are more susceptible to clearance by neutrophils than conventional biofilms.

In terms of mononuclear leukocytes, these host cells typically respond to *C. albicans* infection by phagocytosing invading cells and releasing cytokines [108]. *C. albicans* cells in conventional biofilms are two to three times more resistant to killing by mononuclear leukocytes than cells growing planktonically [103,108]. In addition, *C. albicans* cells growing in conventional biofilms are capable of altering the cytokine profile of attacking mononuclear cells [108]. For example, the presence of a conventional biofilm leads to the downregulation of TNF-α, a pro-inflammatory cytokine produced by mononuclear leukocytes that would normally suppress biofilm formation [103,108,109].

Intriguingly, conventional biofilms that are grown in the presence of mononuclear leukocytes form thicker biofilms, a phenomenon that is thought to be mediated by an unknown soluble factor that is present when the two are co-cultured [108]. Whether or not this process also occurs with sexual biofilms in the presence of mononuclear cells is unknown, but an interesting area for future exploration.

The host response to *C. albicans* infection is typically initiated by the interaction of host pattern recognition receptors and pathogen-associated molecular patterns (PAMPs) and involves secretion of a variety of antimicrobial compounds. Interestingly, several characteristics of conventional and sexual biofilms inhibit the recognition of PAMPs. For example, hyphal cells, a major component of both conventional and sexual biofilms, are able to 'mask' the β-glucan in their cell walls, blocking a key PAMP recognized by many host immune cell types [4,110,111]. In addition, several cell surface and secreted proteins are capable of sequestering and inactivating host complement proteins, and other secreted anti-immune proteins are expressed at higher levels in conventional biofilms than in planktonic cells [3,4,60]. Although studies to date have only examined conventional biofilms, it seems likely that sexual biofilms would also retain some of these host response characteristics. In fact, we know that some cell surface and secreted proteins involved in inactivating the host immune response (e.g., *SAP4, MSB2*) are also upregulated in sexual biofilms [58]. Nonetheless, how sexual biofilms interact with the immune system and how they compare to conventional biofilms in this regard has not been investigated to date.

4.2. Genetic Regulation of Conventional and Sexual Biofilms

Our current knowledge of the regulation of conventional and sexual biofilms is summarized in Figure 1. Given that there are many phenotypic differences between conventional and sexual biofilms, it seems likely that the genetic regulation and transcriptional profiles of these two systems should differ as well. As discussed above, the signaling pathway that triggers the formation of sexual biofilms is a MAPK cascade initiated by the pheromone receptors Ste2 or Ste3 [73–75]. This pathway is unique to sexual biofilms, as a Ras1/cAMP pathway that includes Cdc35, Tpk2, and an unknown receptor has been shown to trigger conventional biofilm formation [59,112,113]. In the conventional biofilm pathway, Ras1 activation results in cAMP production, and increased concentrations of cAMP stimulate PKA to initiate the complex transcriptional network controlling conventional biofilm formation [59,112,113]. When comparing the transcriptional profiles of *MTL*-heterozygous white cells grown planktonically versus in conventional biofilm conditions, and white **a** cells grown in sexual biofilm conditions with and without the presence of α-pheromone, there are 662 genes that are induced twofold or more in conventional biofilms, 486 genes that are induced twofold or more in sexual biofilms, and 128 genes similarly induced twofold or more in both systems (examples include *HWP1, SAP4, SAP5, ALS1*) [58,60]. In addition, 187 genes are repressed at least twofold in conventional biofilms, 355 genes are repressed at least twofold in sexual biofilms, and only 19 genes are similarly repressed at least twofold in both systems [58,60]. The dramatic differences in transcriptomic profiles between sexual and conventional biofilms strongly supports the idea that distinct transcriptional networks regulate the formation of these two structures.

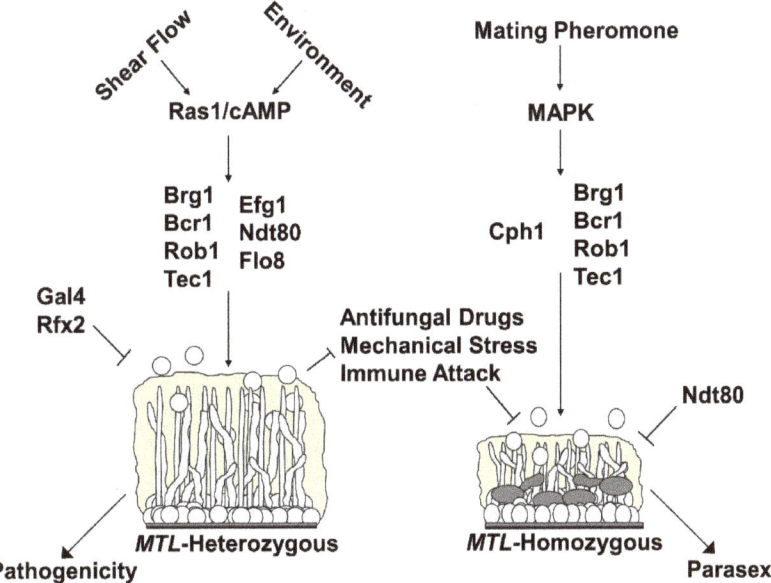

Figure 1. Summary of the regulation of *C. albicans* conventional (mating type-like (*MTL*)-heterozygous) and sexual (*MTL*-homozygous) biofilm formation and their phenotypic characteristics. Arrows with smaller heads indicate activation (e.g., shear flow and environmental conditions activate the Ras1/cAMP pathway). Arrows with large heads indicate the lifestyle each biofilm type facilitates (e.g., *MTL*-heterozygous biofilms facilitate a pathogenic lifestyle). T-bars indicate inhibitory relationships (e.g., Gal4 and Rfx2 inhibit conventional biofilm formation and conventional biofilms inhibit the deleterious effects of antifungal drugs, mechanical stress and immune attack).

The core transcriptional network controlling conventional biofilm formation consists of nine transcription factors: Tec1, Ndt80, Rob1, Brg1, Bcr1, Efg1, Flo8, Gal4, and Rfx2 [60,114]. By screening a mutant library containing 165 strains with homozygous deletions of genes encoding DNA-binding proteins, a transcriptional network of six transcription factors was identified (Tec1, Ndt80, Rob1, Brg1, Bcr1, Efg1), whose deletion hindered conventional biofilm formation in vitro and in vivo [60]. Interestingly, two of these transcription factor mutants were defective in one in vivo model of biofilm formation but not in another (e.g., the *bcr1* mutant was severely defective in the rat catheter model, but formed a decent biofilm in the rat denture model, while the *brg1* mutant formed normal biofilms in the catheter model, but was severely defective in the denture model) [60]. These findings suggest that the genetic regulation of conventional biofilms may be different depending on the environment [60]. Further investigation into the transcriptional regulators of conventional biofilm formation in a temporal biofilm study revealed three additional core regulators: Flo8, Gal4 and Rfx2 [114]. Interestingly, deletion of *GAL4* and *RFX2* resulted in generally enhanced conventional biofilms relative to wildtype, indicating that they may serve as negative regulators of the network [114]. In order to understand how these transcription factors regulate conventional biofilm formation, genome-wide chromatin immunoprecipitation and microarray experiments were performed on each transcription factor and transcription factor mutant, respectively. These experiments revealed that each of the nine transcription factors contribute to the formation of a complex network that encompasses about 1000 downstream "target" genes [60]. Furthermore, extensive binding between the nine transcription factors and their respective *cis*-regulatory regions highlights a complex set of regulatory feedback loops within the core of the biofilm regulatory network [60,114,115]. Overall, the majority of TFs involved in the conventional biofilm network act as both positive and negative regulators of various downstream target genes, with the exception of Tec1, which seems to act primarily as an activator [60]. Although the core transcriptional network regulating conventional biofilm formation has been identified, many additional transcription factors have been found to regulate certain aspects of conventional biofilm formation. For example, Rlm1 and Zap1 are both involved in the regulation of the extracellular matrix [116–118]. As we continue research on biofilms into the future, there will certainly be additional regulators identified to play important roles in different aspects of conventional biofilm formation, as well as an increase in our knowledge of the core regulators of sexual biofilm formation.

Sexual biofilms are currently known to rely on four of the nine core transcription factors involved in the conventional biofilm network: Bcr1, Rob1, Brg1, and Tec1 [58]. Deletion of any of these four transcription factors results in a significant decrease in sexual biofilm thickness relative to wildtype [58]. Deletion of *EFG1* does not hinder sexual biofilm formation [58]; rather, the *efg1* mutant appears to form equally thick sexual biofilms relative to wildtype, indicating that *EFG1* is not required for sexual biofilm formation [58]. Interestingly, the *ndt80* mutant forms thicker sexual biofilms than wildtype, although this may not be due to Ndt80 acting as a negative regulator of sexual biofilm formation since deletion of *NDT80* leads to the misregulation of cell separation genes, specifically *SUN41* and *CHT3* [58]. This could consequently result in thicker sexual biofilms as an artifact of enhanced cell clumping and/or reduced cell dispersion during sexual biofilm formation. The fact that this does not occur in conventional biofilms, and that Ndt80 is in fact required for conventional biofilm formation, is an intriguing area for future research. The roles of the other three core transcription factors involved in regulating conventional biofilm formation—Flo8, Gal4 and Rfx2—have not yet been explored in terms of sexual biofilm formation and is another area of interest for future research. Finally, the transcription factor Cph1, which is not required for conventional biofilm formation, plays a central role in the regulation of sexual biofilm formation [58,60]. Deletion of *CPH1* results in the complete obliteration of sexual biofilm formation, and it has been hypothesized that Cph1 is the terminal transcription factor activated by the MAPK cascade in both white and opaque cells responding to pheromone [58]. These ideas have been challenged, where another group found that although the same GPCR (Ste2/3), MAPK cascade (Ste11, Hst7, Cek1/2) and scaffolding protein (Cst5) are used in both white and opaque cell pheromone responses, there are cell type differences in the terminal transcription factors that are activated by pheromone [74]. In opaque cells, their findings suggest that Cph1 is activated for mating, while in white cells, Tec1 is activated for sexual biofilm formation [74,119,120]. The discrepancies between these two findings may be partially explained by differences in growth conditions utilized by the two groups [11,12,58,74,86]. In fact, the different conditions lead to the formation of sexual biofilms with distinct structural features, and one possibility is that different transcription networks may be involved in the two conditions that depend on distinct environmental cues. Given this information, the terminal transcription factor(s) activated by pheromone-stimulated MAPK signaling in white cells remain to be conclusively determined.

The transcriptional network regulating conventional biofilms has been shown to have evolved fairly recently [60]. By determining the master regulators of sexual biofilm formation and its accompanying transcriptional network, we will be able to explore how two seemingly unrelated transcriptional networks and signaling pathways have evolved to interact with one another. If Cph1 is the terminal transcription factor of the pheromone response in white cells, this would indicate that a conserved signaling cascade and its transcriptional regulator evolved to control a novel set of genes during pheromone activation. We can envision two scenarios where this could occur. First, genes associated with biofilm formation may have come under the direct control of Cph1 by the addition of Cph1 recognition sequences to their promoters. Alternatively, one or several regulators of biofilm formation may have come under the control of Cph1 [115]. In the latter scenario, deemed the "regulator-first" model of the evolution of transcription networks [115], Cph1 would have been directly inserted into the older conventional biofilm network, gaining control of several downstream genes associated with biofilm formation, while adding many of the genes that it previously regulated to the network. This model could account for the large size of transcriptional networks (e.g., the conventional biofilm network comprises approximately 20% of the genome), and the reason why complex transcriptional networks include such large numbers of seemingly extraneous target genes [58,60,115]. Since white cells are unable to mate, their main purpose is to form biofilms in response to pheromone, thus reason dictates that they have no need to express genes involved in mating when stimulated by pheromone. Yet, the expression of mating genes has been observed in white cells responding to mating pheromone, where there is a clear induction of genes involved in cell fusion, karyogamy and other aspects of mating (e.g., *FUS1* and *KAR4*) [58]. This regulator-first model is consistent with the hypothesis that Cph1 is the terminal transcription factor activated by the MAPK cascade in both white and opaque cells responding to pheromone. In the alternative hypothesis, Tec1, whose expression is only induced in conventional biofilms via Efg1, may have come under direct control of a novel signaling pathway, namely the pheromone response MAPK cascade. In this scenario, Tec1 would still regulate many of the genes it traditionally regulated and the transcriptional profile of the white cell pheromone response would look similar to conventional biofilm formation. Given that we see a dramatic change in transcriptional profiles between the two biofilm systems and the activation of so many extraneous genes involved in mating in white cells responding to pheromone, we favor the regulator-first model for the evolution of the sexual biofilm transcriptional network.

5. Conclusions

Sexual biofilms represent a specialized kind of biofilm formed by *MTL*-homozygous cells responding to mating pheromone. The physical characteristics of sexual biofilms differ dramatically from conventional biofilms; indeed, they appear to lack the major characteristics that contribute to the highly pathogenic nature of conventional biofilms. The molecular differences that result in such distinct phenotypes between the two systems remain to be determined. The significance of the unusual characteristics of sexual biofilms and their roles in the lifecycle of *C. albicans* is also not clearly understood. The low frequency of *MTL*-homozygous strains observed in nature and the apparent lack of opaque-specific niches outside of the laboratory led to questions about the existence of a parasexual lifecycle in *C. albicans* in nature. However, it is now appreciated that sexual biofilms may serve as a permeable and penetrable, yet protective, microenvironment that promotes mating in *C. albicans*. Although no in vivo model has been established to investigate the relevance of sexual biofilms in the host, the apparent disadvantageous properties of sexual biofilms for survival in the host may be outweighed by their ability to promote parasexual mating. Future work on the genetic regulation and molecular mechanisms of sexual biofilm formation will improve our understanding of the significance of sexual biofilms as well as the relevance of phenotypic switching and parasexual mating in the lifecycle of *C. albicans* in nature. Overall, the molecular and genetic regulation of conventional and sexual biofilm formation is quite different between the two systems. Conventional biofilms are modulated by the Ras1/cAMP signaling pathway, whereas sexual biofilms are modulated by a MAP kinase pathway; each activating a largely distinct set of transcription factors and likely different transcriptional networks. Understanding how these two transcriptional networks regulate their target genes to give rise to similar yet distinct phenotypes will also provide a basis for studies on the evolution of biofilm formation. Current and future research into sexual biofilms should provide a wealth of knowledge into the molecular genetics, pathogenesis, and evolutionary history of one of the most pervasive fungal pathogens of humans.

Funding: This research was funded by the National Institutes of Health (NIH) National Institute of Allergy and Infectious Diseases (NIAID) and National Institute of General Medical Sciences (NIGMS) awards R21AI125801 and R35GM124594, respectively, to C.J.N., and by a Pew Biomedical Scholar Award from the Pew Charitable Trusts to C.J.N. This work was also supported by the Kamangar family in the form of an endowed chair to C.J.N. A.D.H. acknowledges funding from the NIH NIAID award R15AI379755.

Acknowledgments: The authors thank all members of the Nobile and Hernday labs for insightful discussions on the manuscript as well as the anonymous reviewers for their insightful comments on the manuscript.

Conflicts of Interest: Clarissa J. Nobile is a cofounder of BioSynesis, Inc., a company developing inhibitors and diagnostics of biofilm formation. The company has no role in the manuscript. The funders had no role in the design of the study, in the collection, analyses, or interpretation of data, in the writing of the manuscript, or in the decision to publish the results.

References

1. Hall-Stoodley, L.; Costerton, J.W.; Stoodley, P. Bacterial biofilms: From the natural environment to infectious diseases. *Nat. Rev. Microbiol.* **2004**, *2*, 95–108. [CrossRef] [PubMed]
2. Kolter, R.; Greenberg, E.P. Microbial sciences: The superficial life of microbes. *Nature* **2006**, *441*, 300–302. [CrossRef] [PubMed]
3. Lohse, M.B.; Gulati, M.; Johnson, A.D.; Nobile, C.J. Development and regulation of single-and multi-species *Candida albicans* biofilms. *Nat. Rev. Microbiol.* **2018**, *16*, 19–31. [CrossRef] [PubMed]
4. Gulati, M.; Nobile, C.J. *Candida albicans* biofilms: Development, regulation, and molecular mechanisms. *Microbes Infect.* **2016**, *18*, 310–321. [CrossRef] [PubMed]
5. Nobile, C.J.; Johnson, A.D. *Candida albicans* biofilms and human disease. *Annu. Rev. Microbiol.* **2015**, *69*, 71–92. [CrossRef] [PubMed]
6. Wenzel, R.P. Nosocomial Candidemia: Risk Factors and Attributable Mortality. *Clin. Infect. Dis.* **1995**, *20*, 1531–1534. [CrossRef] [PubMed]
7. Rex, J.H.; Walsh, T.J.; Sobel, J.D.; Filler, S.G.; Pappas, P.G.; Dismukes, W.E.; Edwards, J.E. Practice Guidelines for the treatment of candidiasis. *Clin. Infect. Dis.* **2000**, *30*, 662–678. [CrossRef]
8. Calderone, R.A.; Fonzi, W.A. Virulence factors of *Candida albicans*. *Trends Microbiol.* **2001**, *9*, 327–335. [CrossRef]
9. Kullber, B.J.; Oude Lashof, A.M. Epidemiology of opportunisitic invasive mycoses. *Eur. J. Med. Res.* **2002**, *7*, 183–191.
10. Weig, M.; Gross, U.; Mühlschlegel, F. Clinical aspects and pathogenesis of *Candida* infection. *Trends Microbiol.* **1998**, *6*, 468–470. [CrossRef]
11. Daniels, K.J.; Srikantha, T.; Lockhart, S.R.; Pujol, C.; Soll, D.R. Opaque cells signal white cells to form biofilms in *Candida albicans*. *EMBO J.* **2006**, *25*, 2240–2252. [CrossRef] [PubMed]
12. Park, Y.N.; Daniels, K.J.; Pujol, C.; Srikantha, T.; Soll, D.R. *Candida albicans* forms a specialized "sexual" as well as "pathogenic" biofilm. *Eukaryot. Cell* **2013**, *12*, 1120–1131. [CrossRef] [PubMed]
13. Ganguly, S.; Mitchell, A.P. Mucosal biofilms of *Candida albicans*. *Curr. Opin. Microbiol.* **2011**, *14*, 380–385. [CrossRef] [PubMed]
14. Kumamoto, C.A. *Candida* biofilms. *Curr. Opin. Microbiol.* **2002**, *5*, 608–611. [CrossRef]
15. Kumamoto, C.A. Inflammation and gastrointestinal *Candida* colonization. *Curr. Opin. Microbiol.* **2011**, *14*, 386–391. [CrossRef]
16. Kennedy, M.J.; Volz, P.A. Ecology of *Candida* albicans gut colonization: Inhibition of *Candida* adhesion, colonization, and dissemination from the gastrointestinal tract by bacterial antagonism. *Infect. Immun.* **1985**, *49*, 654–663. [CrossRef]
17. Köhler, J.R.; Casadevall, A.; Perfect, J. The Spectrum of Fungi That Infects Humans. *Cold Spring Harb. Perspect. Med.* **2014**, *5*, a019273. [CrossRef]
18. Lohse, M.B.; Johnson, A.D. White-opaque switching in *Candida albicans*. *Curr. Opin. Microbiol.* **2009**, *12*, 650–654. [CrossRef]
19. Slutsky, B.; Staebell, M.; Anderson, J.; Risen, L.; Pfaller, M.; Soll, D.R. "White-opaque transition": A second high-frequency switching system in *Candida albicans*. *J. Bacteriol.* **1987**, *169*, 189–197. [CrossRef]
20. Huang, G.; Yi, S.; Sahni, N.; Daniels, K.J.; Srikantha, T.; Soll, D.R. N-acetylglucosamine induces white to opaque switching, a mating prerequisite in *Candida albicans*. *PLoS Pathog.* **2010**, *6*, e1000806. [CrossRef]
21. Xie, J.; Tao, L.; Nobile, C.J.; Tong, Y.; Guan, G.; Sun, Y.; Cao, C.; Hernday, A.D.; Johnson, A.D.; Zhang, L.; et al. White-Opaque Switching in Natural MTLa/α Isolates of *Candida albicans*: Evolutionary Implications for Roles in Host Adaptation, Pathogenesis, and Sex. *PLoS Biol.* **2013**, *11*, e1001525. [CrossRef] [PubMed]
22. Tuch, B.B.; Mitrovich, Q.M.; Homann, O.R.; Hernday, A.D.; Monighetti, C.K.; de La Vega, F.M.; Johnson, A.D. The transcriptomes of two heritable cell types illuminate the circuit governing their differentiation. *PLoS Genet.* **2010**, *6*, e1001070. [CrossRef]
23. Lan, C.Y.; Newport, G.; Murillo, L.A.; Jones, T.; Scherer, S.; Davis, R.W.; Agabian, N. Metabolic specialization associated with phenotypic switching in *Candida albicans*. *Proc. Natl. Acad. Sci. USA* **2002**, *99*, 14907–14912. [CrossRef]
24. Tsong, A.E.; Miller, M.G.; Raisner, R.M.; Johnson, A.D. Evolution of a Combinatorial Transcriptional Circuit: A Case Study in Yeasts. *Cell* **2003**, *115*, 389–399. [CrossRef]

25. Ene, I.V.; Lohse, M.B.; Vladu, A.V.; Morschhäuser, J.; Johnson, A.D.; Bennett, R.J. Phenotypic profiling reveals that *Candida albicans* opaque cells represent a metabolically specialized cell state compared to default white cells. *MBio* **2016**, *7*, e01269-16. [CrossRef] [PubMed]
26. Si, H.; Hernday, A.D.; Hirakawa, M.P.; Johnson, A.D.; Bennett, R.J. *Candida albicans* White and Opaque Cells Undergo Distinct Programs of Filamentous Growth. *PLoS Pathog.* **2013**, *9*, e1003210. [CrossRef]
27. Dumitru, R.; Navarathna, D.H.M.L.P.; Semighini, C.P.; Elowsky, C.G.; Dumitru, R.V.; Dignard, D.; Whiteway, M.; Atkin, A.L.; Nickerson, K.W. In vivo and in vitro anaerobic mating in *Candida albicans*. *Eukaryot. Cell* **2007**, *6*, 465–472. [CrossRef] [PubMed]
28. Huang, G. Regulation of phenotypic transitions in the fungal pathogen *Candida albicans*. *Virulence* **2012**, *3*, 251–261. [CrossRef] [PubMed]
29. Ramírez-Zavala, B.; Reuß, O.; Park, Y.; Ohlsen, K.; Morschhäuser, J. Environmental Induction of White–Opaque Switching in *Candida albicans*. *PLoS Pathog.* **2008**, *4*, e1000089. [CrossRef] [PubMed]
30. Huang, G.; Srikantha, T.; Sahni, N.; Yi, S.; Soll, D.R. Report CO(2) Regulates White-to-Opaque Switching in *Candida albicans*. *Curr. Biol.* **2009**, *19*, 330–334. [CrossRef]
31. Alby, K.; Bennett, R.J. Stress-Induced Phenotypic Switching in *Candida albicans*. *Mol. Biol. Cell* **2009**, *20*, 3178–3191. [CrossRef] [PubMed]
32. Geiger, J.; Wessels, D.; Lockhart, S.R.; Soll, D.R. Release of a Potent Polymorphonuclear Leukocyte Chemoattractant Is Regulated by White-Opaque Switching in *Candida albicans*. *Infect. Immun.* **2004**, *72*, 667–677. [CrossRef] [PubMed]
33. Miller, M.G.; Johnson, A.D. White-opaque switching in *Candida albicans* is controlled by mating-type locus homeodomain proteins and allows efficient mating. *Cell* **2002**, *110*, 293–302. [CrossRef]
34. Lockhart, S.R.; Pujol, C.; Daniels, K.J.; Miller, M.G.; Johnson, A.D.; Pfaller, M.A.; Soll, D.R. In *Candida albicans*, white-opaque switchers are homozygous for mating type. *Genetics* **2002**, *162*, 737–745.
35. Hull, C.M.; Johnson, A.D. Identification of a Mating Type–Like Locus in the Asexual Pathogenic Yeast *Candida albicans*. *Science* **1999**, *285*, 1271–1275. [CrossRef]
36. Huang, G.; Wang, H.; Chou, S.; Nie, X.; Chen, J.; Liu, H. Bistable expression of WOR1, a master regulator of white-opaque switching in *Candida albicans*. *Proc. Natl. Acad. Sci. USA* **2006**, *103*, 12813–12818. [CrossRef]
37. Hernday, A.D.; Lohse, M.B.; Fordyce, P.M.; Nobile, C.J.; DeRisi, J.L.; Johnson, A.D. Structure of the transcriptional network controlling white-opaque switching in *Candida albicans*. *Mol. Microbiol.* **2013**, *90*, 22–35.
38. Pendrak, M.L.; Yan, S.S.; Roberts, D.D. Hemoglobin regulates expression of an activator of mating-type locus α genes in *Candida albicans*. *Eukaryot. Cell* **2004**, *3*, 764–775. [CrossRef]
39. Pendrak, M.L.; Yan, S.S.; Roberts, D.D. Sensing the host environment: Recognition of hemoglobin by the pathogenic yeast *Candida albicans*. *Arch. Biochem. Biophys.* **2004**, *426*, 148–156. [CrossRef]
40. Sun, Y.; Gadoury, C.; Hirakawa, M.P.; Bennett, R.J.; Harcus, D.; Marcil, A. Deletion of a Yci1 Domain Protein of *Candida albicans* Allows Homothallic Mating in MTL Heterozygous Cells. *MBio* **2016**, *7*, e00465-16. [CrossRef]
41. Hirakawa, M.P.; Martinez, D.A.; Sakthikumar, S.; Anderson, M.Z.; Berlin, A.; Gujja, S.; Zeng, Q.; Zisson, E.; Wang, J.M.; Greenberg, J.M.; et al. Genetic and phenotypic intra-species variation in *Candida albicans*. *Genome Res.* **2015**, *25*, 413–425. [CrossRef] [PubMed]
42. Magee, B.B.; Magee, P.T. Induction of mating in *Candida albicans* by construction of MTLa and MTLalpha strains. *Science* **2000**, *289*, 310–313. [CrossRef] [PubMed]
43. Forche, A.; Abbey, D.; Pisithkul, T.; Weinzierl, M.A.; Ringstrom, T.; Bruck, D.; Petersen, K.; Berman, J. Stress alters rates and types of loss of heterozygosity in *Candida albicans*. *MBio* **2011**, *2*, e00129-11. [CrossRef] [PubMed]
44. Ou, T.Y.; Chang, F.M.; Cheng, W.N.; Lara, A.; Chou, M.L.; Lee, W.F.; Lee, K.C.; Lin, C.T.; Lee, W.S.; Yu, F.L.; et al. Fluconazole induces rapid high-frequency MTL homozygosity with microbiological polymorphism in *Candida albicans*. *J. Microbiol. Immunol. Infect.* **2017**, *50*, 899–904. [CrossRef] [PubMed]
45. Hilton, C.; Markie, D.; Corner, B.; Rikkerink, E.; Poulter, R. Heat shock induces chromosome loss in the yeast *Candida albicans*. *Mol. Gen. Genet.* **1985**, *200*, 162. [CrossRef]
46. Berman, J.; Hadany, L. Does stress induce (para) sex? Implications for *Candida albicans* evolution. *Trends Genet.* **2012**, *28*, 197–203. [CrossRef]
47. Hull, C.M. Evidence for Mating of the "Asexual" Yeast *Candida albicans* in a Mammalian Host. *Science* **2000**, *289*, 307–310. [CrossRef]

48. Bennett, R.J.; Johnson, A.D. Completion of a parasexual cycle in *Candida albicans* by induced chromosome loss in tetraploid strains. *EMBO J.* **2003**, *22*, 2505–2515. [CrossRef]
49. Bennett, R.J. The parasexual lifestyle of *Candida albicans*. *Curr. Opin. Microbiol.* **2015**, *28*, 10–17. [CrossRef]
50. Alby, K.; Schaefer, D.; Bennett, R.J. Homothallic and heterothallic mating in the opportunistic pathogen *Candida albicans*. *Nature* **2009**, *460*, 890–893. [CrossRef]
51. Soll, D.R.; Lockhart, S.R.; Zhao, R. Relationship between switching and mating in *Candida albicans*. *Eukaryot. Cell* **2003**, *2*, 390–397. [CrossRef] [PubMed]
52. Lockhart, S.R.; Zhao, R.; Daniels, K.J.; Soll, D.R. α-pheromone-induced "shmooing" and gene regulation require white-opaque switching during *Candida albicans* mating. *Eukaryot. Cell* **2003**, *2*, 847–855. [CrossRef] [PubMed]
53. Lockhart, S.R.; Daniels, K.J.; Zhao, R.; Wessels, D.; Soll, D.R. Cell Biology of Mating in *Candida albicans*. *Eukaryot. Cell* **2003**, *2*, 49–61. [CrossRef]
54. Forche, A.; Alby, K.; Schaefer, D.; Johnson, A.D.; Berman, J.; Bennett, R.J. The parasexual cycle in *Candida albicans* provides an alternative pathway to meiosis for the formation of recombinant strains. *PLoS Biol.* **2008**, *6*, e110. [CrossRef] [PubMed]
55. Hickman, M.A.; Paulson, C.; Dudley, A.; Berman, J. Parasexual ploidy reduction drives population heterogeneity through random and transient aneuploidy in *Candida albicans*. *Genetics* **2015**, *200*, 781–794. [CrossRef] [PubMed]
56. Guan, G.; Tao, L.; Yue, H.; Liang, W.; Gong, J.; Bing, J.; Zheng, Q.; Veri, A.O.; Fan, S.; Robbins, N.; et al. Environment-induced same-sex mating in the yeast *Candida albicans* through the Hsf1–Hsp90 pathway. *PLoS Biol.* **2019**, *17*, e2006966. [CrossRef]
57. Sahni, N.; Yi, S.; Pujol, C.; Soll, D.R. The white cell response to pheromone is a general characteristic of *Candida albicans* strains. *Eukaryot. Cell* **2009**, *8*, 251–256. [CrossRef]
58. Lin, C.H.; Kabrawala, S.; Fox, E.P.; Nobile, C.J.; Johnson, A.D.; Bennett, R.J. Genetic Control of Conventional and Pheromone-Stimulated Biofilm Formation in *Candida albicans*. *PLoS Pathog.* **2013**, *9*, e1003305. [CrossRef]
59. Yi, S.; Sahni, N.; Daniels, K.J.; Lu, K.L.; Srikantha, T.; Huang, G.; Garnaas, A.M.; Soll, D.R. Alternative mating type configurations (a/α versus a/a or α/α) of *Candida albicans* result in alternative biofilms regulated by different pathways. *PLoS Biol.* **2011**, *9*, e1001117. [CrossRef]
60. Nobile, C.J.; Fox, E.P.; Nett, J.E.; Sorrells, T.R.; Mitrovich, Q.M.; Hernday, A.D.; Tuch, B.B.; Andes, D.R.; Johnson, A.D. A recently evolved transcriptional network controls biofilm development in *Candida albicans*. *Cell* **2012**, *148*, 126–138. [CrossRef]
61. Dignard, D.; El-Naggar, A.L.; Logue, M.E.; Butler, G.; Whiteway, M. Identification and characterization of MFA1, the gene encoding *Candida albicans* a-factor pheromone. *Eukaryot. Cell* **2007**, *6*, 487–494. [CrossRef] [PubMed]
62. Bennett, R.; Uhl, M.A.; Miller, M.G.; Johnson, A. Identification and characterization of a *Candida albicans* mating pheromone. *Mol. Cell. Biol.* **2003**, *23*, 8189–8201. [CrossRef]
63. Panwar, S.L.; Legrand, M.; Dignard, D.; Whiteway, M.; Magee, P.T. MFα1, the Gene Encoding the α Mating Pheromone of *Candida albicans*. *Eukaryot. Cell.* **2003**, *2*, 1350–1360. [CrossRef] [PubMed]
64. Julius, D.; Brake, A.; Blair, L.; Kunisawa, R.; Thorner, J. Isolation of the putative structural gene for the lysine-arginine-cleaving endopeptidase required for processing of yeast prepro-α-factor. *Cell* **1984**, *37*, 1075–1089. [CrossRef]
65. Newport, G.; Agabian, N. KEX2 influences *Candida albicans* proteinase secretion and hyphal formation. *J. Biol. Chem.* **1997**, *272*, 28954–28961. [CrossRef] [PubMed]
66. Julius, D.; Blair, L.; Brake, A.; Sprague, G.; Thorner, J. Yeast α factor is processed from a larger precursor polypeptide: The essential role of a membrane-bound dipeptidyl aminopeptidase. *Cell* **1983**, *32*, 839–852. [CrossRef]
67. Bautista-Muñoz, C.; Hernández-Rodríguez, C.; Villa-Tanaca, L. Analysis and expression of STE13ca gene encoding a putative X-prolyl dipeptidyl aminopeptidase from *Candida albicans*. *FEMS Immunol. Med. Microbiol.* **2005**, *45*, 459–469. [CrossRef]
68. Bennett, R.J.; Johnson, A.D. The role of nutrient regulation and the Gpa2 protein in the mating pheromone response of *Candida albicans*. *Mol. Microbiol.* **2006**, *62*, 100–119. [CrossRef]
69. Chen, P.; Sapperstein, S.K.; Choi, J.D.; Michaelis, S. Biogenesis of the *Saccharomyces cerevisiae* Mating Pheromone a-Factor. *J. Cell Biol.* **1997**, *136*, 251–269. [CrossRef]

70. Magee, B.B.; Legrand, M.; Alarco, A.M.; Raymond, M.; Magee, P.T. Many of the genes required for mating in *Saccharomyces cerevisiae* are also required for mating in *Candida albicans*. *Mol. Microbiol.* **2002**, *46*, 1345–1351. [CrossRef]
71. Raymond, M.; Dignard, D.; Alarco, A.M.; Mainville, N.; Magee, B.B.; Thomas, D.Y. A Ste6p/P-glycoprotein homologue from the asexual yeast *Candida albicans* transports the a-factor mating pheromone in *Saccharomyces cerevisiae*. *Mol. Microbiol.* **2002**, *27*, 587–598. [CrossRef] [PubMed]
72. Schaefer, D.; Côte, P.; Whiteway, M.; Bennett, R.J. Barrier activity in *Candida albicans* mediates pheromone degradation and promotes mating. *Eukaryot. Cell* **2007**, *6*, 907–918. [CrossRef] [PubMed]
73. Chen, J.; Chen, J.; Lane, S.; Liu, H. A conserved mitogen-activated protein kinase pathway is required for mating in *Candida albicans*. *Mol. Microbiol.* **2002**, *46*, 1335–1344. [CrossRef] [PubMed]
74. Yi, S.; Sahni, N.; Daniels, K.J.; Pujol, C.; Srikantha, T.; Soll, D.R. The Same Receptor, G Protein, and Mitogen-activated Protein Kinase Pathway Activate Different Downstream Regulators in the Alternative White and Opaque Pheromone Responses of *Candida albicans*. *Mol. Biol. Cell* **2008**, *19*, 957–970. [CrossRef] [PubMed]
75. Lin, C.H.; Choi, A.; Bennett, R.J. Defining pheromone-receptor signaling in *Candida albicans* and related asexual *Candida* species. *Mol. Biol. Cell* **2011**, *22*, 4918–4930. [CrossRef] [PubMed]
76. Dignard, D.; André, D.; Whiteway, M. Heterotrimeric G-protein subunit function in *Candida albicans*: Both the α and β subunits of the pheromone response G protein are required for mating. *Eukaryot. Cell* **2008**, *7*, 1591–1599. [CrossRef]
77. Yi, S.; Sahni, N.; Daniels, K.J.; Lu, K.L.; Huang, G.; Garnaas, A.M.; Pujol, C.; Srikantha, T.; Soll, D.R. Utilization of the Mating Scaffold Protein in the Evolution of a New Signal Transduction Pathway for Biofilm Development. *MBio* **2011**, *2*, e00237-10. [CrossRef]
78. Rastghalam, G.; Omran, R.P.; Alizadeh, M.; Fulton, D.; Mallick, J.; Whiteway, M. MAP Kinase Regulation of the *Candida albicans* Pheromone Pathway. *mSphere* **2019**, *4*, e00598-18. [CrossRef]
79. Scaduto, C.M.; Kabrawala, S.; Thomson, G.J.; Scheving, W.; Ly, A.; Anderson, M.Z.; Whiteway, M.; Bennett, R.J. Epigenetic control of pheromone MAPK signaling determines sexual fecundity in *Candida albicans*. *Proc. Natl. Acad. Sci. USA* **2017**, *114*, 13780–13785. [CrossRef]
80. Dohlman, H.G.; Song, J.; Apanovitch, D.M.; DiBello, P.R.; Gillen, K.M. Regulation of G protein signalling in yeast. *Semin. Cell Dev. Biol.* **1998**, *9*, 135–141. [CrossRef]
81. Ramírez-Zavala, B.; Weyler, M.; Gildor, T.; Schmauch, C.; Kornitzer, D.; Arkowitz, R.; Morschhäuser, J. Activation of the Cph1-Dependent MAP Kinase Signaling Pathway Induces White-Opaque Switching in *Candida albicans*. *PLoS Pathog.* **2013**, *9*, e1003696. [CrossRef] [PubMed]
82. Roberts, R.L.; Fink, G.R. Elements of a single map kinase cascade in *Saccharomyces cerevisiae* mediate two developmental programs in the same cell type: Mating and invasive growth. *Genes Dev.* **1994**, *8*, 2974–2985. [CrossRef] [PubMed]
83. Herskowitz, I. MAP Kinase Pathways in Yeast: For Mating and More. *Cell* **1995**, *80*, 187–197. [CrossRef]
84. Hartwell, L.H. Synchronization of haploid yeast cell cycles, a prelude to conjugation. *Exp. Cell Res.* **1973**, *76*, 111–117. [CrossRef]
85. Nantel, A.; Dignard, D.; Bachewich, C.; Harcus, D.; Marcil, A.; Bouin, A.P.; Sensen, C.W.; Hogues, H.; van het Hoog, M.; Gordon, P.; et al. Transcription Profiling of *Candida albicans* Cells Undergoing Yeast-to-Hyphal Transistion. *Mol. Biol. Cell* **2002**, *13*, 3452–3465. [CrossRef] [PubMed]
86. Daniels, K.J.; Park, Y.N.; Srikantha, T.; Pujol, C.; Soll, D.R. Impact of Environmental Conditions on the Form and Function of *Candida albicans* Biofilms. *Eukaryot. Cell* **2013**, *12*, 1389–1402. [CrossRef]
87. Uppuluri, P.; Chaturvedi, A.K.; Srinivasan, A.; Banerjee, M.; Ramasubramanian, A.; Köehler, J.; Kadosh, D.; Lopez-ribot, J.L. Dispersion as an Important Step in the *Candida albicans* Biofilm Developmental Cycle. *PLoS Pathog.* **2010**, *6*, e1000828. [CrossRef]
88. Mukherjee, P.K.; Chandra, J.; Kuhn, D.M.; Ghannoum, M.A. Mechanism of Fluconazole Resistance in *Candida albicans* Biofilms: Phase-Specific Role of Efflux Pumps and Membrane Sterols. *Infect. Immun.* **2003**, *71*, 4333–4340. [CrossRef]
89. LaFleur, M.D.; Kumamoto, C.A.; Lewis, K. *Candida albicans* biofilms produce antifungal-tolerant persister cells. *Antimicrob. Agents Chemother.* **2006**, *50*, 3839–3846. [CrossRef]
90. Tao, L.; Cao, C.; Liang, W.; Guan, G.; Zhang, Q.; Nobile, C.J.; Huang, G. White Cells Facilitate Opposite- and Same-Sex Mating of Opaque Cells in *Candida albicans*. *PLoS Genet.* **2014**, *10*, e1004737. [CrossRef]

91. Lohse, M.B.; Johnson, A.D. Differential phagocytosis of white versus opaque *Candida albicans* by *Drosophila* and mouse phagocytes. *PLoS ONE* **2008**, *3*, e0001473. [CrossRef] [PubMed]
92. Kean, R.; Delaney, C.; Rajendran, R.; Sherry, L.; Metcalfe, R.; Thomas, R.; Mclean, W.; Williams, C.; Ramage, G. Gaining Insights from *Candida* Biofilm Heterogeneity: One Size Does Not Fit All. *J. Fungi* **2018**, *4*, 12. [CrossRef] [PubMed]
93. Fox, E.P.; Cowley, E.S.; Nobile, C.J.; Hartooni, N.; Newman, D.K.; Johnson, A.D. Anaerobic bacteria grow within *Candida albicans* biofilms and induce biofilm formation in suspension cultures. *Curr. Biol.* **2014**, *24*, 2411–2416. [CrossRef]
94. Tsui, C.; Kong, E.F.; Jabra-Rizk, M.A. Pathogenesis of *Candida albicans* biofilm. *Pathog. Dis.* **2016**, *74*, ftw018. [CrossRef] [PubMed]
95. Lin, Y.J.; Alsad, L.; Vogel, F.; Koppar, S.; Nevarez, L.; Auguste, F.; Seymour, J.; Syed, A.; Christoph, K.; Loomis, J.S. Interactions between *Candida albicans* and Staphylococcus aureus within mixed species biofilms. *Bios* **2013**, *84*, 30–39. [CrossRef]
96. Peters, B.M.; Ovchinnikova, E.S.; Krom, B.P.; Schlecht, L.M.; Zhou, H.; Hoyer, L.L.; Busscher, H.J.; van der Mei, H.C.; Jabra-Rizk, M.A.; Shirtliff, M.E. *Staphylococcus aureus* adherence to *Candida albicans* hyphae is mediated by the hyphal adhesin Als3p. *Microbiology* **2012**, *158*, 2975–2986. [CrossRef]
97. Peters, B.M.; Jabra-Rizk, M.A.; Scheper, M.A.; Leid, J.G.; Costerton, J.W.; Shirtliff, M.E. Microbial interactions and differential protein expression in *Staphylococcus aureus-Candida albicans* dual-species biofilms. *FEMS Immunol. Med. Microbiol.* **2010**, *59*, 493–503. [CrossRef]
98. Kong, E.F.; Tsui, C.; Kucharíková, S.; Andes, D.; van Dijck, P.; Jabra-Rizk, M.A. Commensal Protection of *Staphylococcus aureus* against Antimicrobials by *Candida albicans* Biofilm Matrix. *MBio* **2016**, *7*, e01365-16. [CrossRef]
99. Graham, C.E.; Cruz, M.R.; Garsin, D.A.; Lorenz, M.C. *Enterococcus faecalis* bacteriocin EntV inhibits hyphal morphogenesis, biofilm formation, and virulence of *Candida albicans*. *Proc. Natl. Acad. Sci. USA* **2017**, *114*, 4507–4512. [CrossRef]
100. Lindsay, A.K.; Hogan, D.A. *Candida albicans*: Molecular interactions with *Pseudomonas aeruginosa* and *Staphylococcus aureus*. *Fungal Biol. Rev.* **2014**, *28*, 85–96. [CrossRef]
101. Ramage, G.; Saville, S.P.; Wickes, B.L.; López-ribot, J.L. Inhibition of *Candida albicans* Biofilm Formation by Farnesol, a Quorum-Sensing Molecule. *Appl. Environ. Microbiol.* **2002**, *68*, 5459–5463. [CrossRef] [PubMed]
102. Morales, D.K.; Grahl, N.; Okegbe, C.; Dietrich, L.E.P.; Jacobs, N.J.; Hogan, A. Control of *Candida albicans* Metabolism and Biofilm Formation by *Pseudomonas aeruginosa* Phenazines. *MBio* **2013**, *4*, e00526-12. [CrossRef] [PubMed]
103. Kernien, J.F.; Snarr, B.D.; Sheppard, D.C.; Nett, J.E. The interface between Fungal Biofilms and Innate Immunity. *Front. Immunol.* **2018**, *8*, 1968. [CrossRef]
104. Brown, G.D. Innate Antifungal Immunity: The Key Role of Phagocytes. *Annu. Rev. Immunol.* **2011**, *29*, 1–21. [CrossRef] [PubMed]
105. Urban, C.F.; Reichard, U.; Brinkmann, V.; Zychlinsky, A. Neutrophil extracellular traps capture and kill *Candida albicans* and hyphal forms. *Cell. Microbiol.* **2006**, *8*, 668–676. [CrossRef] [PubMed]
106. Johnson, C.J.; Cabezas-Olcoz, J.; Kernien, J.F.; Wang, S.X.; Beebe, D.J.; Huttenlocher, A.; Ansari, H.; Nett, J.E. The Extracellular Matrix of *Candida albicans* Biofilms Impairs Formation of Neutrophil Extracellular Traps. *PLoS Pathog.* **2016**, *12*, e1005884. [CrossRef] [PubMed]
107. Xie, Z.; Thompson, A.; Sobue, T.; Kashleva, H.; Xu, H.; Vasilakos, J.; Dongari-Bagtzoglou, A. *Candida albicans* biofilms do not trigger reactive oxygen species and evade neutrophil killing. *J. Infect. Dis.* **2012**, *206*, 1936–1945. [CrossRef]
108. Chandra, J.; McCormick, T.S.; Imamura, Y.; Mukherjee, P.K.; Ghannoum, M.A. Interaction of *Candida albicans* with adherent human peripheral blood mononuclear cells increases *C. albicans* biofilm formation and results in differential expression of pro- and anti-inflammatory cytokines. *Infect. Immun.* **2007**, *75*, 2612–2620. [CrossRef]
109. Rocha, F.A.C.; Alves, A.M.C.V.; Rocha, M.F.G.; Cordeiro, R.D.A.; Brilhante, R.S.N.; Pinto, A.C.M.D.; Nunes, R.D.M.; Girão, V.C.C.; Sidrim, J.J.C. Tumor necrosis factor prevents *Candida albicans* biofilm formation. *Sci. Rep.* **2017**, *7*, 1206. [CrossRef]
110. Gantner, B.N.; Simmons, R.M.; Underhill, D.M. Dectin-1 mediates macrophage recognition of *Candida albicans* yeast but not filaments. *EMBO* **2005**, *24*, 1277–1286. [CrossRef]

111. Chen, T.; Wagner, A.S.; Tams, R.N.; Eyer, J.E.; Kauffman, S.J.; Gann, E.R.; Fernandez, E.J.; Reynolds, T.B. Lrg1 Regulates β (1,3)-Glucan Masking in *Candida albicans* through the Cek1 MAP Kinase Pathway. *MBio* **2019**, *10*, e01767-19. [CrossRef]
112. Inglis, D.O.; Sherlock, G. Ras signaling gets fine-tuned: Regulation of multiple pathogenic traits of *Candida albicans*. *Eukaryot. Cell* **2013**, *12*, 1316–1325. [CrossRef] [PubMed]
113. Huang, G.; Huang, Q.; Wei, Y.; Wang, Y.; Du, H. Multiple roles and diverse regulation of the Ras/cAMP/protein kinase A pathway in *Candida albicans*. *Mol. Microbiol.* **2019**, *111*, 6–16. [CrossRef] [PubMed]
114. Fox, E.P.; Bui, C.K.; Nett, J.E.; Hartooni, N.; Mui, M.C.; Andes, D.R.; Nobile, C.J.; Johnson, A.D. An expanded regulatory network temporally controls *Candida albicans* biofilm formation. *Mol. Microbiol.* **2015**, *96*, 1226–1239. [CrossRef] [PubMed]
115. Sorrells, T.R.; Johnson, A.D. Making sense of transcription networks. *Cell* **2015**, *161*, 714–723. [CrossRef]
116. Nobile, C.J.; Nett, J.E.; Hernday, A.D.; Homann, O.R.; Deneault, J.; Nantel, A.; Andes, D.R.; Johnson, A.D.; Mitchell, A.P. Biofilm Matrix Regulation by *Candida albicans* Zap1. *PLoS Biol.* **2009**, *7*, e1000133. [CrossRef]
117. Nett, J.E.; Sanchez, H.; Cain, M.T.; Ross, K.M.; Andes, D.R. Interface of *Candida albicans* Biofilm Matrix-Associated Drug Resistance and Cell Wall Integrity Regulation. *Eukaryot. Cell* **2011**, *10*, 1660–1669. [CrossRef]
118. Nett, J.E.; Sanchez, H.; Cain, M.T.; Andes, D.R. Genetic Basis of *Candida Biofilm* Resistance Due to Drug-Sequestering Matrix Glucan. *J. Infect. Dis.* **2010**, *202*, 171–175. [CrossRef]
119. Daniels, K.J.; Srikantha, T.; Pujol, C.; Park, Y.N.; Soll, D.R. Role of Tec1 in the development, architecture, and integrity of sexual biofilms of *Candida albicans*. *Eukaryot. Cell* **2015**, *14*, 228–240. [CrossRef]
120. Sahni, N.; Yi, S.; Daniels, K.J.; Huang, G.; Srikantha, T.; Soll, D.R. Tec1 mediates the pheromone response of the white phenotype of *Candida albicans*: Insights into the evolution of new signal transduction pathways. *PLoS Biol.* **2010**, *8*, e1000363. [CrossRef]

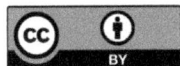

© 2020 by the authors. Licensee MDPI, Basel, Switzerland. This article is an open access article distributed under the terms and conditions of the Creative Commons Attribution (CC BY) license (http://creativecommons.org/licenses/by/4.0/).

MDPI
St. Alban-Anlage 66
4052 Basel
Switzerland
Tel. +41 61 683 77 34
Fax +41 61 302 89 18
www.mdpi.com

Journal of Fungi Editorial Office
E-mail: jof@mdpi.com
www.mdpi.com/journal/jof

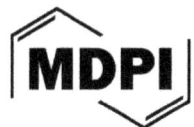

www.ingramcontent.com/pod-product-compliance
Lightning Source LLC
LaVergne TN
LVHW070626100526
838202LV00012B/735